A HISTORY OF THE BIRTH CONTROL MOVEMENT IN AMERICA

A HISTORY OF THE BIRTH CONTROL MOVEMENT IN AMERICA

PETER C. ENGELMAN

Healing Society: Disease, Medicine, and History
John Parascandola, Series Editor

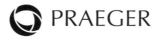 PRAEGER

AN IMPRINT OF ABC-CLIO, LLC
Santa Barbara, California • Denver, Colorado • Oxford, England

Library of Congress Cataloging-in-Publication Data

Engelman, Peter.
    A history of the birth control movement in America / Peter C. Engelman.
        p. cm. — (Healing society : disease, medicine, and history)
    Includes bibliographical references and index.
    ISBN 978-0-313-36509-6 (hardcopy : alk. paper) — ISBN 978-0-313-36510-2 (ebook)
1. Birth control—United States—History. 2. Birth control—United States—Political aspects. 3. Birth control clinics—United States—History. I. Title.
    HQ766.5.U5E54   2011
    363.9'60973--dc22   2010050979

ISBN: 978-0-313-36509-6
EISBN: 978-0-313-36510-2

15 14 13 12 11   1 2 3 4 5

This book is also available on the World Wide Web as an eBook.
Visit www.abc-clio.com for details.

Praeger
An Imprint of ABC-CLIO, LLC

ABC-CLIO, LLC
130 Cremona Drive, P.O. Box 1911
Santa Barbara, California 93116-1911

This book is printed on acid-free paper ∞

Manufactured in the United States of America

for Kendall

CONTENTS

SERIES FOREWORD

The Praeger series *Healing Society: Disease, Medicine, and History* features individual volumes that explore the social impact of particular illnesses or medically related conditions or topics for a broad audience. The object is to publish books that offer reliable overviews of particular aspects of medical and social history while incorporating the most up-to-date scholarly interpretations. The books in the series are designed to engage readers and educate them about important but often neglected aspects of the social history of medicine. Disease and disability have significantly influenced the course of human history, and the books in this series will examine various aspects of that influence.

A History of the Birth Control Movement in America is not concerned with a disease or disability, but with another health-related topic, pregnancy and efforts to prevent it. The book provides an excellent example of how social, political and economic forces affect health issues. Peter Engelman has written an informative and fascinating account of the birth control movement in America, with emphasis on the period when the movement became established (between the First and Second World Wars).

The book in by no means a biography of Margaret Sanger, but as the primary force behind the early birth control movement, her work is central to the story. Sanger has been a hero to some and a villain to others, and Engelman provides an objective account of her contributions and her failings. In general, he has produced an authoritative, balanced and accessible account of what he calls "one of the few women-led social movements in American history." It is a story that involves "an unlikely alliance of radicals, socialites, and professionals who successfully confronted the moral condemnation of birth control and broke down successive social and legal barriers."

In spite of the fact that a number of excellent scholarly historical and biographical works on the birth control movement have been published in recent years, there was still a need for an accessible history that was not a biography of Sanger or based solely on secondary sources, a book that could be recommended to an interested nonspecialist reader. *A History of the Birth Control Movement in America* has filled that gap in the literature. It is a book that will be of interest to historians, health professionals, social activists, politicians, and members of the general public who want to learn more about the history of this important issue.

John Parascandola

ACKNOWLEDGMENTS

This book is in many ways an extension of my work on the Margaret Sanger Papers Project at New York University. I must begin by thanking the Project's editor and director, Esther Katz, who not only trained me to become a documentary editor, but also shaped my understanding of the birth control movement more than anyone else. Esther has always encouraged me to take on other challenges and has helped me to become a better writer. My other colleague on the Sanger Papers, Cathy Moran Hajo, has contributed to this work far more than she may realize. I benefitted from her constructive advice on how to tackle a long research and writing project, and her own scholarship proved indispensible. Both Esther and Cathy gave me useful comments on the manuscript and made this a stronger and more accurate book. I feel fortunate for their intellectual support and friendship.

Most of the research for the book was conducted in the Sophia Smith Collection, Smith College, where I have worked closely over the last two decades with the rich collections of birth control material housed there. I am indebted to Sophia Smith Collection Director, Sherrill Redmon, and staff: Amy Hague, Maida Goodwin, Susan Boone, Susan Barker, Margaret Jessup, Karen Kukil, Joyce Follet, Burd Schlessinger, and Kelly Anderson. And thanks also to College Archivist Nanci Young and Deborah Richards. I can't emphasize enough how much I appreciate the friendship and support I have been given. I owe a special debt of gratitude to Amy Hague, the Curator of Manuscripts, for reading the manuscript and making some insightful suggestions.

Thanks also to the Smith College Library reference and interlibrary loan staffs, especially Pam Skinner, for tracking down obscure sources and giving me helpful research advice.

I am grateful to the many other archivists and librarians, too numerous to list, who have given their time and assistance at the following institutions: Countway Library of Medicine at Harvard Medical School (especially Jack Eckert); Houghton Library, Harvard University; Library of Congress; National Archives; Schlesinger Library, Radcliffe Institute, Harvard University; Bobst Library, New York University (especially Andrew Lee); New York Public Library; Beinecke Rare Book and Manuscript Library, Yale University; Boston Public Library; New York Academy of Medicine; Archives and Special Collections, Amherst College Library; Duke University Medical Center Library (especially Louis Wiethe); W.E.B. Du Bois Library, University of Massachusetts, Amherst; Brooklyn Public Library; Multnomah County Library, Portland, Oregon; New York State Archives.

This book would not have come about if not for author and historian John Parascandola, the Healing Society series editor at Praeger, who approached me in 2008 to write a history of the birth control movement. John made sure I was moving in the right direction, and I thank him for his comments on the manuscript. Brian Foster helped me get started at Praeger, Michael Millman guided me through the editing process, and Lori Pierelli at Cadmus oversaw production.

Special thanks to Jimmy Wilkinson Meyer, who read the manuscript in her dual roles as editor and historian. Her sound advice and assertive red pen significantly improved my narrative. And I greatly appreciate the camaraderie offered by Manon Parry at the National Library of Medicine, who read several chapters and, through our discussions, strengthened my arguments in the last chapter. Kevin McClearey's research on Sanger's 1916 speaking tour was extremely helpful and led me to a number of sources, and I thank him for generously sharing it. There are many scholars, researchers and students who have shared ideas and resources over the years. They are too numerous to list here, but I greatly benefitted from their interest and enthusiasm.

Finally, friends and family certainly give more than they get with a project such as this, and I appreciate their support and patience. I regret that my father, Fred Engelman, a historian and writer early on in his career, did not live to see this book in print, though I am grateful we were able to share with each other many stories about the process of research and writing. My mother, Joyce Wieland, has always expressed confidence in my decisions and abilities, and I welcome this opportunity to say an indelible thank you to her for her love and encouragement. She made sure that I grew up with respect for and an understanding of women's gifts and burdens. I am also grateful to her for reading and commenting on the first draft of the manuscript.

Writing mostly at home meant that my daughters, Waverley and Grace, were a constant presence—my spirited muses and my biggest diversions. Knowing they will read this someday was a constant motivation. My wife, Kendall Clark, was unfailingly supportive and made sure that I had the space and time to write. To her I express my gratitude and love in the dedication of this book.

ABBREVIATIONS

ABCL	American Birth Control League
ACLU	American Civil Liberties Union
AMA	American Medical Association
BCCRB	Birth Control Clinical Research Bureau
BCFA	Birth Control Federation of America
BCLNY	Birth Control League of New York
BCR	Birth Control Review
CMH	Committee on Maternal Health
CRB	Clinical Research Bureau
CTCA	Commission on Training Camp Activities
FSL	Free Speech League
IWW	Industrial Workers of the World
NBCL	National Birth Control League
NCFLBC	National Committee on Federal Legislation for Birth Control
NYWPC	New York Women's Publishing Company
PPFA	Planned Parenthood Federation of America
VPL	Voluntary Parenthood League
YMCA	Young Men's Christian Association

INTRODUCTION

The most important force in the remaking of the world is a free motherhood.[1]
—Margaret Sanger, 1920

On a late spring evening in 1914, Margaret Sanger gathered together in her New York City apartment a small group of radical friends that comprised her informal staff for *The Woman Rebel*, the militant-feminist monthly that addressed gender oppression, prostitution, marriage inequities, women and labor, and the link between population growth and war, among other issues. The feisty paper called on working-class women to rise up against all oppressors and dedicate their lives to social and economic emancipation. Though Sanger seemed intent on printing a wide range of anarchist thought—like an angry protester throwing every rock she could find—her central aim was to highlight a woman's need to control her own fertility.

Sanger made it clear in the first issue, published that March, that she would "advocate the prevention of conception" and "impart such knowledge in the columns of this paper." The decision could have resulted in her arrest for violating the Comstock Act, the series of prohibitions passed beginning in 1873 that banned the circulation of a wide range of materials considered obscene, including contraceptive information. Well aware of the potential consequences of her actions and outright daring the government to interfere, Sanger sought an attention-getting phrase, clear and unequivocal, to express the concept of voluntary parenthood without sounding too indirect or technical. She wanted the name to "convey to the public the social and personal significance of the idea." Sanger queried her close-knit group of supporters, a colorful assortment of Greenwich Village radicals who had worked on various leftist publications. They included: Edward Mylius, a thickly-set former British journalist who gained notoriety for being convicted of libeling the King of England; Otto Bobsien, a young and idealistic writer and activist; Robert Parker, a polio-stricken editor and drama critic; and John Rompapas, a swarthy Greek tobacco importer and anarchist publisher who had entered into an affair with Sanger the previous year. One or two other activists may have also been present when Sanger challenged them to find "a distinctive name."[2]

They reviewed the popular terms used in marriage manuals and medical journals, or that had been bandied about for years: conception control, family limitation, pregnancy prevention, limitation of offspring, regulation of reproduction, preventive arts, neo-Malthusianism (after followers of English demographer Thomas Malthus), and voluntary parenthood or voluntary motherhood. The group considered more original phrases, such as "conscious" or "constructive generation" and the antiseptic-sounding "prevenception," favored by Dr. William Robinson, an outspoken early medical proponent of fertility control. *Contraception* had been used sparingly in scientific literature but sounded both illicit and disapproving. Then, as Sanger remembered it, her friends called out in succession: "'family control' and 'race control' and 'birth-rate control,'" and, Sanger recalled, "finally it came to me out of the blue—'Birth Control!'" At least one other participant remembered that the writer Robert Parker was the one to seize on the final name, not Sanger. Nevertheless, the group unanimously accepted those simple and assertive words—maybe the most controversial phrase in the English language since Darwin introduced *natural selection* in 1859.[3]

The coining of the term *birth control* and its emergence in print set into motion a series of free speech battles that launched the American birth control movement. The phrase remains commonplace today, even though the organization that Sanger founded and has become synonymous with reproductive rights dropped *birth control* for the more family-friendly *planned parenthood* in 1942. That year roughly marks the end of the social movement chronicled in this book.

The campaign that Sanger started in 1914 to challenge antiobscenity laws grew into one of the most far-reaching social reform movements in American history. The movement emphatically declared a distinction between sex and procreation, as it helped to turn the use of contraception into an acceptable social practice. It contributed more than any other factor to validating women's sexual expression and to making sexual satisfaction for both men and women a central component of marriage.

Is there any other social movement that has so fundamentally altered women's roles or affected, in one way or another, all of our lives? I need look no further than my own planned and well-spaced family. My paternal and maternal grandparents—who started their families in the 1920s and 1930s respectively—each had two children, my parents had two children, and my wife and I have two children. My wife's side of the family parallels mine, with the exception that her paternal grandparents had three children. This family trend, a direct consequence of safe, effective, and available reproductive control, is by no means uncommon today but would have been relatively rare a century ago except among the educated and the upper class. The last three generations of women on both sides of our families balanced motherhood with interests and needs outside of the home, taking advantage of educational and employment opportunities that were simply unavailable and impractical for most women who came of childbearing age before World War I.

Many developments affected women's roles and changing attitudes about sex and childbearing in the 20th century, but birth control was the most powerful underlying force in moving women toward sexual, social, and political equality. And it has contributed more than any other factor to the birth rate decline that precipitated the demographic revolution in which we find ourselves in today. The U.S. birth rate now stands at roughly replacement level (about 2.1 children per woman), while much of the rest of the developed world is entering a depopulation phase (less than two children per woman).[4]

Yet the history of the birth control movement is still not widely known in this country. Some educators are reluctant to cover the movement in public schools for fear of instigating a debate on abortion and stirring up social conservatives who vehemently oppose any classroom consideration of sexuality that does not promote abstinence. Contemporary discussions about abortion rights and reproductive choice too often identify the 1960s—the sexual revolution, the advent of the birth control pill, and the campaign to repeal abortion laws—as the starting point for organized advocacy of reproductive control, rather than the World War I era. Moreover, controversy and confusion surrounding the birth control movement's objectives have complicated efforts to present this history in textbooks, the media, and public forums.

In the last decade especially, opponents of reproductive rights have highlighted the birth control movement's association with eugenics—the flawed science of human betterment that influenced social policy from the late 19th century through the 1920s and that was used to justify Nazi atrocities during World War II—and condemned the pioneer birth control activists, Margaret Sanger in particular, as racist. A number of books published in the last 20 years and scores of Internet sites feature incendiary quotes, misappropriated or taken out of context, as evidence that the movement used coercive racist policies, advocated the extermination of blacks and Jews, and carried out millions of abortions. Some reproductive rights supporters have chosen to side-step the controversy and depict a movement that never strayed from its early feminist and humanitarian intentions. Ideologues on both sides have failed to either evaluate the documentary record of the movement or carefully consider the historical context.[5]

Margaret Sanger's writings lie at the center of this controversy over the birth control movement's eugenic policies. Attacks on her legacy from fringe sources have fueled critical commentary in the right wing media and spilled over into the mainstream press, onto biographical Web sites and even into congressional hearings. (In April 2009, Secretary of State Hillary Clinton, who had recently received Planned Parenthood's Margaret Sanger Award, found herself on the defensive when questioned by a Congressman about Sanger's legacy of racism.) It has become more challenging for students and the general public to find reliable information that is not spun out by individuals or groups with a political agenda. All of this attention has created a demand for more resources on the movement, especially for authoritative accounts that are not driven by extreme political or religious views.

Fortunately there are a number of excellent scholarly and biographical works on birth control in America. Linda Gordon's *Moral Property of Women: A History of Birth Control Politics in America* (2002) offers maybe the most comprehensive treatment on women's struggle for reproductive autonomy. James Reed's fine history, *The Birth Control Movement and American Society: From Private Vice to Public Virtue* (1978), presents interwoven biographical studies of the key players. Carole R. McCann's *Birth Control Politics in the United States, 1916–1945* (1994) closely examines the alliances and compromises that shaped the movement's agenda in the interwar years. Andrea Tone's *Devices and Desires: A History of Contraceptives in America* (2001) is the best single source on the business (both licit and illicit) of birth control. David J. Garrow's monumental *Liberty & Sexuality: The Right to Privacy and the Making of Roe v. Wade* (1994), though concerned with the later history of reproductive rights, is indispensible for understanding the legal ramifications of the birth control movement's law-defying activism. Ellen Chesler's *Woman of Valor: Margaret Sanger and the Birth Control Movement in America* (1992, 2007) is far and away the most accurate and insightful biography of Sanger. And the documentary edition, *The Selected Papers of Margaret Sanger* (Volumes 1 through 3, 2003, 2006, 2010; Volume 4 is forthcoming), edited by Esther Katz, Cathy Moran Hajo, and myself, is the only reliable published source of Sanger's writings and the most complete scholarly treatment of her life.

I know many of these works inside and out, and yet I still struggle to suggest one source to a curious student or a journalist on deadline, or anyone looking for an accessible history rather than a scholarly treatment or a biography of one of the movement leaders. I want to recommend the type of readable narrative history that I have found compelling and informative when delving for the first time into a subject outside of my area of expertise, but there is nothing on the birth control movement that satisfies this need. That explains how this project came about.

First and foremost, this book tells the story of one of the few women-led social movements in American history and an unlikely alliance of radicals, socialites, and professionals who successfully confronted the moral condemnation of birth control and broke down social and legal barriers. The movement turned repeated attempts to silence speech into opportunities to educate the public, convincing a large majority of Americans that married couples should have access to contraception and that birth control was a necessary component of women's health care. Arrests and indictments, clinic raids, imprisonments, courtroom dramas, religious condemnation, public debates, bootlegging, and, of course, sex—from sexual regulation to sexual revolution—make for one of the more sensational and engaging chapters in social history.

I have tried my best to let this engrossing and at times astonishing story unfold in a chronological fashion with a minimum of interruptions and digressions. When I do depart from the narrative, it is in an effort to explain important background information, supply some necessary technical knowledge about contraception, or wrestle with some of the complexities and contradictions of the movement—as in a discussion of birth control and eugenics at the end of Chapter 3.

Chapter 1 surveys the history of birth control and summarizes contraceptive techniques, knowledge, trends, and prohibitions in America through the 19th century. It focuses on the legal and medical reaction to growing contraceptive use and the changing attitudes toward sexuality in American society after the Civil War. Chapter 2 relates the early free speech battles between the government and Emma Goldman, Margaret Sanger, William Sanger, and other activists and covers the emergence of a viable movement out of the pre-World War I radicalism of New York's Greenwich Village. Chapter 3 recounts the opening and police shut-down of the country's first birth control clinic in 1916 and its legal repercussions, and ends with the establishment of the first permanent contraceptive clinic in 1923. It also explains how Sanger, in the late 1910s and early 1920s, steered the movement away from its radical, feminist beginnings in an attempt to gain medical and scientific approval for the health and eugenic benefits of birth control. Chapter 4 measures the widespread acceptance of birth control and, in a less detailed fashion than in Chapters 2 and 3, traces the organizational growth and medicalization of the movement up until the incorporation of the Birth Control Federation of America in 1939 and its name change to the Planned Parenthood Federation of America (PPFA) in 1942. The new name provides an apt bookend for this narrative, which starts with the coining of the phrase *birth control*. However, it is more than an arbitrary ending point. By dispensing with that powerful phrase, birth control, the leadership of PPFA sought to close the era of birth control activism that was so closely tied to Margaret Sanger, radical feminism, and defiance of the law. By 1942 the once militant cause had become an institution.

I make an important distinction between the early protest movement that formed in 1914, led by Sanger and defined by its activism, and the later clinic movement and institutionalization of birth control starting in the mid-1920s. Social movements tend to develop through three stages—emergence, coalescence, and bureaucratization—before coming to some end result: a failure and breakup, cooption by a larger movement, or a successful integration into mainstream society, which is the case here. In this history I devote more attention to the first two stages, the emergence and coalescence of the movement. I try to be comprehensive in tracing the leaders' activities from 1914 to the early 1920s, the years during which the movement achieved its greatest accomplishment in making birth control acceptable to the public. Other scholars point to public opinion polls in the late 1930s that followed medical and legal approval of birth control as confirmation of society's acceptance. However, a number of indications leave me no doubt that birth control was widely used and widely accepted by a majority of Americans more than a decade earlier.[6]

I also distinguish between the birth control movement and the reproductive rights movement that began in the 1960s. The short conclusion to this book attempts to bridge the two movements and clarify the evolution of privacy rights.

This book is tightly focused on national organizations based in New York City and the leadership of the movement. I regret I do not have the space and time to say a little more about birth control activism and clinic organization in other cities and states. Nor can I cover but a few of the hundreds of advocates—nurses, midwives, social workers, community leaders, and many others—who courageously broke the law for what they believed. They included women like Fannie Walton in Kalamazoo, Michigan, who in 1919 quit her job as a librarian and joined the board of the local YWCA so she would have a safe place to advise women and supply them with contraceptive suppositories. She helped form the first birth control committee in that city in the early 1930s and organized a group of local doctors to volunteer their services. For years Walton escorted women to the doctor's office to be fitted for diaphragms. She was active in family planning into her nineties. Each year I learn about a few more Fannie Waltons, whose stories remain untold.[7]

The reader will quickly identify Margaret Sanger as the central figure in this narrative. Much of the book revolves around her actions and leadership. Few social reformers in history have so dominated—or led lives as intertwined with—a cause. Her early activism has received varying degrees of treatment in other histories, but none of them offers the level of detail found here. I also devote considerable attention to William Robinson, William Sanger, Mary Ware Dennett, Robert Dickinson, and lesser-known figures who are pushed to the fringe in some other studies.

Finally, this book is written for a general audience. It should appeal to students and be ideal for classroom use. I hope historians, public health professionals, and others whose field of work or interest intersects in some way with the history of birth control and reproductive rights will add it to their shelves and find it useful both as an accurate history and a resource for tracing some of the primary materials that I relied on. Not only have I enjoyed unparalleled access over the last two decades to the manuscript and records collections that provide the documentation for this important history, but because of the recent and rapid digitization of newspapers and other serials, I also have been able to uncover press reports on the early events of the movement from all corners of the country, and evidence of the ubiquity of the term *birth control* in American society in the first decade of the movement's existence. These and other sources have come to light through new Internet search capabilities. The early, nationwide press coverage I document in Chapters 2 to 4 demonstrates that the movement's rationales for family limitation reached a broad population in a relatively brief span of time. Newspapers delivered the concept of safe and effective contraception to breakfast tables across the nation, largely erasing the stigma of obscenity within just a few years.

ONE

BEFORE "BIRTH CONTROL"

Few persons are aware how extensively this "destruction of unborn life" is carried on even in what are considered the better classes of society. But the "arts of prevention" which are also being extensively employed are a far more dangerous foe, not only to the family, but to the virtue and purity of the community. They open in a covert way the flood-gates of iniquity. If violations of law are encouraged in married life, and found to be safely practiced there, the same things will be attempted outside and the primary object of marriage will be defeated.[1]
—Dr. N. Allen, "The New England Family," 1882

It has been a little less than 100 years since the words *birth control* first appeared in print, but birth control, as a social practice, is as old as human history. Since the beginning of civilization, women were expected to produce children from marriage to menopause, in a constant battle to birth more children than died in utero, in infancy, or of childhood disease. Yet women in every era and culture, acting alone or with their husbands or lovers, sought ways to delay childbearing or reduce the odds of pregnancy. They did so in spite of cultural and religious prohibitions or societal pressures to increase the size of the tribe. Couples attempted family limitation for reasons that included their own health and sanity and the well-being of their existing children, economic benefits of a smaller family, to reduce the population in times of disease or famine, and because of particular circumstances of time and place.

Besides contraception, two other deliberate methods of family limitation, abortion and infanticide, have also been practiced throughout history, sometimes rarely and at other times with far greater frequency than contraception. However, neither act, occurring after fertilization and birth respectively, is considered a form of birth control in the context of this narrative. (In this text, the terms *birth control* and *contraception* are used interchangeably.) While infanticide is usually viewed as a most extreme form of population control and is universally condemned in the modern era, perceptions about abortion have changed repeatedly over time. Abortion has been conflated with contraception in the past, and strong debate continues as to whether it should be considered an acceptable and legal form of reproductive control. It is worth noting that the birth control movement of the early 20th century, which evolved into a reproductive rights movement that vowed to make and keep abortion legal, set out initially to end the practice of abortion, which was then illegal.

A SHORT HISTORY OF BIRTH CONTROL METHODS

With few exceptions, the birth control strategies and methods couples resorted to and often relied on throughout history did not change significantly until the 20th century. The chief means of family limitation over the centuries might more accurately be described as avoidance techniques: abstinence and withdrawal. Abstinence, either by delaying marriage or avoiding intercourse for protracted periods, has always been the most effective form of birth control, though among the most unsatisfactory. Withdrawal (coitus interruptus), the deliberate act of withdrawing the penis from the vagina prior to ejaculation, is less effective, male-reliant, and viewed in many cultures as at best a lusty male indulgence and at worst a mortal sin: the wider the separation between a sexual act and the potential for procreation, the more likely that the act is fraught with turpitude. Withdrawal is often synonymous with any practice of "spilling the seed"—the act that led God to strike down Onan, withdrawal's unwitting poster-boy—whether by masturbation, oral sex, or any other form of extravaginal sexual contact. Another so-called natural method is extended nursing. Lactation can delay, for a time, the resumption of menstruation. Women have long depended on this natural respite from childbearing, though it is highly unreliable.[2]

Contraceptives, the tools and materials used to prevent conception, have also been around at least as long as humans have recorded their activities. We do not know if contraceptives were widely used in ancient times, but historians and anthropologists suspect that in many regions women employed several types of contraception. There is evidence that some women in the ancient world used suppositories or pessaries: substances or removable objects inserted in the vagina before intercourse to block or kill sperm or reduce sperm motility. Recipes for vaginal plugs and pastes have been found on Egyptian papyrus. The ingredient lists include gum and honey, crocodile dung (animal dung was used in many cultures), the tips of the acacia shrub and other substances that were naturally spermicidal or occlusive—creating a barrier. Depending on the region, women invented and experimented with vaginal plugs made from the roots or pods of certain plants, seaweed, grass, balls of paper, fabric, and other materials. Wool plugs or tampons soaked in a salt solution, or oil or fruit acids were used in ancient Greece and Rome. Aristotle recommended olive oil applied inside the vagina, a method used with some success in recent times. Ancient Jews used natural sponges, possibly soaked in citric acid or a salt solution; French women rediscovered the vaginal sponge in the 18th century and Americans in the late 19th and 20th centuries. Douching or washing carefully after intercourse was employed as a contraceptive method in the ancient world but did not become pervasive until the 1800s. There is even evidence that in preindustrial societies crude surgical sterilizations were performed on both males and females, that women tried the rhythm or safe period method—engaging in intercourse on the days they believed that they were least likely to be fertile—and that trial and error led some enterprising women to devise cervical caps and interuterine devices similar to their modern counterparts.[3]

Other methods that we think of as recent discoveries, such as the oral contraceptive, have earlier, though somewhat suspect, precedents. Most of the drugs, potions, teas, and tinctures that were taken orally and distributed by midwives or passed from woman to woman, were either harmless herbal concoctions or poisons that served as sometimes effective but often harmful abortifacients—substances that cause abortion. There is a long history of women seeking sterility by drinking water boiled with copper or from the blacksmith's cooling bucket; certain metals create a harmful environment for sperm. Several 19th- and 20th-century medical explorers and anthropologists were dazzled by the contraceptive success experienced by Fijian women who regularly consumed a tea made from the roots of the kakaula plant or roqa tree. Handling a sample sent to her by an eccentric naturalist in the late 1930s, Margaret Sanger thought she might be holding the catalyst for the "magic pill" that she hoped would finally liberate women from unwieldy methods and devices. However, the herb proved ineffective in laboratory tests. Russian researchers discovered around 1900 that they could create an immune response to sperm by injecting women subcutaneously with either animal or human semen. These so-called "spermatoxins" looked extremely promising by the 1930s, but scientists could not reliably produce a contraceptive effect. (Fertility specialists today are revisiting these studies and have made significant strides toward developing a birth control vaccine or immunocontraceptive.) Native Americans ingested an infusion made from *lithospermum*, a desert plant in the Southwest that suppresses the estrous cycles in females by acting on the pituitary gland. Other plants and fruits—the papaya for one—contain hormonal compounds that can alter a woman's cycle. Even with our advanced medicine of the 21st century, we are not too far removed from relying on nature to furnish contraceptives.

Wild Mexican yams supplied the steroid hormone that was synthesized to create that "magic pill" Sanger had long envisioned, the first effective oral contraceptive that revolutionized birth control and helped usher in the sexual revolution in the 1960s.[4]

Condoms derive from the early modern period, though various sheaths were worn before then, mostly as a hygienic covering and a barrier to insects. The condom was not developed as a contraceptive but as a prophylactic, to prevent against venereal disease. It became associated almost immediately with prostitution, hindering its potential as a form of marital birth control. Condoms in the 16th through 18th centuries were made of linen or animal skins and bladders, but they were expensive to produce and uncomfortable for both partners. The vulcanization of rubber in the 1840s led to the mass production of the condom, cheaper prices, and increased use as a contraceptive. In fact, though much maligned, the condom became the most popular contraceptive in the United States in the mid-20th century. But it has always been an imperfect method for women who do not wish to rely on men for fertility control.[5]

REPRODUCTIVE CONTROL IN EARLY AMERICA

The methods of reproductive control favored by early Americans did not differ markedly from their European forebears. High fertility rates suggest that married couples either rarely tried or were unable to prevent pregnancies. When couples did decide to limit fertility, they most often turned to withdrawal and abstinence, while relying on extended breastfeeding to help space births. Yet the indelicate subject rarely entered public discussion. Although there were no laws against fertility control until the 19th century, what we know about early American birth control practices comes mainly from legal cases stemming from acts of adultery and fornication.

Plymouth Governor William Bradford wrote in his journal about the predicament of a young wife whose pastor approved her for marriage to another man only after the pastor himself had tested her sexual suitability. The pastor, who likely had prior experience of using his sanctified pedestal to launch sexual assaults, took precautions and "endeavored to hinder conception"; in other words he withdrew in a timely fashion. Abortion, by all accounts, was more common than contraception in colonial America and legal if performed in the early stages of pregnancy, before "quickening" (detectable fetal movement). Herbal concoctions that incorporated savin, pennyroyal, rue, and other known natural abortifacients were taken to trigger miscarriage and used to varying degrees of success. Desperation drove some women to attempt mechanical abortion (the insertion of an instrument into the cervix) or employ other physical means to try to end a pregnancy. In many cases a woman chose this route or was coerced into doing so to conceal an illicit sexual relationship.[6]

American women emerged from the colonial period with a greater desire to control fertility, to time and space births. After the American Revolution, there was less moral oversight of private lives, more freedom in the selection of a spouse and a greater emphasis on personal needs and contentment. Although it is impossible to know for sure, heading into the 19th century, it seems likely that a relatively small number of married couples deliberately tried to control family size. But that number was increasing. For most Americans there were few economic incentives for small families. Agrarian communities especially relied on large families to run farms and preserve them for the next generation. Even so, fertility rates gradually began to decline. After several hundred years of relatively stable birth rates, the United States experienced a demographic transition from larger to smaller families that began around 1800 and lasted until World War II. The fertility rate dropped an astounding 50 percent from 1800 to 1900, from slightly more than seven to about three-and-a-half children per couple. No physiological reasons, such as a high incidence of venereal disease or lack of proper nutrition, could explain such a drop. The reduction in family size was more pronounced among the middle- and upper-classes, particularly in the Northeast. Birth rates held steadier in many rural areas, frontier regions, and among slaves and new immigrants. But a definite trend had developed. The fact that women ceased childbearing at an increasingly earlier age tells us that the overall birth rate decline was due to increased use of birth control.[7]

19TH-CENTURY BIRTH CONTROLLERS

Urbanization and industrialization in the mid- to late 19th century profoundly affected the American family and gave new impetus to fertility control. However, the trend toward smaller families was evident decades before this massive economic growth and migration of jobs from rural farms to urban factories. Birth rate declines began before technological innovation, increased mobility, and, notably, before public health campaigns reduced infant mortality rates. Historians have offered a great deal of speculative logic rather than a singular explanation. Improvements in education and literacy rates, secularization, more open attitudes about sexuality, a greater emphasis on love and intimacy in marriage, and an emerging small family ideal modeled by the wealthy—all of these changes may have played a role in motivating couples to limit family size. But the biggest factor may have been the growth of a middle class that led to women's emergence from domestic confinement. Because women have been the chief instigators of fertility control, it stands to reason that women were exerting greater autonomy to reduce domestic burdens, define themselves outside of their circumscribed roles as mothers and wives, and achieve more control over their lives—and over their sexuality.[8]

Though an increasing number of early-19th-century women and couples may have sought safe birth control and abortion, the whole issue, as historian Janet Brodie has written, was "clothed in secrecy" and "just beginning to emerge into the public domain." Reliable sources of contraceptive information were scarce, and most Americans remained ambivalent about nonprocreative sexuality. The ubiquitous marital and hygiene guides and religious pamphlets of the day mainly focused on sexual excess and other forms of moral depravity. Many set forth strategies for controlling the sexual impulse. Men and women seeking to control conception confronted social and religious conventions that condemned such behavior and severely inhibited sexual expression of any kind. With limited access to information, it is likely that they practiced withdrawal, chose to endure periods of marital chastity, or opted for abortion. It must be emphasized just how bleak these last two options were for most people, which helps explain, in part, the popularity of withdrawal. This method required no cost or special preparation or instruction and offered at least some degree of sexual satisfaction for both partners. However, moral leaders maligned withdrawal as an unnatural and physically harmful act, the same way as they viewed masturbation. Though far less common, some parents committed infanticide, a method of last resort typically for the very poor.[9]

Two groundbreaking American tracts on birth control, first published in the early 1830s, helped to lift the veil of secrecy and instigate a public and legal debate over contraception. Freethinker (someone who rejected state authority and church dogma) Robert Dale Owen (1801–1877), a newspaper editor and writer, published *Moral Physiology; or, A Brief and Plain Treatise on the Population Question* in 1831. In the long essay, Owen considers human reproduction to be "the most social and least selfish of all our instincts" and recommends ways to achieve sexual "gratification" without having more children. He presents social and economic arguments for family limitation, followed by a reasoned explanation of the virtues of withdrawal, including some of the first case studies ever published to prove the efficacy of Owen's preferred method. He also briefly discusses the pros and cons of the vaginal sponge and the French *baudruche*, or condom, made of fine animal skin or silk. Owen advanced the idea that sexual pleasure removed from procreation should be viewed without compunction and is, in fact, desirable. The book stayed in print for 40 years and sold over 70,000 copies. It also inspired Dr. Charles Knowlton (1800–1850) to write *Fruits of Philosophy*, first published anonymously in 1832 and subtitled *The Private Companion of Young Married People*, a more influential book than Owen's tract and one that landed the author in prison.[10]

An ambitious country doctor in western Massachusetts, Knowlton was inspired by Owen's social reasoning. And, like Owen, his work was shaped by Francis Place, the English social reformer whose *Principles of Population* (1822) and series of handbills distributed among the English working class promoted withdrawal, as well as the vaginal sponge and plug. Knowlton largely rejected these methods and instructed his married women readers to douche, "syringing the vagina, soon after the male emission into it, with some liquid, which will not merely dislodge nearly all the semen, as simple water would do . . . but which will destroy the fecundating property of any portion of semen that may remain." He recommended a douching solution of alum, a readily available preservative and baking powder ingredient, but found bicarbonate of soda, vinegar, salt water, and other solutions to be effective as well. Knowlton was the first American marriage advice writer to endorse a contraceptive device (a syringe) that placed women in control, although the method had a fairly high failure rate. Knowlton also laid out the terms of the debate over birth control that would extend well into the 20th century. Those opposed to contraception, he wrote, believed it was an unnatural act and would lead to immoral behavior. But Knowlton responds by asking rhetorically, "What is civilized life but one continual warfare against nature? The high prerogative of man consists in his power to counteract and to control nature." He points out that women were just as capable of losing their chastity without the knowledge of contraception and with the fear of pregnancy. Moreover, he believed that birth control, what he called the "anti-conception art," would reduce prostitution, limit excessive population growth, and ease poverty. Anticipating the role that eugenics, the study of how to improve human heredity, would play in the 20th century birth control movement, Knowlton held that contraceptive practice would eventually prevent hereditary diseases and lead to a stronger and healthier race.*[11]

Knowlton sold over 9,000 copies of *Fruits of Philosophy* before the end of the 1830s. Many of those books were probably passed on to other interested readers, making for an impressive audience at that time. With its success, the book raised the moral hackles of local clergy and more than a few fellow physicians in Massachusetts. Some opponents complained to the authorities about the dangerous advice that Knowlton doled out in his frank and friendly manner. Others may have been more alarmed over Knowlton's explicit descriptions of human sexual anatomy and sexual functioning than the fact that he advocated contraception. Between 1832 and 1835, Knowlton was prosecuted three times on obscenity charges; the second case resulted in a three-month sentence to hard labor. He was the first, but by no means the last, birth controller to go to prison. No rabble-rouser, Knowlton quietly served his sentence before returning to his respectable medical practice in the small farming town of Ashfield, Massachusetts. Although he has been called "the founder of American contraceptive medicine"—and the popularity of contraceptive douching through the 19th and into the 20th century can be directly linked to his multiple editions of *Fruits*—Knowlton had no interest in becoming a crusader. His book, however, like Owen's, lent an air of legitimacy to conception control and began to move a private matter into the public light. It also inspired activism long after the author's death in

---

* The term *race*, as used by birth controllers and eugenicists, commonly referred to the human race as a whole.

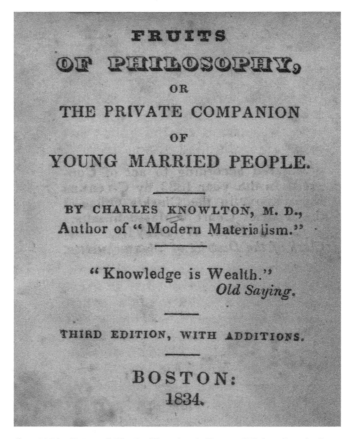

Title page of an 1834 edition of Charles Knowlton's *Fruits of Philosophy*, which was published anonymously in 1832. It was the most detailed contraceptive guide of its time and landed the author in prison. (Courtesy of the Duke University Medical Center Library.)

1850 and led, indirectly, to the establishment of the first organization in the world formed to promote family limitation.[12]

In England in 1877, the lawyer and social reformer Charles Bradlaugh and fellow freethinker Annie Besant reprinted *Fruits of Philosophy* with the intent to challenge attempts by the British government to suppress contraceptive information. They were arrested for violating Britain's Obscene Publication Act, and the ensuing trial ended on appeal with a dismissal of the charges. The case created enormous publicity and popular support for the free discussion of birth control, and resulted in the formation in England of the Malthusian League in 1878, established by neo-Malthusians Charles Robert Drysdale and his wife Alice Vickery. The neo-Malthusians adapted the central theory of economist and demographer Thomas Malthus (1766–1834). Malthus contended that the rate of population would continue to rise exponentially because of the human sex drive. He claimed that population growth would eventually exceed the means of subsistence, resulting in poverty and other forms of human distress. Malthus doubted that societies could regulate population growth and argued that human disasters such as war, famine, or disease were the only limiting factors. The only concept of birth control that he advocated was moral restraint. However, the neo-Malthusians believed in finding positive means of controlling population and became strong advocates of contraception. They also subscribed to many of the beliefs held by the economist, philosopher, and women's rights advocate, John Stuart Mill, who, though he did not explicitly discuss methods, emphasized the improvements that family limitation would bring to the lives of the working class. The Malthusian League's chief aim was to lower the birth rate of the poor and improve their standard of living. Though it operated more as a think tank than an outlet for practical information, the League guided the creation of similar organizations throughout Europe and inspired Dutch physician Aletta Jacobs to open the world's first contraceptive clinic in Amsterdam in 1882.[13]

THE PROLIFERATION OF CONTRACEPTIVE LITERATURE AND DEVICES

The Bradlaugh-Besant trial kicked up sales of reprint editions of *Fruits of Philosophy* in the United States, where it achieved new notoriety. In the years since it first appeared, the book had been joined by an array of sex guides and hygiene books. Itinerant sex educators (both male and female) crisscrossed antebellum America speaking on issues related to fertility and sexual health, dispensed birth control advice, and peddled their publications. Some were charlatans; many were legitimate doctors selling their own wares or publications. Frederick Hollick, a young English-born physician, filled lecture halls with talks on sexual diseases, sexual functioning, and ways to avoid conception by following a safe-period method—charting when a woman was most likely to conceive according to the date of her ovulation. It is not clear how many women successfully followed Hollick's method, since no one had yet pinned down the correct timing of a women's cycle, but his calculations were picked up by other advice mavens. Hollick used his well-attended lectures, enlivened by impressive life-like, pull-apart models of the human torso, to peddle a series of publications that became even more popular following his arrest and acquittal on obscenity charges in the mid-1840s.[14]

One quasi-quack, A. M. Mauriceau of New York, charged customers an exorbitant $10 to send them the "French secret," probably an alum powder douching solution that he advertised in his pamphlets. Mauriceau (the alias was meant to evoke

French sexual expertise and savoir-faire) was actuality Joseph Trow. He probably worked with his sister, Ann Trow Lohman, better known as the infamous New York City abortionist, Madame Restell. He (or they) wrote another sought-after guide, *The Married Woman's Private Medical Companion*—much of it taken verbatim from Owen's work—which was published in at least nine editions in the 15 years before the Civil War. It included advertisements for abortion-causing drugs, condoms, and douches that were available through the mail or at a Manhattan office that performed abortions. Although much of the information on reproductive control was untrustworthy, by mid-century it was pervasive in these books and others. In the absence of legal regulation before 1873, this information reached many working-class Americans, even in rural areas. However, poor women were still more likely to resort to abortion than middle-class or wealthier women, who generally had access to more effective contraception.[15]

The process of rubber manufacturing was perfected in the early 1850s, leading to a boom in the production of inexpensive rubber goods, most notably condoms, which had previously been made from animal intestines and imported from Europe. Often referred to as "French rubber goods," condoms were easily obtainable and widely advertised in newspapers and flyers to prevent disease. A whole array of rubber devices for women, including pessaries and rubber syringes for douching, were offered in pharmacies, and through mail-order businesses and independent rubber goods vendors. Some of these devices had other medical uses, but mainly they were sold as contraceptives. In fact, every contraceptive that was available in mid-20th-century America had also been for sale in pre-Civil War-America, except for the modern diaphragm. A kind of expanded cervical rubber cap, the diaphragm was possibly created by Dr. Edward Bliss Foote in the 1860s and improved by the German physician Wilhelm Mensinga in the 1880s, but was not widely used until years later.[16]

The growing consumer demand for contraceptives and abortifacients encouraged doctors, midwives, druggists, and other entrepreneurs to enter this burgeoning trade. In 1856, Dr. William Alcott, a prolific hygiene writer and social observer, raised the alarm that the "general disposition to avoid conception and pregnancy seems to me greatly increasing." He commented on the ubiquity of *Fruits of Philosophy* and several other advice books, which had sales in the hundreds of thousands, and expressed great concern about the public tolerance of abortion, which retained common-law protection if done before quickening. By mid-century there was an upsurge in both the use of abortifacients, widely available through mail-order firms and often even sold over the counter, and the number of doctors who devoted their practices to performing abortions. One of the first medical specializations in the country, abortion then carried less risk than childbirth. Many daily newspapers ran ads for cure-alls and remedies (the word *abortion* was not used) that were marketed as pregnancy preventatives. Classified listings for "Dr. Duponco's French Periodical Golden Pills" promised that its medicine would "prevent pregnancy to those ladies whose health will not permit an increase in family." Ads for "Cherokee Pills," a "female regulator" available through a mail-order firm in New York City, appeared with a sales pitch disguised as a warning: if the pills were used during the first three months of pregnancy, "the unfailing nature of their action would infallibly prevent pregnancy." Hygiene and medical publications were available from dubious outfits such as the "New York Benevolent Infirmary," which sold the "Ladies Medical Friend" and the "Gentlemen's Medical Companion," guaranteed to have all of the answers on pregnancy "cures" and venereal disease. These and other publications were also advertised in many newspapers.

As contraceptive information became more widely available, much of the advice literature also became more direct, dispatching with euphemism and delicacy and launching into frank discussions of reproductive anatomy and conception control. F. Barham Zincke, an English clergyman who toured America in 1867 to 1868, noted the increasing prevalence of small families and later wrote "There is no secret as to the various means resorted to for carrying out these unnatural resolutions. They are advertised in every newspaper, and there are professors of the art in abundance . . . in every city." He found that though "many denounce it . . . still it spreads; and we cannot expect that it will die away, as long as the motives which prompt it continue to be felt as strongly as they are at present."[17]

What were those motives? The purveyors of contraceptive devices and information generally stuck to the rationale of improving women's health, although some urged birth control for economic reasons or to avoid passing on a disease or deformity. At the most basic level, however, men and women wished to enjoy sexual union without the concern of pregnancy, regardless of whatever other reasons they may have had to limit childbearing. Reflecting changing attitudes about sexuality, the medical advice literature emphasized pleasure and happiness and the importance of physical intimacy to a sound marriage. Anticipating modern marketing practices, the self-help industry, which took off in the latter half of the 19th century, promoted contraception as a means to forge stronger marriages and gain greater self-control. Marriage manuals and advice tracts idealized sexual union and often labeled abstinence unnatural.

The one extant survey of the sexual habits of 19th-century women confirms that sexual intimacy and pleasure had become an acknowledged cornerstone of marriage and that the regular use of birth control made this goal attainable. Between 1892 and 1912, 47 wives of professional men filled out Dr. Clelia Mosher's extensive questionnaire covering their sexual experiences dating from a few years before the Civil War to the early years of the 20th century (most of the respondents were born before 1870). Though the sample was small, it indicates that these middle- and upper-class women used birth control often. Forty-three of the 47 women said they employed some form of fertility control. Douching was by far the most common method, with nearly twice as many users as withdrawal or the safe period. A smaller number relied on condoms or pessaries, and many used methods in combination. At a minimum, half of the women had to have procured a contraceptive, either from a store or mail-order firm. The numbers alone tell us that women were actively taking control of their fertility, with or without their husbands' involvement. The women's comments on the survey leave no doubt that a majority viewed marital sex as pleasurable and could disengage sex from its procreative function, though they still viewed reproduction as the primary purpose of marital intercourse.[18]

OPPOSITION TO REPRODUCTIVE CONTROL

Surprisingly, the upsurge in abortions and contraceptive use did not arouse a noticeable increase in opposition to family limitation or advocacy of moral reform from the religious community. Clerical disapproval of reproductive control, evident during the first decades of the 19th century, amounted to little more than background noise after the 1830s, with the exception of a few vociferous Protestant opponents. The Western Massachusetts moralist and Congregational minister, Reverend John Todd, wrote bitterly in 1868 about the shameless, unnamed "fashion"—family limitation— that was destroying the American family and "threatens to desolate our land." Even in the last decades of the century, religious leaders across the denominations rarely spoke about reproductive control, except to warn of Onan's sin (withdrawal).

Instead, by mid-century, physicians became the main oppositional force and moral arbiters on issues related to birth control and especially abortion. Doctors grew more outspoken in deploring abortion on moral grounds; more of them acknowledged a belief that abortion at any stage of gestation amounted to the destruction of human life. The nascent medical establishment was more conflicted over contraception. Some doctors conflated it with abortion; others approved of natural methods like the safe period but condemned "unnatural" rubber devices. Physicians disagreed about the effectiveness and safety of various methods. Most doctors simply avoided the subject, at least publicly. But with considerable self-interest at stake, a growing number of physicians aimed to crack down on the rampant quackery inside the profitable contraception and abortion trades to improve the reputation of the medical profession. In the 19th century a fine line often separated an educated doctor from either the charlatans who dispensed panaceas or folk healers and midwives. Ostensibly, doctors expressed concern over the health risks of abortion, and to a lesser extent, mechanical contraceptives. However, their opposition to family limitation was steeped in conservative values, centered on preserving a traditional concept of sexuality wed to reproduction, and focused on limiting female sexual independence and keeping women from taking control over their own reproductive lives. Speaking out about the dangers of birth control and abortion helped lift doctors to a higher position of moral authority in American society and distance them from abortionists and other "irregular" practitioners. The organization of the medical community and the establishment of medical standards coincided with medicine's growing opposition to all forms of reproductive control. The American Medical Association, founded in 1847 to professionalize doctors, became a leading force behind the passage of the nation's most restrictive abortion laws starting in the 1860s. Before then, a majority of states had enacted limitations on abortion chiefly to regulate providers but not to oppose the practice, as long as it occurred before quickening. Between 1860 and 1890, 40 U.S. states and territories passed antiabortion statutes that either criminalized abortion at any stage of pregnancy or imposed severe restrictions. The new laws also limited advertising and, more significantly, shifted the decision-making power if and when to end a pregnancy from woman to doctor.[19]

SOCIAL PURITY

After the Civil War, the medical community was joined in its efforts to reign in the contraceptive and abortion industries by a new morality movement and social purity crusade that emerged largely in reaction to the postwar rise in prostitution, pornography, and venereal disease. The momentous changes taking place in American society added to these concerns: urbanization and the new industrial economy, worker migration, the movement of more women into the workforce, and the flood of immigrants. Increased mobility, isolation, and anonymity weakened the moral authority of the church and family. More single men and women left small towns for cities, where they had to navigate temptation and squalor. Crime rates soared, Gilded Age greed ruled the business world, and corruption defined the politics of the time. Morality was being undermined everywhere.

War-torn America had been fertile ground for sexual commerce, which continued to thrive after the war. Cheap pornographic pulp novels, prints, and photographs were widely available by mail-order and in train stations, pool halls, and other places where men congregated. In most urban centers, professional and casual prostitution flourished, and dance halls and massage parlors were commonplace. As historian James Reed has written: "Prostitution symbolized the degradation of woman through the separation of sex from both love and procreation." Pornography and alcohol only flamed the fire, driving more men to seek sexual expression outside of the home. "The men who committed such crimes," Reed continues, were seen as "poor fathers, poor citizens, and a danger to innocent wives and infants who might become infected with syphilis or gonorrhea. A just society in which healthy mothers could flourish depended on the suppression of male vice."[20]

The purity movement was a loose coalition led by women's rights activists and Protestant moral reformers. It was energized by middle-class women who looked to control male sexual desire as a way of gaining more autonomy and to enforce the same sexual standard for men and women. Purity advocates had established their reform credentials in movements for women's rights, temperance in matters of alcohol, and the abolition of slavery, or from experience with Protestant missions, anti-prostitution crusades, law-enforcement leagues, and moral education groups. They had different political agendas and often worked at cross purposes but shared the goal of restricting sexuality to the private sphere, to the marital bed, and ridding the urban environment of sexual depravity and corruption. Contraception was implicated in the perceived growth of moral decay by its association with a freer sexual climate, though it was not the main target of reform. By restricting sexual expression to the home, purity crusaders hoped to reassert the reproductive function of sexuality and the spiritual nature of the marriage bond. Some called this merged social movement the *new abolitionism*. The zealotry at times reached an evangelical fervor as reformers focused on what they deemed a moral crisis in the nation's cities.

Although the medical profession and law enforcement generally sought to contain prostitution through regulation, women's rights and purity advocates wanted it stamped out to protect families from the threat of syphilis and gonorrhea, which were both then incurable. In waging a battle over the regulation of prostitution and obscenity, these reformers logically extended their campaign to the suppression of birth control devices and information, which further drove the divide between sex for reproduction and sex for pleasure. Medical conservatives and religious fundamentalists—those most dead set against contraception—were particularly alarmed about the declining birth rate and the potential for fertility control to empower women. However, many women reformers who looked to restrict the sexual freedom of men—and sexual expression in general—did not always rule out birth control, though they generally refused to condone devices viewed as tools of the sex trade, such as condoms. Their preference was to abstain from sex except when trying to become pregnant. Feminists confirmed that women had sexual desires (something of a revelation at the time), and they wanted to give women more control over marital sexuality—to be able to decide when and how often to engage in intercourse—as well as reproduction. Many women reformers also respected the small family ideal that was spreading in industrialized America. Vehemently opposed to abortion, their concerns over contraception were muted. Nevertheless, when the sweep of moral reform extended to encompass reproductive control, women purity advocates, even those who expressed ambivalence about contraception, did not stand in the way.[21]

COMSTOCKERY

An emphatic federal legal response to controlling sexual vice came less than a decade after the Civil War, with the passage in Congress in 1873 of the "Act for

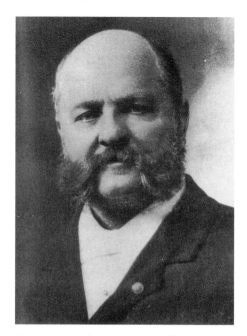

Undated portrait of Anthony Comstock at the height of his career as America's foremost anti-vice crusader. (Courtesy of the Sophia Smith Collection, Smith College.)

the Suppression of Trade in, and Circulation of Obscene Literature and Articles of Immoral Use," Section 211 of the U.S. Criminal Code.* Better known as the Comstock Act, named after the notorious vice crusader, Anthony Comstock, this repressive legislation was part of a larger postal bill that Congress passed during a flurry of legislative activity, without significant debate. The new law prohibited the mailing of lewd and obscene publications, prints or pictures, and "any article or thing designed or intended for the prevention of conception or procuring of abortion," as well as any type of advertisement for birth control and just about any form of contraceptive information. It also banned the importation of contraceptives. By associating contraception with illicit sex and pornography, the Comstock Act tainted the very idea of birth control.

Anthony Comstock (1844–1915) manifested the moral reform movement's most extreme inclinations to censor and suppress. Not unlike Senator Joseph McCarthy's

---

* Prohibitions specified in the act were also codified in sections 245 and 312 of the Criminal Code and Section 305 of the Tariff Law.

excessive and reckless campaign to ferret out Communists in the 1950s, Comstock took it on himself to identify purveyors of sin, confiscate the goods, and intimidate or arrest the violators. He targeted pornographers, prostitutes, abortionists, and retailers who sold condoms, cervical caps, or other rubber devices, ruining many lives in the process. The product of a conservative Christian upbringing, Comstock exerted a self-righteous, evangelical Puritanism as he set about to protect the young from immoral influences. "Our youth are in danger;" he wrote, "mentally and morally they are cursed by a literature that is a disgrace to the 19th century. The spirit of evil environs them." Making his living as a shipping clerk and then a dry-goods salesman in New York City, Comstock became obsessed with snuffing out pornography dealers large and small. His vigilante work led him into an association with the New York Young Men's Christian Association (YMCA). With backing from a number of wealthy and influential businessmen, the YMCA formed the Committee for the Suppression of Vice in 1872 and named Comstock as its chief special agent. In 1873, he went to Washington to lobby Congress for stronger federal antiobscenity laws, which contained a number of loopholes and were enforced only sporadically. He exhibited to members of Congress some of the assorted contraceptives, sex devices, and pornographic materials that he had seized during raids of New York sex shops, and submitted a draft bill that became his eponymous act, making his name synonymous with censorship and prudery. So taken were some congressmen with Comstock's zealotry and accomplishments that they appointed him a special postal agent to implement the new law. With unprecedented enforcement powers for a clerk with no formal training, Comstock labored mightily—and almost single-handedly at times—for the next 40 years to lessen the blight of immorality that he believed was corrupting the souls of young Americans. He measured his success in numbers of people arrested and tons of obscenity destroyed—over 3,000 and 160, respectively, by the end of his career.[22]

Comstock classed contraceptives with obscenity because both encouraged the sexual impulse, opened the door to sexual relations outside of marriage, and ultimately led to "the degradation of youth." Like many of his contemporaries, he connected artificial birth control with lasciviousness and found it unnatural and ungodly. On his vice hunts Comstock did not discriminate between unsavory rubber vendors, abortionists, or respected doctors who published birth control tracts, although he usually focused his attacks on the seedier elements. Dr. Edward Bliss Foote became the first well-known contraceptive proponent to fall victim to Comstock's purge. In 1874, Comstock used a decoy letter to obtain Foote's *Words in Pearl for the Married*, a 10-cent pamphlet that advocated certain contraceptive techniques to be used by women whose health would be endangered by pregnancy. Foote was prosecuted on charges of sending obscenity through the mail and fined a hefty $3,000. Though he continued his medical practice, he proceeded more cautiously. This arrest and other proscriptive actions brought about by the Comstock Act and earlier antiabortion laws led to the censorship of information on all forms of fertility control. Along with the many "little Comstock" state laws enacted in the latter decades of the 19th century, the restrictions forced contraceptive advocates and commercial interests underground.

Sensational publicity surrounding Comstock's elaborate entrapments and arrests and the sometimes dramatic trials that followed reinforced the danger faced by abortionists, advice writers, and contraceptive dealers. Ann Lohman, the abortionist and contraceptive entrepreneur doing business as Madame Restell, was among Comstock's most notorious victims. In 1878, Comstock paid a visit to the 67-year-old Restell at her posh Fifth Avenue town house (the reproductive control business had been very lucrative), pretending to be destitute and in need of an aid to end his wife's pregnancy. He left with "some implements and remedies." Comstock later returned with two police officers at his side. Restell was arrested and sent to The Tombs, the deplorable holding jail in lower Manhattan. After several weeks she met bail, but the strong likelihood of a lengthy prison sentence sent her into despair. The *New York Times* reported "End of a Criminal Life. Mme. Restell Commits Suicide. She Cuts Her Throat with a Carving Knife, and Is Found Dead in a Bathtub." Despite a chorus of disapproval from the press over Comstock's methods, he summed up the case with a shameless shrug, noting it was "A bloody ending to a bloody life." He bragged that Restell was his fifteenth victim to commit suicide.[23]

Comstockery (the term coined by British playwright George Bernard Shaw to refer to America's fit of extreme moralizing) was fortified by political endorsement and judicial sanction, and it spread outward from its epicenter in New York. Antivice groups sprung up in New England, several cities in the Midwest, and in San Francisco. Agents provocateurs across the country lured in unsuspecting merchants and publishers, and police chased away contraceptive vendors. Relatively few were arrested for giving contraceptive information (only about 5 percent of Comstock's cases involved contraception), and judges often showed a bit more tolerance for birth control offenders than other types of obscenity criminals. But on the whole, the courts legitimized the Comstock Act, hewing to the letter of the law despite uncertainty over the meaning of obscenity and, in some instances, in spite of clear violations of an individual's right to free speech.

After criminalization, the medical profession became even more reluctant to dirty their hands in the matter. By the end of the 19th century, stricter laws in a number of states clearly prohibited doctors from giving contraceptive advice or performing abortions at any time during pregnancy. These laws reinforced the prevalent medical judgment that contraception was physiologically dangerous, aberrant, and immoral. Although the legislation helped reduce the number of medical frauds who competed with professionals, these federal and state laws created confusion for a medical profession that was still working hard to achieve legitimacy and position doctors as standard-bearers of morality. Medical schools, with very few exceptions, had avoided condoning contraception or teaching contraceptive techniques; criminalization ensured that this trend would continue. Doctors struggled to figure out under what circumstances—if any—they *could* prescribe contraception or perform an abortion. Some physicians questioned whether the law restricted their speech with patients and even with colleagues, and they feared sending contraceptive information through the mails or publishing journal articles that discussed the subject. Many doctors did exercise ethical latitude in dispensing contraception and arranging "therapeutic abortions"—legal in a number of states if performed to save a woman's life. As a consequence, middle- and upper-class women, especially in urban areas, often could find and afford a sympathetic private doctor willing to assist them with contraception or take care of an untenable situation, while most poor and working-class women had to resort to inferior birth control and disreputable and unsafe abortion providers. So began a class-based trend that continued until the legalization of abortion in 1973.[24]

UNDERGROUND CONTRACEPTIVE TRADE

Criminalization scared off many of the mainstream publishers of contraceptive advice literature, narrowed the distribution channels, and suppressed respectable authors. The old standbys like Knowlton's *Fruits* and Annie Besant's *Law of Population* continued to circulate but were more difficult to obtain. Other guides disguised, or in some cases omitted, sections on contraceptive advice. To guard against indictment, a few advice authors prefaced their works with warnings about the potential dangers associated with various forms of reproductive control and cut out or reduced the number of contraceptive ads that helped pay for their tracts. Increasingly, it was left to small and more nimble publishing outfits and underground presses to try to fill a growing information void. The net result was a decrease in the quantity and the quality of available contraceptive information.

Under the shadow of the Comstock laws, contraceptive manufacturers continued to sell their products but were forced to adjust to the new realities. It was more difficult to advertise in newspapers and magazines, which took more care in screening ads for unlawful terms such as "prevention of conception." A number of catalogs and stores, including many pharmacies, still carried popular birth control methods, but supplies were unpredictable. For marketing reasons, the industry had already given more appealing names to various preventives, and it now adopted euphemisms for its own protection. Contraceptives became "marital aids" or "hygienic" devices. Manufacturers played up effectiveness and reliability without mentioning reproductive control. Pessaries were advertised as "womb supporters" and "uterine elevators," needed for proper recovery after childbirth. They were used to correct a "tipped" uterus and other supposed female problems, but mainly were sold as contraceptives. Contraceptive sponges were offered as sanitary products. (As historian Andrea Tone has written, it was as if "sperm became a germ.") Syringes and suppositories were labeled for hygienic use and to treat a vast array of gynecological problems. Condoms were marketed as shields, "*capotes*" (an overcoat in French) and gentlemen's "rubber goods." Various abortion concoctions continued to be sold as cure-alls and featured explicit warnings that they might interfere with early pregnancy. Customers knew what they were buying, and surely the authorities recognized deceptive promotion. But it was not easy to prove illicit use of medical products or track down the numerous small-time entrepreneurs who used false names and seldom stayed in one location. Nor were vice agents equipped to confront the well-established, respected, and profitable medical and drug supply businesses, rubber conglomerates like Goodyear and Goodrich, and the mega-catalog retail outlets like Sears & Roebuck. Instead, Comstock and his men concentrated on the smaller mom-and-pop operations, condom outlets, and medical quacks who frequently operated cheek-and-jowl with smut shops in urban prostitution districts.[25]

FREE LOVERS

Comstock also became obsessed with the utopians and anarchists known as free lovers, who rejected the legal constraints of marriage and celebrated a woman's right to sexual pleasure. These civil libertarians, driven to abolish the institution of marriage, were primarily concerned with individual rights. They defended access to birth control information under the mantle of free speech. Prevention of conception was central to their ability to achieve fulfilling sexual relationships and gain equality for women, but it never became their principal cause. Although some of the sexual radicals accepted artificial contraception or practiced withdrawal, many opted for alternative forms of control, primarily coitus reservatus—intercourse whereby the man brings himself close to orgasm, but does not ejaculate and remains engaged until long after his loss of erection. Though the technique was never widely adopted for obvious reasons, this more female-friendly method, generally referred to at the time as male continence or the Magnetation Method, was practiced mid-century in John Humphrey Noyes's utopian Oneida Community in upstate New York. The anarchist and feminist, Ezra Heywood, revisited the idea in his antimarriage tract, *Cupid's Yokes* (1878), as did the physician and advice writer, Alice Stockham, who called it *Karezza* (1896). Free lovers also practiced other variations of male continence, believing that such restraint built character and robust health.

Many at the time, Comstock included, erroneously believed that these sex radicals promulgated a promiscuous lifestyle when, in fact, they discouraged gratuitous sex and accepted monogamy. Free lovers (Comstock called them "free lusters") and social purity reformers, apart from their insuperable differences on marriage, were fairly closely aligned in their views on sexuality: both opposed male sexual dominance, whether manifested through prostitution or within marriage; advocated self-control; and celebrated an exalted, more spiritual love between man and woman. Much of the sex radicals' thinking had become so rooted in the mainstream of late-19th-century attitudes toward sexuality that they might have escaped persecution if not for their commitment to the free discussion of sexuality in public forums. Sexual radicals such as Heywood and the women's rights advocate, publisher, and early proponent of eugenics, Moses Harman, both wrote about or circulated explicit information on sexuality and birth control. Along with several other sex radicals, they became victims of Comstock's campaign. Heywood was hounded by Comstock for years and was tried several times on obscenity charges, serving three years in prison at the end of his life. One charge stemmed from an ad he printed in his anarchist monthly, *The Word*, for a douching device called the "Comstock Syringe," a not-so-subtle taunt. Moses Harman, publisher of *Lucifer, the Light-Bearer*, a radical journal devoted to freeing women from all forms of sex slavery, ran afoul of the Comstock Law in 1890 for publishing a letter about marital rape. Harman served five years in prison and then another in 1906, at age 75, for publishing an article on birth control.

The free lovers, along with groups of antireligious freethinkers, were the only ones in the 19th century to mount a sustained public protest of the Comstock Law. They passed resolutions that called for legislative reform and attacked the law as an enemy of free thought and free expression. Although unsuccessful in changing the law, they provided something of an activist model for the 20th-century birth control movement, which first rallied over free speech concerns. The sex radicals' unequivocal belief in a woman's right to control her own body also prefigured the central feminist rationale for reproductive rights in the 20th century. In 1880, feminist writer Angela Heywood, Ezra Heywood's wife, summarized the emerging feminist contention in regard to the government suppression of contraceptive information:

> . . . any information "article or thing designed or intended to prevent conception" is proscribed by the statute, which thereby affirms the present subjection of woman to man, denying us all discrimination as to when, where, how or by whom we may bear children. . . . This so called "government" now holds woman's person for man's use or abuse as he pleases; and that *her* claim to own even her womb is *criminally* obscene!"[26]

By the end of the 19th century, government, medicine, and public opinion jointly supported state suppression of contraception. Many citizens were clearly disturbed that boundaries confining sex to marriage and reproduction appeared irreparably broken. Contraception had been sullied by its legal association with obscenity and growing popular identification with sexual commerce. Reproductive control was at odds with the glorification of female sexual purity and the sentimentalized ideal of marriage—loving and faithful but in effect sexless—that was central to temperate, moral America as it emerged from one of the greatest periods of transition and social turbulence in its history. Yet we know from the thriving illicit trade in contraceptives, the Mosher survey, and the continuing declines in the birth rate that birth control was prevalent and used not only to restrict family size and for health reasons, but also to increase sexual enjoyment. The 20th-century birth control movement would seize on this contradiction between the private acceptance of, and public opposition to, birth control. Despite their ambivalence about female sexuality and the legitimacy of nonprocreative sex, Americans were increasingly turning to both old and new ways to control reproduction. Although the Comstock Law "had teeth," as Margaret Sanger later wrote, the days of Comstockery were numbered.[27]

TWO

❦

BIRTH CONTROL
AND FREE SPEECH

Pass on this information to your neighbor and comrade workers. Write out any of the following information which you are sure will help her, and pass it along where it is needed. Spread this important knowledge![1]

—Margaret Sanger, 1914

THE FREE SPEECH LEAGUE

"If *The Woman Rebel* were allowed to publish with impunity elementary and fundamental truths concerning personal liberty and how to obtain it, the birth control movement would become a movement of tremendous power in the emancipation of the working class." So wrote Margaret Sanger in a June 1914 article in *The Woman Rebel* in which she first used the phrase *birth control* and first cited the existence of a birth control movement. This was a ploy to attract supporters, as no movement had yet formed beyond the handful of friends and others who worked on the *Rebel* in Sanger's living room.[2]

What did exist was a small but vigorous free speech movement rooted in the campaigns to repeal the Comstock Law, campaigns waged by Ezra and Angela Heywood, Moses Harman, the freethinker and publisher D. M. Bennett, and other late-19th- and turn-of-the-century libertarian radicals, feminists, and atheists. Freethinker organizations such as the National Liberal League and its more radical offshoot, the

National Defense Association, mounted free speech protests and distributed petitions against obscenity laws. Suppression of anarchist speech following the assassination of President McKinley in 1901 prompted the formation of the Free Speech League (FSL) in 1902 (incorporated in 1911). The FSL was a loosely gathered organization that assisted victims of censorship and looked to spread free speech agitation beyond the anarchist community. Fertility control, considered an essential component of free expression by many libertarian radicals, was just one of many free speech issues pursued by the FSL in the first decade of the 20th century. Leadership of the FSL included Dr. Edward Bond Foote (the son of Dr. Edward Bliss Foote), civil rights attorneys Theodore Schroeder and Gilbert Roe, socialist and freethinker Leonard Abbott, and the muckraking journalist Lincoln Steffens, among others.

In one of the League's first acts, it supported Ida Craddock, a spiritualist and marriage advice writer, who was arrested and imprisoned by Comstock. She was charged with sending her quirky and frank, but rather wholesome and conservative (no drinking, touching, or artificial birth control) sex instruction manuals through the mails. In October 1902, between prison sentences, Craddock killed herself, leaving a letter to the public that she hoped would raise questions about Comstock's motives and methods. She wrote, "Perhaps it may be that in my death more than in my life, the American people may be shocked into investigating the dreadful state of affairs which permits that unctuous sexual hypocrite, Anthony Comstock, to wax fat and arrogant, and to trample upon the liberties of the people, invading, in my own case, both my right to freedom of religion and to freedom of the press." Craddock's suicide did spark a backlash against Comstock, not unlike Madame Restell's death over 20 years before, and focused greater attention on the right of free speech. Harman, Foote, and the other radicals who helped coordinate the FSL understood that in creating a debate over free speech they could appeal to a broader public who might be willing to support civil liberties even if they objected to certain other radical ideas. Harman wrote just a few months before Craddock's death that "even among those who will not so much listen to our more extreme views," some "will respond to the plea for free speech. . . ."[3]

EMMA GOLDMAN

The FSL played a role in nearly every major free speech dispute through the end of World War I and was closely associated with defending the speech of anarchist Emma Goldman (1869–1940), the radical leader most active before the war in agitating for birth control. A Russian Jewish immigrant who arrived in the United States in 1885, Goldman became the most recognized and notorious Progressive Era radical. Her particular brand of anarchism developed out of a belief in the unrestricted right of free expression, borrowed from both European and American concepts of

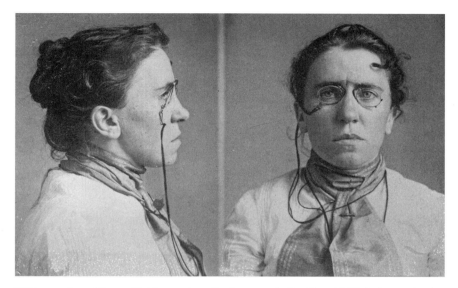

1901 mug shot of Emma Goldman taken after her arrest in President McKinley's assassination case. (Courtesy of the George Grantham Bain Collection, Library of Congress.)

individualism. Goldman also emphasized sexual and reproductive freedom—an unconventional and at times controversial position to embrace within an anarchist community where labor actions and anti-authoritarian campaigns often eclipsed women's issues and matters of self-expression, which many anarchists deemed less important.

Convicted of unlawful assembly in 1893, Goldman spent 10 months in New York's Blackwell's Island prison, where she trained on the job as a prison nurse, work that later led to formal studies in Vienna in obstetric nursing and midwifery. Back in New York, Goldman juggled meetings and speaking engagements with her new profession as a midwife, tending to poor, immigrant women who "lived in continual dread of conception." "When they found themselves pregnant," she wrote, "their alarm and worry would result in the determination to get rid of their expected offspring." Goldman noted the desperate ways in which these women sought to end their pregnancies, by "jumping off tables, rolling on the floor, massaging the stomach, drinking nauseating concoctions, and using blunt instruments. These and similar methods were being tried, generally with great injury. It was harrowing, but it was understandable." Many women asked Goldman to perform abortions, which she refused out of concern about complications. Others asked her to furnish them with birth control information, about which Goldman professed ignorance. When she consulted with physicians about contraception, they were dismissive, blaming the women themselves for their reproductive distress, calling them ignorant and lacking in self control. Goldman soon abandoned nursing, in part because of her own health problems and also to focus on a cross-country lecture tour. Her nursing experience had given her a first-hand understanding of how unwanted pregnancies could destroy women's lives, and it infused her speeches with a stronger emphasis on reproductive freedom.

It was not until several years later that Goldman became educated about the contraceptive choices then available. While in Paris in 1900 to attend the International Revolutionary Congress of the Working People, an anarchist meeting set to coincide with the Paris Exposition, she learned about an underground meeting of neo-Malthusians. The French suppressed the anarchist congress, but Goldman was able to sit in on the first International Conference of Neo-Malthusians, attended by about a dozen delegates from England, Holland, Germany, and France. She heard Charles Robert Drysdale, the president of England's Malthusian League, and others speak on the benefits of small families and demonstrate various preventive methods. "I marveled," Goldman later wrote, "at their ability to discuss such a delicate matter so frankly and in such an inoffensive manner." She came away with literature as well as sample contraceptives. On her return to the states, Goldman folded birth control advocacy into her speeches on marriage, the economic and social inequality of women, and later on the need to starve the military-industrial machine of soldiers and workers. She gave out information when women approached her privately but did not publicly discuss methods, "because the question of limiting offspring represented in my estimation only one aspect of the social struggle and I did not care to risk arrest for it."

Although Goldman decided to avoid a free speech fight over birth control—and there was little impetus from the anarchist community for her to do so—she did not limit her political expression for fear of arrest. Police took her in routinely and suppressed her meetings and rallies, sometimes before she had uttered a word. Goldman's defense of direct action tactics and her association with the terrorist acts of other anarchists had established her notoriety as a dangerous woman, making her public presence alone objectionable to authorities. Charges filed against her seldom stuck. The excitement and press coverage surrounding her arrests bolstered support for free speech rights and organizations in a number of the cities that she visited. Although she even rankled some of her comrades with certain extreme views and her reflexive empathy for perpetrators of political violence, Goldman never let either ideological challenges or attempts to suppress her speech inhibit her passion to fight for unlimited free expression. She did more to advance the issue of free speech than any other figure at that time, especially in New York City, the heart and hotbed of pre-World War I radicalism.[4]

With the FSL operating at times as a kind of ring leader, regular battles over free speech created a spirit of common purpose in the circus-like subculture of radical dissent in Greenwich Village. Historian Christine Stansell writes that "free-speech politics . . . linked artists, writers, and professionals of a progressive bent to working-class militants." Goldman worked closely with the FSL in drawing out support on free speech grounds from radical groups with different political agendas as well as middle-class progressives and left-leaning intellectuals. And though she did not mount a challenge to the Comstock laws in these prewar years, Goldman lent her support to those who did, including Harman, up to his death in 1910, and Margaret Sanger, who was first suppressed by Comstock in 1913.[5]

MARGARET SANGER'S EARLY YEARS

Sanger, 10 years Goldman's junior and a bit of a late-blooming activist, nevertheless followed in a path remarkably similar to Goldman's in terms of her awakening on the issue of birth control, her dramatic flair for self-promotion, and her skill in creating free speech incidents. Although she was the central figure and life-long leader of the birth control movement, Sanger's biography is still not as widely known as Goldman's, despite new scholarship and popular biographical treatments.* Because Sanger's life is so intertwined with the movement she organized, her early years deserve more than a cursory look.

Sanger (1879–1966) was the sixth of 11 children born to a freethinking socialist stone cutter and his Catholic wife, both Irish immigrants, in Corning, New York. Her father, Michael Higgins, a bibulous, soapbox radical, alienated from the church and distrusting of authority, provided Margaret Sanger with daily lessons in independent thinking and defiance of conformity, although he seldom demonstrated constructive means of dissent. Sanger later credited her father with instilling in her a spirit of idealism and teaching her to reject dogma. Anne Higgins, a patient and efficient housekeeper, tolerated her husband's whims and paltry earnings and resigned herself to his bouts of rebellion. She suspended the public practice of her faith and hunkered down to childbearing and domestic duties in a Catholic town, where her little ones were known as "children of the devil." Weakened by each successive pregnancy, she died of tuberculosis at age 50 in 1899. Sanger later stated bluntly that her mother died because "she had too many children and had worked herself to death."

Although well provided for and cared for, the Higgins children grew up with few expectations that any would move beyond the provincialism of Corning, dominated by its famous glass factory. Sanger aspired to something more. She had a passing

---

* See, for instance, Ellen Chesler's biography, *Woman of Valor* (1992; revised 2007), *The Selected Papers of Margaret Sanger*, Vols. 1–3 (2003–2010), and the film documentary, *Margaret Sanger*, that aired on PBS in 1998.

fancy for a stage career before setting her sights on the medical profession. With great sacrifice, her sisters pooled together incomes from various jobs and sent her to Claverack College, a nearby Methodist preparatory school. Sanger then briefly tried her hand at teaching in an elementary school before being called home to care for her dying mother, an experience that strengthened her interest in medicine. In 1900, she entered a nursing program in White Plains, New York, but left after two years to elope with William Sanger, a draftsman and artist in his late twenties whom she had met on a training assignment in Manhattan. Although she suffered from tuberculosis contracted from her mother, Sanger managed to have three children between 1903 and 1910, two boys and a girl, and to make a comfortable home for her family in Hastings, New York, just outside of New York City.

William Sanger, a quixotic painter who for money pieced together drafting work from architectural firms, longed to express his high ideals and burgeoning political passion for working-class empowerment. He became involved in socialist political circles and increasingly shared his radical views with his wife. She seemed to hunger like he did for what she later called the "religion without a name," the new radicalism fermenting in and around Greenwich Village that burst out in causes to emancipate work, art, women, and sex from bourgeois conventions and the rigidity of Victorian-era America. The Sangers moved from the suburbs to upper Manhattan in 1911 to be closer to the action in the Village. They both joined the Socialist Party, and Margaret became a paid lecturer and organizer for the Party's Women's Committee.

She also signed up with a visiting nurse's association and, like Emma Goldman, tended to obstetrical patients in the tenement districts of the Lower East Side. The work revealed a squalor and suffering that Sanger had not previously confronted. Women begged for relief from childbearing, for any means to avoid having more mouths to feed. "Pregnancy was a chronic condition," Sanger wrote. It broke down too many women like a disease and strained family relationships. Sanger knew one woman who had her eighth child with the help of her 10-year-old son: "Under his mother's direction, [he] cleaned the bed, wrapped the placenta and soiled articles in paper, and threw them out of the window into the court below." Women talked of ways to "bring themselves around," Sanger later wrote, by "drinking various herb teas, taking drops of turpentine on sugar, steaming over a chamber of boiling coffee or of turpentine water, rolling down stairs, and finally inserting slippery-elm sticks, or knitting needles, or shoe hooks into the uterus." They also asked Sanger to divulge the secrets of the rich (the Catholic women called them "Yankee tricks"), who managed to keep their families small. Sanger shared her limited knowledge of prevention: the male-controlled methods of withdrawal and the condom. But the women generally did not trust their husbands with this responsibility. Condoms continued to be associated with prostitution, and coitus interruptus was highly undesirable and condemned in religious teachings. Sanger turned to doctors for advice, just as Goldman had, and found them reticent, grudgingly advising abstinence. After treating a number of patients for septicemia, an infectious disease often caused by unsterilized abortion tools, and watching them die, Sanger decided to educate herself on reproductive control. Years later she condensed these desperate cases and her own feelings of helplessness into a single story of one woman's suffering and death following a botched abortion. The story concludes with Sanger's transformation from conscientious nurse to emboldened radical: "I resolved that women should have knowledge of contraception. They have every right to know about their own bodies. I would strike out—I would scream from the housetops. I would tell the world what was going on in the lives of these poor women. I *would* be heard."[6]

VILLAGE RADICALS

In reality, it was not immediately clear to Sanger or to anyone else around her that she would dedicate herself to, as she put it, doing "something to change the destiny of mothers whose miseries were vast as the sky." Sociable but seldom the center of attention at this time, with an ear always out for her young children, Sanger later depicted herself as a supportive wife to her husband's grand ideas and a busy host to the garrulous friends who congregated in their small apartment. "These vehement individualists had to have an audience, preferably a small, intimate one. They really came to see Bill; I made the cocoa." But it did not take long before Sanger was drawn into conversations or debates with the engaging personalities who made up this intimate society of cultural and political renegades. Within a year of their move to the city, the Sangers were regulars at various radical gathering spots, including the Liberal Club in the Village and its basement restaurant, Polly's; the nearby Ferrer Center, founded by Emma Goldman and other anarchists as a cultural and education center, and its Modern School, in which Sanger's oldest child, Stuart, enrolled in 1912; and the Fifth Avenue salon of the arts patron Mabel Dodge. Dodge's "evenings" brought together fashionable uptown moderns and the sartorially-challenged downtown bohemians to flaunt their diversity of opinion on such topics as unionization, class boundaries, Freudian psychology, the sexual impulse, and cubism.[7]

Through these gatherings, Sanger became close to a number of prominent radical figures, including writers John Reed, Upton Sinclair, Walter Lippmann, Max Eastman, and Floyd Dell; artists Rockwell Kent and Robert Henri; labor activists Carlo Tresca, William ("Big Bill") Haywood, and Elizabeth Gurley Flynn; and anarchists Hippolyte Havel, Alexander Berkman, and, of course, Goldman. Goldman helped establish the terms and the tone for the discussion of women's sexual liberty and remained the most knowledgeable of the Village radicals about neo-Malthusian principles. Goldman and Sanger saw each other frequently. As early as 1912, Sanger was dropping in on Goldman's office at *Mother Earth*, the influential anarchist monthly that Goldman began in 1906. But Sanger never warmed to Goldman, who may have, in her mentoring role, treated Sanger with some condescension. Early on, Sanger saw the benefit in contrasting herself with Goldman, who was a theatrical and, at times, intimidating public presence: stout and strong, "glaring through her eyeglasses," "fiery-tongued." The press frequently described Goldman in unflattering, masculine terms. Sanger, on the other hand, was slight, small-featured, and soft-spoken, and had learned to employ a disarming prettiness. Typically, observers encountering her for the first time in public referred to her as "young," "feminine," and "mild-looking." "Mrs. Sanger," wrote a reporter in 1916, "presented anything but the expected radical appearance." Even Goldman had trouble convincing people who had only heard about Sanger but had never met her, that she was really "a little, delicate woman, refined and shrinking." Sanger's gentle look made her approachable and unthreatening, especially to women seeking advice on the most private of matters, and tripped up opponents who underestimated her mettle.[8]

SEXUAL MODERNS

Although Sanger later went to great pains to avoid giving Goldman any credit for guiding her in the pre-World War I years, Goldman's influence on Sanger and others seeking sexual liberation was enormous. In asserting a woman's right to control her body, Goldman played a key role in bridging the 19th-century American sex radicals' vision of women's sexual freedom—their critique of traditional marriage and advocacy of nonprocreative sex—with a new wave of scientific sexual thought emanating from Europe that was being devoured by the new bohemians. Goldman helped introduce New York City radicals to theories about sexual repression introduced by Sigmund Freud. She had heard him lecture in Vienna in 1896 and again in Worcester, Massachusetts, in 1909, just prior to his work being translated into English. Goldman and many other Village intellectuals delved into the writings of the English sexologist, Havelock Ellis, and his monumental, multivolume *Studies in the Psychology of Sex*, published between 1897 and 1910. They also read the work of the Swedish feminist Ellen Key, who linked sex with women's spiritual, psychological, and physical health, and English socialist Edward Carpenter. In his controversial book, *Love's Coming of Age* (1896), Carpenter wrote about sexual liberation for women and homosexuals. These authors viewed sexuality as a natural impulse and a basic need to be understood and fulfilled—even outside of marriage. As historian Linda Gordon has noted, all three "considered sexual liberation to be primarily dependent on women's sexual liberation, which in turn required women's independence and opportunity to seek full, creative lives."

Ellis's groundbreaking studies inspired Sanger more than any other sexual theorist. "Sex lies at the root of life," he began his seven-volume work, "and we can never learn to reverence life until we know how to understand sex." By making sex central to one's identity and by encouraging sexual exploration, Ellis envisioned a new day where sex need not be inhibited by adherence to rigid self-control—as it was through much of the 19th century—defined by marriage or limited to heterosexual monogamy. Ellis emphasized several rationales for birth control, most prominently sexual gratification and women's autonomy. He also became a leading proponent of eugenic improvement through family planning. He confirmed in 1910 what many knew but did not talk about: "The control of procreation by the prevention of conception has . . . become a part of the morality of civilized peoples." Ellis found the condom to be the "safest, the most convenient, and the most harmless method," yet he recognized that even it was too expensive for the very poor. He underscored the birth control movement's later conundrum: how to close the divide between the rich and poor as to contraceptive knowledge and access to methods.[9]

The confluence of new ideas about sexuality in the radical community led to an acceptance of variations in sexual relationships. Village radicals experimented with trial marriages, open marriages, and other means of finding personal sexual fulfillment, even though many of these explorations ended in ruin, destroyed by jealousy, or undermined by instability. They were less oriented toward achieving monogamous bliss than their free-love predecessors and more dedicated to liberating women from traditional gender roles. However, even this enlightened crowd struggled to realize women's autonomy both in the bedroom and in the workplace. These radicals further widened the separation between sex and reproduction and acknowledged that a woman's erotic needs and passions were not so different from a man's. Following Ellis's tenets, they increasingly embraced sex for psychological needs—intimacy, release, assertion of identity, and self-expression. They wrote about sex, used sex for artistic inspiration, and talked about sex in private and public. Though a number of radicals are remembered for their sexual discourse, Sanger rather quickly established a reputation as the most outspoken champion of sexual pleasure. As Mabel Dodge remembered, "It was as if she had been more or less arbitrarily chosen by the powers that be to voice a new gospel of not only sex knowledge in regard to conception, but sex knowledge about copulation and its intrinsic importance. . . . She was the first person I ever knew who was openly an ardent propagandist for the joys of the flesh."

SANGER'S EARLY WRITINGS AND ACTIVISM

Gradually, Sanger worked in talks on "sex hygiene"—information on female sexuality from menstruation to menopause, as well as courting and marriage—when meeting with women's groups. She presented these talks as a Socialist Party lecturer and on her strike assignments with the more inclusive (of women) national labor organization, the Industrial Workers of the World (IWW). She left the Socialist Party in 1912, as did many other disaffected radicals, to join the more militant "Wobblies," as the IWW was known, and became more connected to the anarchist community. The direct action tactics of the IWW, including both nonviolent strikes and violent provocations such as sabotage, came closer than socialism to satisfying Sanger's impatience for change.

With her nursing background, Sanger felt comfortable discussing basic information on sexual functioning, venereal disease, prostitution, and coming of age issues for girls and their mothers. She had started a budding journalism career not long after moving to the city, writing short pieces for *The Call*, the Socialist daily, on the exploitation of women and the working class. The editor of *The Call's* "Women's Sphere" column asked Sanger in the fall of 1911 to write a series of articles on teaching children about sex. "What Every Mother Should Know, or How Six Little Children Were Taught the Truth" was based on lessons Sanger had sketched for her own children. She used everyday observations in the plant and animal world to craft simple stories that presented sexuality in a relaxed and honest fashion, with no admonitions or clumsy morality. The series ran for several months and was published in 1913 as a pamphlet. She followed this with another series, "What Every Girl Should Know," that tackled more sensitive subjects, including masturbation and venereal disease, areas seldom explored in a daily newspaper. The last installment, subtitled "Some Consequences of Ignorance and Silence—Part III," was set to appear in the February 9, 1913, issue of *The Call*. Instead, over the space of two columns, the paper printed vertically in large block letters: "WHAT EVERY GIRL SHOULD KNOW—NOTHING!—BY ORDER OF THE POST-OFFICE DEPARTMENT." The article had contained the words "syphilis and gonorrhea," sufficient justification for Comstock to suppress the piece. He reversed course after many *Call* readers and apparently some city leaders raised objections on free speech grounds. The article was published in its entirety the next month and later in book form. The incident proved fortuitous for Sanger, giving her some instant notoriety among the free speech crowd.

Both of these series read in sharp contrast to the facts-of-life literature of the day, which was usually a cross between a Sunday school lesson and a medical text. Sanger's pieces elicited divergent responses: one reader wrote that *The Call* would have to "be banished from our home circle as a paper unfit to be read by our sons and daughters. Such a revolting article I have never read before." Another wrote, "I am a woman of most 66 years and I have learned more from them than from any books or even from my own life, and I am the mother of eight children!"[10]

Comstock's rapid response to a relatively obscure piece in a socialist paper indicated the level of control that he and other censors wielded over the press and public speech in the decade or so before World War I. The campaign to stamp out prostitution had reached a feverish pitch in these years, and vice crusaders and moralistic social reformers found themselves in agreement that obscene publications influenced the immoral behavior that was at the root of social disease. They also found common ground in justifying the suppression of obscene material. If the crusaders overreached, as in the case with Sanger and many others who published educational material on sex hygiene, it only helped scare other potential perpetrators and create a self-censoring environment. The press ran occasional articles on venereal disease and prostitution but was careful to use vague terminology and to advocate chaste living. Even when editors made it past the censors, their own readers often complained or stopped reading. Seventy-five thousand women cancelled their subscriptions to the *Ladies' Home Journal* after it published a series on venereal disease in 1906. There were exceptions, such as the popular Broadway production of a French play, *Damaged Goods,* in 1913 (later staged for President Wilson and Congress), which focused public attention on the pernicious consequences of sexually transmitted diseases. If this play succeeded in opening the door just a little to a more public discussion of sexuality, it was mainly because it forcefully preached moral responsibility. In the first decade of the 20th century, contraception was rarely mentioned in the press or in mainstream, nonmedical publications. The subject came up in discussions of race suicide—the notion that the "better classes" were dying out because of delayed marriage and fertility control—and reports on neo-Malthusian trends in Europe. But such articles and books never delineated the ways and means of controlling fertility.[11]

It is not clear how often before 1914 Sanger spoke about family limitation, either in radical forums or in the talks she gave to groups of women and strikers. The writer Jacques Rudome, who taught French at the Ferrer Center, remembered that Sanger's attempts to broach sex education issues were often drowned out by heated political discussion, especially among the anarchist crowd. Suffragist Mary Sumner Boyd recalled a speech that Sanger gave to women strikers in which she discussed the need for family limitation among the working class. She was followed on the podium by IWW leader Bill Haywood, who made light of Sanger's message by envisioning a postcapitalist future where women "could have without fear of want all the babies they pleased." Her comrades generally advised Sanger to hold off on the prevention arguments until women got the vote or until socialism prevailed. As Goldman had concluded earlier, the real work of both the social and economic radicals—their pursuit of an egalitarian ideal—was too important to risk with a public birth control campaign and the legal problems that would ensue. Yet the more time Sanger devoted to labor activism, the more she reasoned that birth control was not a subsidiary issue, but the necessary first step in lifting up women, confronting poverty, and improving the lives of working families. She wrote:

> . . . it seemed to me the whole question of strikes for higher wages was based on man's economic need of supporting his family, and that this was a shallow principle upon

which to found a new civilization. Furthermore, I was enough of a Feminist to resent the fact that women and her requirements were not being taken into account in reconstructing this new world about which all were talking. They were failing to consider the quality of life itself.

Sanger also began to see birth control as the only available course by which to change the dynamic of an industrial, imperialist nation reliant on the complicity of women in producing a constant stream of new workers and soldiers. It was a simplistic argument, but it resonated in parts of the radical community. Other women radicals especially understood. They were fed up with the male leadership of the labor movement for failing to discuss the consequences of large families among the working class and for neglecting women's most basic concerns about family and children.[12]

Although Sanger's involvement in labor activism in 1913 left her little time to pursue sex education writing, she stole away from domestic duties whenever she could to search for contraceptive information, visiting several libraries in New York that spring and the Boston Public Library that summer, while her family was camped in Provincetown, Massachusetts. She famously claimed years later that she perused countless books on the sexual function, as well as medical periodicals and texts, but found nothing, not even in the Library of Congress, on practical means of birth control. She said that she could locate only theory and Malthusian arguments, and nothing whatsoever by American writers except fear mongering about race suicide. Yet her personal library belies her suggestion that information was inaccessible.* She had her own copy of Havelock Ellis's *Studies,* which referred to works (some of which she also had) by other European sex theorists, such as Richard von Krafft-Ebing, Enoch Kisch, and Auguste Forel, who all discussed contraception to varying degrees. She had been exposed to Moses Harman's writings in *Lucifer, the Light-Bearer* and could have rounded up a copy of Charles Knowlton's *Fruits of Philosophy* or Annie Besant's *Law of Population*; both tracts merged theory and practice and had been republished multiple times.

Theodore Schroeder's 1918 bibliography of publications on birth control lists scores of sources prior to 1913, including many medical writings. The *Medical World*, a widely circulated publication for physicians, devoted space to forums on contraception. A run of issues in 1897 included discussions on cocoa butter suppositories, zinc sulphate and warm water douches, and a cotton plug saturated with petroleum. The Alkaloidal Clinic in Chicago had published a sex hygiene guide in 1902 in which they surveyed various methods. One of its doctors was particularly fond of sterilized gauze acting as a sort of womb veil, "with a stout cord of floss silk for removal." There

---

* Many volumes are preserved in the Sophia Smith Collection at Smith College.

were more provocative publications as well, such as the 1904 pamphlet, *Love without Danger: Secrets of the Alcove*, supposedly printed in Paris, that offered accurate information with a sense of humor: "A distinguished physician called it [the condom] a bad umbrella that was of little use in a storm, and did not prevent you from getting your feet wet." Surely Emma Goldman, who had acquired contraceptive literature and devices over the years, was also an important resource for Sanger.[13]

DR. WILLIAM ROBINSON

Most noticeably, Sanger makes no mention of William J. Robinson, the outspoken socialist physician well known to the radical community and to Sanger through his lectures and writings, including sex hygiene articles in *The Call*, the same paper that regularly published Sanger from 1911 to 1913. Although Robinson, a urologist and medical writer, did not publish contraceptive information, apart from an early leaflet distributed to other doctors, he often asserted that contraception was the most important force for positive change in the world: "There is no other single measure that would so positively, so immediately contribute towards the happiness and progress of the human race." In letters to the editor and lectures before medical groups and lay audiences, in his 1904 pamphlet, *Limitation of Offspring*, and in his editorials starting in 1903 for the *American Journal of Urology*, and especially in the more mainstream *Critic and Guide*, which he founded and edited, Robinson persistently and unambiguously advocated teaching those means of prevention known by doctors to be safe and reliable. "The important question is," he wrote in 1904, "should we allow the women to continue to use injurious, health-ruining measures to prevent conception, or, what is still worse, hurry themselves to their graves by repeated abortions—or should the knowledge of sage and hygienic anticoncepts—for there are such—be spread broadcast?" Just as often, Robinson called for repeal of the Comstock laws.

Robinson argued that doctors had the right to dispense contraception for both medical indications and socioeconomic reasons. Although he never discussed whether or not he prescribed contraception in his medical practice, it seems certain that he did, and he later admitted to performing some abortions. In speeches and in print, Robinson dispelled the myth that contraception led to sterility and other health problems, and he repeatedly corrected the mistaken notion that contraception resulted in abortion. Remarkably, you can find in Robinson's writings, even before 1913, just about every argument in favor of birth control that was later adopted by the movement, including to reduce infant and maternal mortality; to improve women's health and free women from "enforced motherhood;" to limit abortion; to avoid the neuroses and sexual dysfunction that many physicians attributed to withdrawal and prolonged abstinence; to strengthen marriage; to space births; to control population; to limit disease and defect; to improve the quality of the human race; and to recognize that because sex was a natural instinct and pleasurable, it should not be restricted to procreation only.[14]

Robinson heralded a new era in medical thinking about sexuality. "I speak the language of joy and progress . . . the language of the free scientist," he wrote in 1910. Taking cues from Ellis and Freud, he fought his profession's inclination to deny and contain the sexual impulse, and took on considerable professional risk to publicize his views on birth control. In 1913, he even went so far as to try to produce a play in New York that tackled illegitimacy and family limitation. The production fell apart, but it gave Robinson an opportunity to tell the press that people must be taught "how to regulate the number of their offspring so that they may have only as many children as they want and only when they want them." And unlike the earlier birth control doctor, Edward Bliss Foote, who was derided by many in his profession for his radical and unorthodox views, Robinson retained his professional stature and wielded influence in the medical establishment. He published other doctors' endorsements of birth control, including essays by Edward Bond Foote. In 1912, Robinson convinced the 82-year-old president of the American Medical Association (AMA), Abraham Jacobi, the pioneer of pediatrics, to endorse contraception in his presidential address. Jacobi spoke obliquely about family limitation in the context of economic inequality and concluded his remarks with a harsh eugenic judgment:

> Is there no way to prevent those who are born into this world from becoming sickly both physically and mentally? . . . The resources for prevention or cure are inaccessible to many—sometimes even to a majority. That is why it has become an indispensable suggestion that only a certain number of babies should be born into this world. I often hear that an American family has had 10 children, but only three or four survived. Before the former succumbed, they were a source of expense, poverty, and morbidity to the few survivors. For the interests of the latter, and the health of the community at large, they had better not have been born.[15]

Jacobi's comments shook up the old-line medicos. There was some protestation, but most in the profession did not want to engage the issue at all. It would take another 25 years for the AMA to endorse birth control.

Robinson also wrote about the importance of activism in raising awareness. "Because we cannot perhaps help you today, is no reason why we should not work for the benefit and happiness of the people 10 or 20 years hence. And besides, the agitation itself possesses a very decided value even now, for it makes people inquisitive, it makes them seek for information which eventually they do get in spite of any laws." Though Robinson was unwilling to take the next step, to engage in the kind of unlawful activities that would force the courts to review the obscenity laws, there was no one else before 1914 who pushed birth control as a single-issue reform that would "render all other measures" to help the human race "superfluous." In essence, Robinson laid out a blueprint for Sanger, not only in presenting a series of common-sense justifications for birth control education, but also in explaining that activism and propaganda would erode the effect of the Comstock laws by gradually spreading information. Furthermore, he firmly believed that contraceptive education should come from the medical community, that it is appropriate and necessary for physicians to prescribe contraception, and that the doctor-patient relationship is inviolable. These are positions that before long became the cornerstone of Sanger's argument for the legalization of birth control and medical supervision over access to contraceptives.[16]

Yet Sanger, who was not unaware of Robinson's contributions, failed to credit him for his pioneering work. Part of the explanation is that Sanger and Robinson later feuded over who had the better claim to pioneer status. Consequently, in her auto-biographical writings, Sanger only mentions Robinson's tepid support for her after she had established the movement. But there is more to it than this petty conflict suggests. Once Sanger committed herself to birth control activism, she set about to create an inspiring storyline. She had observed how the most effective labor leaders reduced their argument down to a battle of good versus evil, pitting the underdog, the powerless worker, against a monolithic, greedy corporation. Similarly, Sanger fully embraced the notion that the government and the medical establishment combined to enforce women's bondage. As James Reed has written, "Sanger turned the reluctance of doctors to provide contraceptive information into a symbol of oppression and thus defined a cause for her own." She, too, was a victim of this professional elitism and intransigence: a nurse unable to help her patients, compelled to challenge authority and uncover secrets locked away in medical repositories or encoded in foreign texts. Recognition of a respected physician's tireless advocacy for birth control or the disclosure of a rich body of 19th-century contraceptive literature would challenge the narrative that Sanger relied on to justify her calling and to establish the cause as her own—as something new and fundamentally feminist.[17]

SANGER'S QUEST FOR CONTRACEPTIVES

No doubt it was a challenge for Sanger to find information on effective woman-controlled methods that she thought could be readily used by the poor or methods that satisfied her nurse's instinct for the medically safe and sound. (Sanger never says what sort of birth control *she* used.) Methods were not tested or widely discussed in medical circles, so even doctors lacked a firm grasp on what worked best and, as in the case of the safe period, frequently gave out erroneous information. Female contraceptive devices circulated on the black market, including suppository tablets and various cervical caps, but they were pricey and not everyone knew how to obtain them or felt comfortable with either the stigma or the legal risk. Feminine hygiene aids such as douching syringes were sold in drugstores, but not every woman knew how to use them as a contraceptive. Sanger likely collected more information than she knew how to digest but could not discover that single, woman-controlled method that was affordable, effective, and easy to use. She credits Big Bill Haywood with the suggestion that she make a research expedition to Paris to find practical contraceptive information. American newspapers had been running articles since the turn of the century about France's struggle to stem a plummeting birth rate and the prevalence there of conception control. Sometime in the early summer of 1913 the Sangers decided that a move to Paris would satisfy both Margaret's desire to continue her search and William's dream to have a painting studio on the Left Bank. It was also something of a last ditch effort to save their marriage, a clean break from the combustible free-love scene in the Village that had followed them to Provincetown in the summer of 1913.

Sanger stayed in France for just two months, long enough to partake of some of the ongoing debate about neo-Malthusianism that had spiked after a series of recent birth strikes—organized attempts to encourage the proletariat to cease childbearing—in France and Germany. She found the French much more open to discussing family limitation than Americans. In this aspect of their lives, as in others, the French expressed, in Sanger's words, their "predilection for quality rather than quantity." Yet politically speaking, only a segment of the Left fervently backed birth control, chiefly the anarcho-syndicalists, part of the labor branch of the European anarchist movement. This group had strong ties to neo-Malthusian organizations and viewed birth control as an important weapon in the class struggle. Victor Dave, a veteran of French syndicalism who had helped Emma Goldman in 1900, acted as Sanger's tour guide. She was joined by Haywood and his current lover, the lawyer and feminist Jessie Ashley, whose stay in Paris overlapped with Sanger's. Together they visited bookstalls and pharmacies, met with midwives and druggists, even chatted with people on the street, and came away with a sampling of contraceptive devices and information. Many recipes for suppositories were passed down from mother to daughter, and Sanger found that soap douches were widely used. It is unclear if she discovered anything particularly new or insightful, though she did forge, through Dave, many important European contacts. Overall, she came away from her Paris sojourn even more radicalized than when she left the United States, energized by the revolutionary spirit and social unrest evident in crowded Paris meetings and street rallies. Sanger returned to the United States more convinced than before that family limitation must play a central role in lifting up working people, especially women, to overcome the inequalities of the capitalist system.[18]

THE WOMAN REBEL

Back in New York with the children, Sanger rejoined her anarchist circle of friends that included John Rompapas, a Greek importer and radical publisher who had begun an affair with Sanger in 1913; the Belgian-born, radical journalist and British expatriate Edward Mylius; and the colorful and combative Hippolyte Havel. A true Bohemian, Havel was born of a gypsy mother and Czech father, and had his hand in nearly every pre-war anarchist publication in the United States. Havel, once Emma Goldman's lover, had accompanied her to Paris in 1900 when she attended the neo-Malthusian conference.

Sanger sifted through all of the information she had collected to prepare for writing an informational tract on contraception. William Sanger, who remained in Paris to paint, funneled additional literature to his wife that he collected from Victor Dave and other friends in Europe. In mid-February Sanger set aside her book project and decided to publish a monthly newspaper. Rompapas, Mylius, and Havel had all worked together on the militant weekly, *The Social War*, and at least the latter two had a wealth of experience in editing and publishing radical journals. Whether or not they pushed Sanger in this direction is not clear, but they may have recognized the need to tie birth control to working-class concerns and convince the radical community of its urgency. In all likelihood Rompapas helped fund this new endeavor with earnings from his importing business. Sanger also set about collecting, in advance, $1 subscription fees from socialists and trade union members. In just a few weeks, working from her dining room table and with help from several other radical friends, Sanger laid out the first issue of *The Woman Rebel*.[19]

The eight-page paper that appeared in mid-March ran the gamut of radical interests, delivering its news and "rebel thoughts" with an angry and feminist edge. For the masthead, Sanger used the IWW slogan "No Gods, No Masters," and she prodded her readers to "look the whole world in the face with a go-to-hell look in the eye; to have an ideal; to speak and act in defiance of convention." Over the first few issues she emphasized the causes of women's oppression: "I believe that woman is enslaved by the world machine, by sex conventions, by motherhood and its present necessary child-rearing, by wage slavery, by middle-class morality, by customs, laws and super-stitions." Liberation could be achieved through women's participation in a worker revolution, when women rise up and fight the "outrageous suppression" whereby they have no "control of the function of motherhood." Sanger later called the *Rebel* "anti-capitalist soapbox oratory," but it was more than an angry attack on establishment. She also took on other radicals whom she deemed to be too passive, especially the so-called "new feminists." Sanger saw the more moderate lot of educated women professionals as part of a middle-class movement wholly invested in suffrage as a sure fix

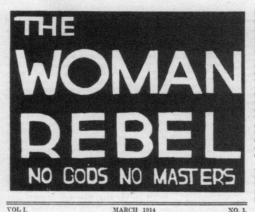

VOL I.   MARCH 1914   NO. 1.

THE AIM

This paper will not be the champion of any "ism."

All rebel women are invited to contribute to its columns.

The majority of papers usually adjust themselves to the ideas of their readers but the WOMAN REBEL will obstinately refuse to be adjusted.

The aim of this paper will be to stimulate working women to think for themselves and to build up a conscious fighting character.

An early feature will be a series of articles written by the editor for girls from fourteen to eighteen years of age. In this present chaos of sex atmosphere it is difficult for the uncertain age to know just what to do or really what constitutes clean living without prudishness. All this slushy talk about white slavery, the man painted and described as a hideous vulture pouncing down upon the young, pure and innocent girl, drugging her through the medium of grape juice and lemonade and then dragging her off to his foul den for other men equally as vicious to feed and fatten on her enforced slavery — surely this picture is enough to sicken and disgust every thinking woman and man, who has lived even a few years past the adolescent age. Could any more repulsive and foul conception of sex be given to adolescent girls as a preparation for life than this picture that is being perpetuated by the stupidly ignorant in the name of "sex education"?

If it were possible to get the truth from girls who work in prostitution to-day, I believe most of them would tell you that the first sex experience was with a sweetheart or through the desire for a sweetheart or something impelling within themselves, the nature of which they knew not, neither could they control. Society does not forgive this act when it is based upon the natural impulses and feelings of a young girl. It prefers the other story of the grape juice procurer which makes it easy to shift the blame from its own shoulders, to cast the stone and to evade the unpleasant facts that it alone is responsible for. It sheds sympathetic tears over white slavery, holds the often mythical procurer up as a target, while in reality it is supported by the misery it engenders.

If, as reported, there are approximately 35,000 women working as prostitutes in New York City alone, is it not sane to conclude that some force, some living, powerful, social force is at play to compel these women to work at a trade which involves police persecution, social ostracism and the constant danger of exposure to venereal diseases. From my own knowledge of adolescent girls and from sincere expressions of women working as prostitutes inspired by mutual understanding and confidence I claim that the first sexual act of these so-called wayward girls is partly given, partly desired yet reluctantly so because of the fear of the consequences together with the dread of lost respect of the man. These fears interfere with mutuality of expression —the man becomes conscious of the responsibility of the act and often refuses to see her again, sometimes leaving the town and usually denouncing her as having been with "other fellows." His sole aim is to throw off responsibility. The same uncertainty in these emotions is experienced by girls in marriage in as great a proportion as in the unmarried. After the first experience the life of a girl varies. All these girls do not necessarily go into prostitution. They have had an experience which has not "ruined" them, but rather given them a larger vision of life, stronger feelings and a broader understanding of human nature. The adolescent girl does not understand herself. She is full of contradictions, whims, emotions. For her emotional nature longs for caresses, to touch, to kiss. She is often as well satisfied to hold hands or to go arm in arm with a girl as in the companionship of a boy.

It is these and kindred facts upon which the WOMAN REBEL will dwell from time to time and from which it is hoped the young girl will derive some knowledge of her nature, and conduct her life upon such knowledge.

It will also be the aim of the WOMAN REBEL to advocate the prevention of conception and to impart such knowledge in the columns of this paper.

Other subjects, including the slavery through motherhood; through things, the home, public opinion and so forth, will be dealt with.

It is also the aim of this paper to circulate among those women who work in prostitution; to voice their wrongs; to expose the police persecution which hovers over them and to give free expression to their thoughts, hopes and opinions.

And at all times the WOMAN REBEL will strenuously advocate economic emancipation.

THE NEW FEMINISTS

That apologetic tone of the new American feminists which plainly says "Really, Madam Public Opinion, we are all quite harmless and perfectly respectable" was the keynote of the first and second mass meetings held at Cooper Union on the 17th and 20th of February last.

The ideas advanced were very old and time-worn even to the ordinary church-going woman who reads the magazines and comes in contact with current thought. The "right to work," the "right to ignore fashions," the "right to keep her own name," the "right to organize," the "right of the mother to work"; all these so-called rights fail to arouse enthusiasm because to-day they are all recognized by society and there exist neither laws nor strong opposition to any of them.

It is evident they represent a middle class woman's movement; an echo, but a very weak echo, of the English constitutional suffragists. Consideration of the working woman's freedom was ignored. The problems which affect the and stuck on identity issues rather than working for basic freedoms. While these bold women fought for "the right to ignore fashions" and to keep their "own name" in marriage, Sanger dismissed such petty matters and claimed for all women "The Right to destroy" and "to create," an early, uncompromising position on reproductive rights that she would soften in the years to come. *The Woman Rebel* also included articles on labor strife, marriage, prostitution, and notable woman rebels of the past; contributions by anarchist writers, including Emma Goldman; and editorials by Sanger on subjects ranging from labor issues and military conflicts, to a few short pieces on sexuality, birth control, and abortion.

Although Sanger stated that one of the aims of *The Woman Rebel* would be "to advocate the prevention of conception and to impart such knowledge in the columns of this paper," she held off on printing any substantive articles on contraception. She clearly wanted to draw the government's attention without getting shut down and arrested too quickly. She notified her audience and the censors in the first issue: "Is it not time to defy this law? And what fitter place could be found than in the pages of the WOMAN REBEL!" Sanger's first article on birth control, "Prevention of Conception," focused on class difference: "The woman of the upper middle class have [sic] all available knowledge and implements to prevent conception. The woman of the lower middle class is struggling for this knowledge . . . left in ignorance of this information." She attacked the "blood-sucking men with M.D. after their names" who performed abortions that most working-class women could not afford. "It's far cheaper to have a baby," Sanger wrote, "though God knows what it will do after it gets here." She reminded her largely pro-labor audience that smaller families create a smaller workforce and increased wages.[20]

Despite the lack of any content that was even remotely obscene, Sanger's militant tone and taunting of authority prodded the post office into action. On April 2, New York Postmaster Edward Morgan informed Sanger by letter that the first issue of *The Woman Rebel* was unmailable under Section 211 (the Comstock Act) of the Criminal Code and would be confiscated, presumably because of the article on prevention, although the letter did not specify. "Woman's Magazine Barred from Mail," read the headline in the *New York Tribune*. Similar articles appeared in April in the *New York Times, Washington Post* (Sanger believes "large families among the poor are responsible for many of the present day evils"), and smaller out-of-town papers like the *Pawtucket* (Rhode Island) *Evening Times* ("Peppery Feminist Paper Slips Into the Mail Bags"), creating overnight publicity for Sanger and her theory of "race control," as the *Times* phrased it. Some in the press attacked *The Woman Rebel*. The *Pittsburgh Sun* concluded an editorial with the line: "The thing is nauseating." But the flurry of publicity, negative and positive, aroused free speech support for Sanger, and she began to seek advice from FSL attorneys.

Cleverly, Sanger and her helpers had disguised individual copies by wrapping them in other publications and dropping them into different mailboxes across the city. Many copies made it through to a mailing list that eventually reached about 2,000. They also sent bulk copies by freight to various radical organizations and labor groups. In Chicago, Emma Goldman received a bundle and requested more, but noted "it would be almost impossible for you to continue the 'Woman Rebel,' if the authorities place their damnable seal upon it." Goldman set up Sanger with news agents in various cities who agreed to sell the *Rebel*.

Sanger teased the censors in the April issue—"the WOMAN REBEL, humbled and repentant, curtseys coyly to the Postmaster and apologizes for the expression of any opinion that is unmailable . . ."—before the post office suppressed the May issue, confiscating 200 copies. The offending articles included Sanger's "Abortion in the United States," which concludes: "Abortions, with their horrible consequences, are quite needless and unnecessary when the subject of preventive means shall be open to all to discuss and use." Surprisingly, authorities let the June issue circulate despite the first use of the term *birth control* in print and a lengthy article on neo-Malthusianism. In all, five of the seven *Rebel* issues published were suppressed. "If only the authorities were not so stupid," Goldman wrote Sanger in June, "they would realize that they are doing you more good by holding up the paper than any amount of money could do. The 'Woman Rebel' is the best seller of anything we've got, just because it is known that the paper has been held up." Indeed, word spread quickly that *The Woman Rebel* was contraband, explosive and ready to land its editor in jail. Sanger showed no sign of backing down. "My plan is to continue to the end," she wrote to a supporter in April, "regardless of what views and actions our moral censors may take. . . ."[21]

INDICTMENTS

The July issue announced the formation of the Birth Control League of America, which existed on paper only, included a short piece on the safety of contraceptives, and featured a jarring article "In Defense of Assassination" by a little-known free speech activist. It incensed postal officials, troubled a number of radicals, and momentarily diverted attention away from birth control. On August 18, two postal inspectors paid a visit to Sanger to inform her that they would seek criminal charges. Five days later a grand jury returned a series of indictments against her for publishing articles on birth control, abortion, and sexuality as well as the subversive assassination piece and a short attack on the institution of marriage. Once again the story made some of the big city papers, including the *Boston Journal* and *Philadelphia Inquirer*. Sanger was arraigned and given an October court date, enough time to get out a final issue of the *Rebel* in which she included a sampling of over 10,000 letters she claimed to have received—an inflated number to be sure, but the beginning of a lifelong stream of inquiries from women and men in need of contraceptive and sexual advice.

One letter closed, "Perhaps it is illegal for you to send it, but in God's name send us some knowledge of how to prevent this awful curse of too many children."

Neither Sanger nor her FSL attorneys considered the *Rebel* articles listed in the indictments to be in violation of the law since she only discussed birth control but did not give contraceptive advice. The weakness of the indictments posed a problem if she wanted to create a test case and force the government to substantiate the link between contraception and obscenity. One attorney she contacted was afraid that Sanger would have difficulty forcing the kind of public hearing she desired: "if you are choked off without getting a hearing for the real issue, the cause gains nothing, and you lose your liberty for no real good." It is every martyr's fear, and Sanger did not like her odds. Moreover, she had already decided that she would drop an even bigger bomb than she could muster in the pages of the *Rebel*. She hinted at it several times, telling the postal officials to hold off because "there will be plenty of good material if they wait a little." A month later she wrote to author Upton Sinclair that she was almost ready to put out something "to really indict me on." She was referring to *Family Limitation*, her pamphlet on contraceptive methods that she had started on her return from France, before embarking on *The Woman Rebel*. She had finished it that summer and convinced Schroeder to tap into a free speech defense fund that had been left by Edward Bond Foote to Schroeder and the FSL. He allocated enough money to pay a portion of the printing cost, and Sanger scrambled to find a printer willing to take a sizable risk. She was turned down by more than a dozen before William Shatoff, a Russian-born IWW organizer, Ferrer Center regular, and a linotype operator agreed to the underground job. As Sanger later remembered, she had hoped to "swing the indictment around" to the contraceptive pamphlet so that "going to jail might have had some significance," but the pamphlet was not ready until late October.

So Sanger delayed. When her court appearance came up on the docket, she was a no-show, claiming that she had not received proper notification. She appeared in court two weeks later and requested a lengthy postponement that was denied by the judge. A firm trial date was set for October 20, but Sanger again stayed away, informing the judge and a patient prosecution that she had not properly prepared her case. FSL attorneys advised Sanger to either bargain her way out of a prison sentence or fight her charges on free speech grounds even though she had not published contraceptive advice. Facing the real possibility that she would be cornered into defending objectionable speech—the articles on assassination and marriage—that had nothing to do with birth control and still have to serve a multi-year prison sentence, Sanger chose another option. She fled the country, leaving the three children with William Sanger, who had returned from Paris that summer. "Jail has not been my goal," she wrote on the eve of her departure on October 28 to her "Comrades and Friends" on *The Woman Rebel* mailing list. "There is special work to be done and I shall do it first

. . . I shall attempt to nullify the law by direct action and attend to the consequences later. Over 100,000 working men and women in U.S. shall hear from me."[22]

FAMILY LIMITATION

Before leaving by train to Canada and then sailing to England, Sanger bundled and left with friends 100,000 copies of *Family Limitation* that were then distributed to labor groups, mill and mine workers, local radical organizations, and trusted contacts across the country. The 16-page pamphlet condensed the information she had acquired over the past year on the most available and effective contraceptive methods: douching, condoms, pessaries, sponges, and vaginal suppositories. Even more daring, Sanger advised using the abortifacient quinine shortly after sex if a woman thought conception may have taken place or if she was late in getting her period. This was the first and last time that Sanger would recommend an abortion procedure in print. She also included an illustration of how to insert a pessary, along with drawings of a French pessary (looks like a bowler hat) and a coiled and cobra-like "fountain syringe" for douching. Using accessible, no-nonsense language, Sanger resisted both clinical terminology and the frilly wrappings and euphemisms that other sex advice writers relied on to reach blushing middle-class brides who consulted marriage guides before their wedding night. Her advice is explicit, and her tone throughout is insistent and slightly impatient—a busy nurse with a lot of work to do:

> There is no need for anyone to explain to the working men and women in America what this pamphlet is written for or why it is necessary that they should have this information. They know better than I could tell them, so I shall not try. (2)

> It seems inartistic and sordid to insert a pessary or a suppository in anticipation of the sexual act. But it is far more sordid to find yourself several years later burdened down with half a dozen unwished for children, helpless, starved, shoddily clothed, dragging at your skirt, yourself a dragged out shadow of the woman you once were. (2)

> Don't wait to see if you do *not* menstruate (monthly sickness) but make it your duty to see that you *do*. (4)

> The trouble is women are afraid of their own bodies, and are of course ignorant of their physical construction. They are silly in thinking the pessary can go up too far, or that it could get lost, etc., etc., and therefore discard it. It cannot get into the womb, neither can it get lost. The only thing it can do is to come out. (12)

She addresses an audience that is strictly working class and presumably socialist, positing birth control as something of an equalizer in the class struggle:

> It is only the workers who are ignorant of the knowledge of how to prevent bringing children in the world to fill jails and hospitals, factories and mills, insane asylums and

premature graves, and who supply the millions of soldiers and sailors to fight battles for financiers and the ruling class. The working class can use direct action by refusing . . . to populate the earth with slaves. (3)

Nothing as practical and as revolutionary in its capacity to transform women's lives had been so widely circulated in the United States or anywhere in the world. At least 18 English-language editions were published over the next 20 years. The pamphlet was later translated into more than a dozen languages and influenced marriage manuals and contraceptive guides for several decades. In fact, no other publication covered as much ground on methods of birth control until the 1920s. On its release in 1914 and for many years thereafter, the pamphlet was shared, often copied by hand, and passed on from one woman to another. It likely exposed many women and men to not only their first dose of contraceptive information but also their first accurate understanding of sexual intercourse and human reproduction. And Sanger went so far as to emphasize the importance of women's sexual satisfaction, advising couples that the condom in particular helps delay the male orgasm, giving the woman a bit more time to reach hers. It was a stunning bit of advice to put into print in 1914.

> There are few men and women so perfectly mated that the climax of the act is reached together. It is usual for the male to arrive at this stage earlier than the female, with the consequence that he is further incapacitated to satisfy her desire for some time after. . . . The condom will often help with this difficulty. (11)

Many women could not easily obtain the French or Mizpah pessary, the type Sanger preferred among those sometimes available in the United States, but there were a number of other choices in *Family Limitation* that were relatively easy to come by. Sanger was never particularly fond of the condom since it required so much trust on the woman's part, but she thought it "one of the best protectors against both conception and venereal disease." She offered several recipes for suppositories, some to be mixed by a druggist and some at home, such as "Boric Acid, 10 grains/Cocoa butter, 20 grains." One recipe she brought back from France consisted of gelatine, water, glycerine, and quinine, made into a paste, spread out and allowed to solidify and then cut into cubes. Similarly, she listed eight different douching solutions, from Lysol and water to "potassium permanganate" to basic salt or vinegar solutions, and added a number of douching tips, such as, "Do not be afraid to assist the cleansing by introducing the first finger with the tube and washing out the semen from the folds of the membrane." She also gave advice on where to find various products. Many were sold in drugstores under the guise of menstrual needs, feminine hygiene, or "womb supporters." Later editions of the pamphlet included manufacturer's names and addresses.[23]

Sanger claimed she sent a copy of *Family Limitation* to the judge and prosecutor in her case, "as though to say, 'Make the most of it.'" But there is no indication that

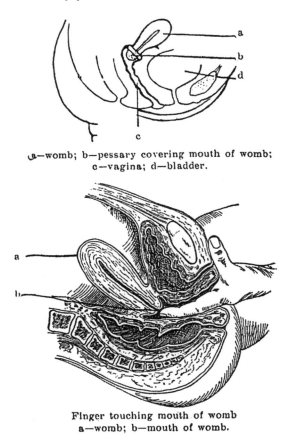

a—womb; b—pessary covering mouth of womb;
c—vagina; d—bladder.

Finger touching mouth of womb
a—womb; b—mouth of womb.

Illustration from the first edition of Margaret Sanger's *Family Limitation* (1914) showing the placement of a pessary. (Courtesy of the Sophia Smith Collection, Smith College.)

the prosecution took the bait. Harold Content, the assistant U.S. attorney on the case, was "annoyed" at Sanger's abrupt disappearance but made no attempt to adjust the charges pending against her or, it seems, any effort to track her down. It would not have been easy if he had tried. Sanger traveled under an alias, "Bertha Watson," arriving in England in mid-November 1914, just as Europe descended into World War I.

SANGER'S EXILE

Over the next 11 months, Sanger used her *Woman Rebel* notoriety and list of contacts given to her by Victor Dave and other radical friends to form associations and, in some cases, life-long friendships with leading neo-Malthusians, sex theorists, educators, Fabian socialists, writers, and feminists in England and the mainland. She met Edith How-Martyn, one of the few English feminists and suffragettes to advocate birth control, who would partner with Sanger years later in organizing an international movement. She struck up a friendship with future rival Marie Stopes, the paleobotanist turned sex advice maven who was in the midst of revising *Married Love*, her groundbreaking treatise on marriage equality and sexual satisfaction. Stopes turned to birth control activism after meeting Sanger in the spring of 1915. Sanger also met a number of the authors she had been reading and excerpting in *The Woman Rebel*, including Edward Carpenter, Havelock Ellis, and the head of the Malthusian League, Charles Vickery Drysdale, who steadily promoted a small family ideal. Although the League was a shadow of its past, Drysdale, his wife Bessie, and his mother, League founder Alice Vickery, continued to cooperate with neo-Malthusian leagues in Western Europe. They sent Sanger off to the Netherlands with a letter of introduction to leaders of their Dutch counterpart.

In Amsterdam, home to the first birth control clinic in the world, opened in 1882, and some of the lowest infant and maternal mortality rates in Europe, Sanger met in February 1915 with Dr. Johannes Rutgers, an officer in the Dutch Neo-Malthusian League. He and Dr. Aletta Jacobs, the first Dutch woman to receive a medical degree, were largely responsible for developing the Dutch system of small contraceptive clinics staffed mainly by trained midwives and lay nurses. The Dutch League, and Rutgers especially, sought to reach working people and educate them to pass on contraceptive knowledge to others. This approach was more in line with Sanger's thinking than the British birth controllers, who believed in a trickle-down strategy: establish family planning practices among the middle and upper classes and the poor will learn by example. Although Jacobs would not meet with Sanger because she lacked medical credentials, Rutgers allowed Sanger to participate in an instruction course for fitting a Mensinga diaphragm, a larger pessary with a spring rim that created a full barrier in the vaginal canal rather than simply capping the cervix. Because of its effectiveness, the Mensinga would become Sanger's method of choice, largely supplanting smaller pessaries and cervical caps by the 1920s. However, it had to be properly fitted by a doctor, midwife, or nurse to maximize comfort and effectiveness, adding a level of medical control over the process. Although it ran counter to the do-it-yourself mentality of *Family Limitation*, Sanger realized that medical supervision was the best way to increase safety and efficacy. The diaphragm had the added benefit of ensuring that women learned about their anatomy and sexual functioning and had regular contact with medical professionals who could detect venereal disease or address other health problems. Sanger's three weeks in the Netherlands, combined with her research in England, convinced her that the Dutch clinic system should be emulated in America.[24]

Of all the of people Sanger met during her exile, Havelock Ellis had the most profound influence on expanding and clarifying her intellectual rationale for birth control and in giving scientific validation to the importance of women's sexual fulfillment. In a matter of days, the two developed a comfortable rapport that eased into a sexual relationship, opening the way for intimate discussions about sexual practices and proclivities, and the "spiritual essence" of sexual pleasure that was central to Ellis's approach to the subject. He directed Sanger's several weeks of research at the British Library, helping her to pull together additional material on contraception that led to three more birth control pamphlets to supplement *Family Limitation*. *English Methods of Birth Control* focused on birth control safety and included sections of the Malthusian League's *Hygienic Methods of Family Limitation* (1913). *Dutch Methods of Birth Control* was an edited, English translation of a Dutch Neo-Malthusian League publication. The conclusion to the series, *Magnetation Methods of Birth Control*, consisted of various strategies for pursuing intercourse without ejaculation, such as the Karezza method, and illustrated French-made methods of contraception, mostly pessaries and syringes. These pamphlets were published in the spring and summer of 1915 and eventually sent to *Woman Rebel* subscribers. (Several thousand copies went down on the British liner *Arabic*, when it was sunk by a German U-boat in August, limiting the distribution of the series.) Especially in *English Methods*, Sanger continued to develop her feminist argument for birth control, envisioning women as an equal partner in sexual relations and emphasizing the need to better ensure women's sexual gratification through family limitation:

> There has been among men a common idea that woman had little or no sex desire or interest, and that marriage sanctioned a union which made of woman a recipient but not a mutual partner in the sex life. Fortunately this idea is giving way, and men of ideals and fine temperaments dislike the idea of the relation when it is not mutual. That is one of the reasons that the use of preventive measures has come to play so important a part in the lives of both men and women, and why it must sooner or later receive the fullest attention from the medical profession, as well as from society at large.

Ellis also instilled in Sanger an understanding and appreciation for birth control's eugenic potential, the key role it should play in the voluntary control of inherited disease and in limiting human misery by reducing family size and population levels. "Substituting the ideal of quality," he had written a few years earlier, "for the vulgar ideal of mere quantity, is now generally accepted, alike by medical pathologists, embryologists, and neurologists, and by sociologists and moralists." Ellis had an almost blind faith in the power of science to create a better and stronger human race, and he conveyed this confidence to Sanger. But what made his views on what he called "race regeneration" more palatable to Sanger, who was just beginning to explore eugenic thought, was Ellis's expectation that women's sexual autonomy would bring about voluntary motherhood. When motherhood is a choice, he reasoned, rather than a result of accident or compulsion, children fare better and society benefits. "The women will solve the question of mankind," wrote Ellis, quoting the playwright Henrik Ibsen, "and they will do it as mothers." Ellis's imperative was: women must assert control over their sexual lives, and this could only be realized through the prevention of conception.[25]

WILLIAM SANGER'S ARREST

Sanger's will to remain in exile was tested mightily in late January 1915 when she received word that Anthony Comstock had arrested William Sanger at his Manhattan studio for handing an undercover vice agent a copy of *Family Limitation.* Though William Sanger did not seek this legal entanglement or moment of notoriety, Margaret resented him for getting "mixed up in my work" and putting himself in exactly the position that *she* had hoped to be in—fighting for the right to give out contraceptive information on free speech grounds in a case that was uncomplicated by other charges and issues. Sanger believed William's arrest was little more than a trap set by Comstock to lure her back to New York. She refused to "go meekly like a lamb to slaughter." Nor did the FSL lawyers advise her return, fearing her immediate arrest. Moreover, she had not prepared a coherent defense strategy. With the children safely with friends, Sanger decided to remain in Europe until William's trial was over.

"I think that this may become a famous case," wrote Leonard Abbott, now the president of the FSL, to Mabel Dodge in February 1915 about the prosecution of William Sanger. And, indeed, the arrest marked something of a threshold moment in the formation of the birth control movement. Much more than the *Woman Rebel* indictments, the resulting publicity from William Sanger's case expanded the public discussion of birth control. In early March, the year-old liberal magazine, the *New Republic,* offered a nearly unconditional endorsement of birth control, asserting, "The relief which it would bring to the poor is literally incalculable. The assistance it would lend all effort to end destitution and fight poverty is enormous." In April, the more moderate *Harper's Weekly* kicked off the first of more than a dozen articles on birth control it published in 1915 because "the subject insists on coming up, as many Americans are not willing to be kept in tutelage on a matter so freely treated in Europe." Written by the journalist Mary Alden Hopkins, the series covered the issue from numerous viewpoints and included medical and religious concerns, an analysis of the birth rate and a discussion of large families and poverty. "So at last birth control—that matter about which men, and especially women, have thought so much and have dared talked so little and then furtively—is to be brought out into the open," the *New York Tribune* stated in May. Coverage of the story made it into middle

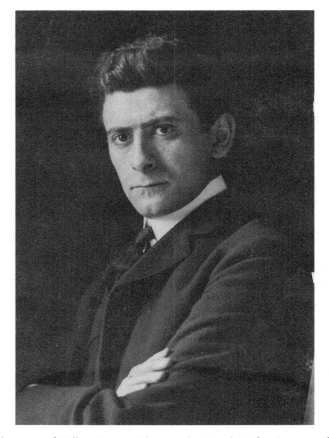

An undated portrait of William Sanger. (Photographer: Frank Forfey. Courtesy of the Sophia Smith Collection, Smith College.)

America as well: "William Sanger and Mrs. Sanger, his wife . . . are being hounded, prosecuted and doubtless, persecuted by Comstock and others in the metropolis," ran an editorial in the Biloxi, Mississippi, *Daily Herald*; "Birth Control A Problem," read the headline in the *Kansas City Star*, in a report on agitation in New York. Across the country, many Americans were exposed for the first time to arguments in favor of legalizing birth control as they read the details of what would be Comstock's last great conquest and, because of the publicity perhaps his greatest failure.[26]

William Sanger's arrest also galvanized a dedicated group of radical activists, feminists, and medical proponents of birth control and aroused the interest of a number of more moderate supporters. Within a few weeks, factions of New York's radical community, sensing a free speech martyr in their midst, began banding together to form a defense fund and, soon after, a birth control group. The FSL put it into perspective: "The Sanger case involves much more than Mr. Sanger and his wife. It involves broad social questions . . . issues of personal liberty and of a free press. It raises squarely the questions: How much longer will liberty-loving men and women submit to 'Comstockery'?" The response to William Sanger's arrest was far more impressive than the halfhearted efforts to drum up support for Margaret Sanger following her departure in the fall of 1914. In fact, Margaret had lashed out against Goldman's *Mother Earth* and the radical press in general for failing to advance solidarity over her case or raise funds to support her in exile. (She survived on FSL contributions, odd jobs, and the generosity of her English friends.)

William Sanger filled a better victim profile: struggling artist, abandoned husband, and single father—an unwitting accomplice entrapped by the crafty vice crusader. He drew the attention of a broader swath of Village radicals. Some of them—the new feminists in particular—were primed for a birth control campaign but had been put off by Margaret Sanger's political extremism and belittling attacks against them in *The Woman Rebel*. William Sanger's case also attracted some support from outside the radical community, from progressive society women who would, within two years, become the bedrock of the movement. The FSL leadership, especially Abbott, Gilbert Roe, and Theodore Schroeder, went into high gear, recognizing that they had a much stronger test case with William than with his wife. They also found it easier to raise money. "This Sanger case is proving to be a veritable gold-mine," Abbott wrote to Theodore Schroeder. "Considerably more than the $500 we asked for has come in." The FSL raised bail, sent out flyers and form letters, and explored the best legal strategy.[27]

THE NATIONAL BIRTH CONTROL LEAGUE AND REGIONAL GROUPS

In March after attending a William Sanger defense meeting, a small group of liberals, including the suffragist Mary Ware Dennett, FSL vice-president Lincoln Steffens, the feminist attorney and Sanger friend Jessie Ashley, and Otto Bobsien, who had been part of Sanger's small *Woman Rebel* staff, formed the National Birth Control League (NBCL), the first American birth control organization to have more than a nominal existence. Dennett quickly asserted leadership of the new League and embraced the cause of birth control as her own. This move underscored the rapid evolution of birth control agitation—from anarchist noise to an issue that was beginning to capture the attention of moderate progressive reformers. The wellborn Dennett (1872–1947), a recognized figure in the Arts and Crafts movement and a veteran women's suffrage organizer, seemed like a slightly eccentric, buttoned-down matron in contrast with Sanger. Yet her interest in social welfare had led her to embrace the single-tax and aspects of socialism, and her steadfast commitment to individual rights and civil liberties allowed her to bump shoulders with the free speech crowd and some of the more revolutionary types in Greenwich Village. Like Sanger, Dennett's marriage had grown sour, resulting in a drawn-out divorce and custody dispute that left her virtually penniless. And like a number of women reformers who gravitated to the birth control cause, Dennett had been rebuffed by doctors when she inquired about birth control, after excruciating childbirth experiences.

At the first NBCL meeting, Dennett spoke with confidence that the "time is ripe" to take action, because the cause for birth control had expanded beyond the anarchist community. "There has been marked unanimity on one point," she said, that it is "the absolute conviction of each individual," from "the most cramped conservative to the freeist radical . . . that correct information about birth control should be freely attainable." The NBCL announced that it was formed to "create an intelligent public demand for the repeal of all laws prohibiting the giving out of information concerning methods of birth control" and "to distribute accurate information on the subject of birth control after it has become legal to do so." But the League had no intention of defying the law.[28]

William Sanger's arrest and the circulation of *Family Limitation* led to a flurry of organizing activity in the spring of 1915. Birth control leagues were started in San Francisco in February; in Portland, Oregon, in March; and in Seattle and Los Angeles later in the year. The IWW and other radical groups joined efforts to help the William Sanger defense fund, encourage protest mailings, and distribute pamphlets. Henrietta Rodman, maybe the most recognizable feminist in New York, joined with Dr. William Robinson in creating a Committee on Birth Control to organize a meeting held at the New York Academy of Medicine on May 26, 1915. An overflowing crowd of more than 2,000 attended to hear Dr. Abraham Jacobi, Robinson, Dr. Lydia Allen DeVilbiss, a rising public health physician, and several other speakers give their support for allowing doctors greater discretion in prescribing contraception. Sensing the changing times, Jacobi remarked, "We have come here as a nucleus around which democratic men and women may gather, and in a year or two public opinion will veer about and people will wonder how they could have been so stupid and callous. What is now a crime will be considered a beneficial measure." The organizers passed out petition cards and compiled a list with which to build an organizational base and quickly rally support. The event was widely covered in the press and, though the organizers failed to get the state legislature to propose an amendment to the penal code, a goal of the meeting, they demonstrated that the interest in birth control legalization went beyond the libertarian base of the cause.[29]

BIRTH CONTROL OPPOSITION AND RACE SUICIDE

"Are we to have homes or brothels?" Comstock ranted in response to the birth control agitation. "Can't poor people learn self-control? Can't everybody, whether rich or poor, learn to control themselves?" Apart from Comstock, opposition to birth control at this stage was unorganized and scattershot. Much of the country was simply unsure of what it all meant and preferred to keep the issue private. But gradually, the sexually liberating spirit of Greenwich Village had wafted across America through books, films, plays, and lectures, often covered in newspaper and magazine articles and reviews. The idea of sex for pleasure was becoming more conventional and expressed more often in popular culture. As John D'Emilio and Estelle Freedman concluded, many Americans at the onset of World War I "were prepared to accept revised notions of female sexuality and to reassess the place that sexual expression held in a happy life." And the increasing numbers of women seeking higher education and entering the workforce brought about a practical tolerance of family planning.

Nevertheless, as birth control publicity increased, opposition voices, though few in number, grew louder. Some continued to equate contraception with abortion and associate birth control with promiscuity and other forms of social degeneration. With more young people delaying marriage and the birth rate in steady decline, one outspoken physician quipped, "We have plenty of birth control already without teaching any of it." Another well known doctor, Howard A. Kelly, the chief gynecologist at Johns Hopkins University, made something of a sideline opposing birth control. He stated in 1915, "All meddling with the sexual relation to secure facultative sterility degrades the wife to the level of a prostitute . . . there is no right or decent way of controlling births but by total abstinence." A number of conservative voices expressed their disappointment that such a delicate issue had been thrust before the public but, muffled by their own sense of decency and uneasiness with the subject, they were reluctant to engage in debate. In a newspaper interview, Josephine Jewell Dodge (better known as Mrs. Arthur M.), the notable antisuffragist, thought the fear of pregnancy "the last barrier against immorality" and did not want anyone to have access to contraceptive information. "Instead of giving it to the poorer classes," she said, "I feel it should be taken away from the well-to-do people." Grace Strachan, a New York school superintendent, called the public discussion of birth control "indelicate" but overcame her discomfiture to ask, "By what right or authority does any group of people set itself up to regulate God's or nature's laws?" She wondered how many great men would be lost if the average family size continued to contract. She also believed the legalization of contraception would bring about promiscuity and a dangerous decrease in population.

After the war, the Catholic Church grabbed hold of the issue. But up until then the Church was loath to publicly air its views on an issue it relegated to the confessional booth, and few Catholic clerics spoke out in public. One exception, Father John A. Ryan, who would help lead the Catholic side of the debate over the next two decades, published a letter he wrote to the NBCL in the spring of 1915: "I regard the practice which your organization desires to promote as immoral, degrading, and stupid. The so-called contraceptive devices are intrinsically immoral because they involve the unnatural use, the perversion of a human faculty . . . Such conduct is quite as immoral as self mutilation or the practice of solitary vice."[30]

The strongest anti-birth control sentiment continued to come from traditionalists and a growing number of eugenicists who were convinced that the so-called "native stock," the lineage of the Protestant Yankee, was rapidly dying out because the more educated and affluent had adopted family planning practices. The Sanger prosecutions, along with the escalation of the European war, reinvigorated race suicide arguments and increased concerns that America was becoming more like France, viewed by many Americans as a decadent and weakened country focused on individual comforts rather than the common good. The chief spokesperson for the race suicide alarmists, Theodore Roosevelt, had been banging the same drum since the early years of his presidency, scolding middle- and upper-class American women for restricting births as he raised fears about America's future. "The Truth is self-evident," he said in 1914, "that if the average married couple . . . only has two children, the whole race will disappear in a very few generations." He encouraged each couple to have four or more children. For Roosevelt and many Progressive Era eugenicists, birth control represented "a reckless and brutal selfishness" that put the country at great risk. Not only was America producing fewer soldiers, it was also, as Harvard economist Thomas Nixon Carver phrased it in 1915, gradually allowing its "true American stock" to be submerged by "triumphant immigrants" and the "force of their greater virility as revealed in their much higher birth rates." The race suicide theorists had a full quiver of arrows with which to attack not only birth control and the differential fertility rate between the rich and poor, but also feminism, individualism, pacifism, and immigration. Thus their specific arguments against family limitation were sometimes obscured by more overarching concerns about the nation's security and a changing family dynamic, brought on by women's increasing social freedoms and a new abundance of leisure time.[31]

GOLDMAN AND REITMAN

The frequent warnings about the deleterious consequences of birth control both in the individual and society did little to thwart the momentum of the burgeoning movement. Apart from organizational work on both coasts, another significant contribution to the diffusion of information came from Emma Goldman and Dr. Ben Reitman (1879–1942), the flamboyant Chicago anarchist and "hobo" doctor to the poor, who joined Goldman in love and on the lecture circuit starting in 1908. "We have taken up an important movement," Reitman announced in March 1915. "It is to limit the production of humanity." After years of carefully avoiding a free speech fight over birth control and with Margaret Sanger in exile, Goldman seized the public platform, recognizing that the time was ripe to push defiance of the Comstock laws to the limit. In at least one New York appearance she arrived with an overnight bag for prison and took the stage to explain how to use a diaphragm. She was inexplicably spared arrest and continued the practice in other cities, speaking in Pittsburgh, Cleveland, Detroit, Chicago, Minneapolis, Denver, Portland, and Los Angeles in the summer and fall of 1915. Reitman proved to be a masterful manager and promoter, drawing large audiences to hear Goldman give talks on birth control and other issues. He distributed thousands of contraceptive pamphlets, including *Why and How the Poor Should Not Have Many Children*, a fold-over, four-page summary of contraceptive choices probably written by Reitman and reminiscent of William Robinson's earlier flyer for doctors. They also sold Sanger's *Family Limitation* every chance they could. Reitman wrote that fall in *Mother Earth*:

> O brave Margaret Sanger! You can be glad even if they hang you or send you to the penitentiary for life, your pamphlet has found its way into nearly every hamlet or village in America, and dozens of other men or women have republished your pamphlet or similar ones and scattered them broadcast throughout the land and Anthony Comstock, though aided by all the powers of government or hell, cannot stop this stupendous movement.

Goldman and Reitman marched through their ninth lecture tour together unscathed by the law until they came to Portland, Oregon, in early August. Just as Goldman concluded her speech on August 6, she saw Reitman and a police officer headed for the stage. "Here comes an officer to arrest me now," she yelled out to the crowd. The two were charged with "circulating literature of an illegal character" and taken to the city jail. The five-month-old Portland Birth Control League turned out a crowd at the courthouse that sighed audibly when the deputy city attorney declined to read aloud the offending pamphlet. Goldman and Reitman were fined $100 and appealed the case to the Circuit Court. There Judge William Gatens dismissed it, noting, "Ignorance and prudery are the millstones about the neck of progress. Everyone knows that we are all shocked by things publicly stated that we know privately ourselves." News of the arrests hit most Western papers and increased interest in birth control in the remaining cities on Goldman's tour.[32]

WILLIAM SANGER'S TRIAL AND THE DEATH OF COMSTOCK

A few weeks later, William Sanger's case finally came to trial before three judges of the Court of Special Sessions in New York, following several unsuccessful attempts on the part of FSL lawyers to secure a jury trial. Convinced that "an acquittal with a lawyer—only meant an anticlimax" and offered little publicity, at the last minute Sanger dismissed his attorney, Gilbert Roe, and decided to go it alone. The decision injected some added drama into the proceedings. William Sanger claimed that Comstock offered him a suspended sentence if he pled guilty, but he refused because he believed that there was nothing indecent about *Family Limitation*. The trial was a chaotic scene and entertaining fare for the tabloids. The gallery was filled with anarchists, suffragists, and socialists, including Alexander Berkman, Elizabeth Gurley Flynn, Carlo Tresca, and Leonard Abbott. A bit too "anarchistic," William thought, for the "Reds," as they were referred to in the newspapers, scared off the "safe folk." However, Gertrude Minturn Pinchot, an NBCL member and a philanthropist well known in New York society circles, stood out from the radical crowd and was prominently mentioned in press reports. Following preliminaries, Sanger was confronted by Comstock, who took the stand to summarize the entrapment that resulted in William Sanger's arrest. Sanger then began to read a lengthy statement, admitting that he broke the law, but declaring that it was "the law" that was on trial, "not I." He was interrupted by the presiding Judge, James McInerney, a devout Catholic and father of six, who inserted his own views into the record, calling William Sanger a "menace to society," and "crazy." An agitated Comstock also interrupted without the permission of the court to accuse Sanger of lying about Comstock's offer of a plea agreement. Sanger read only a short portion of his statement before the judges cut him off and convened to find him guilty. "In my opinion," McInerney told Sanger in delivering the verdict, "the pamphlet is both indecent and immoral. Your crime violates not only the laws of the state, but the laws of God." William Sanger was sentenced to a fine of $150 or 30 days in prison. He chose the latter, and police hustled him into a holding pen. A *New York Tribune* reporter described the scene that ensued:

> At this the storm that had been gathering in the crowded courtroom broke. It began with a volley of hand-clapping and ended in a medley of shouts and cries. Men and women stood on the benches and waved their hats and handkerchiefs. The three Justices, their faces red with anger, stood at the bench. The gavel of the Chief Justice went on pounding, which only marked time for the din of the room. The court attendants, reinforced by policemen, finally succeeded in getting the anarchists into the corridor.[33]

Comstock took ill with a fever shortly after witnessing the commotion in the court room and never recovered, developing pneumonia that led to his death 10 days later. By the time of his demise, he had already become a relic of a bygone era. His power had waned, and to many Americans he had become either a tiresome bore or a target of ridicule. *The Masses* magazine ran a political cartoon in September 1915 by the artist Robert Minor, who had sat in on the William Sanger trial, which depicted a rotund Comstock before a judge, clutching a young mother, saying "Your honor, this woman gave birth to a naked child!" Increasingly in Progressive Era America, intelligent people were disturbed by sexual ignorance—the lack of knowledge concerning venereal disease, sexual exploitation, birth control, and women's sexuality—more than sexual expression. Comstock's arrest scorecard and hodgepodge collection of confiscated indecency was looking more like a time capsule that marked the era of Victorian prudery. He would live on, but only because the Comstock Law survived and the birth control movement continued to prop him up as a symbol of repressive morality.[34]

William Sanger's 30 days in The Tombs were uneventful, and he quickly exited the public stage, returning to his studio. Historians and commentators on the early years of the birth control movement have generally glossed over his contribution, viewing him as little more than a proxy for his wife's cause. After all, his trial was really a condemnation of *Family Limitation* rather than a judgment on his innocuous act. But by extending his legal battle for nearly eight months and standing up with gritty resolve to Comstock and a trio of intractable judges, he emboldened others outside of anarchist and socialist circles to come forward in support. Moreover, as William noted in a prison letter to Margaret, the case helped make "Birth Control—a household term." When William Sanger declared in court, "I deny the right of the State to encroach on the rights of the individual by invading the most private and fundamental relations of men and women"—words that were printed in a number of U.S. publications and in *The Malthusian* in England—he joined his wife and Emma Goldman in being among the first Americans to defend reproductive rights.

When William Sanger entered the courtroom in early September 1915, it had been a little more than a year since the *Woman Rebel* indictments were handed down against Margaret Sanger. Yet in that relatively short time, public silence over birth control had been broken, leagues had been created on both coasts, and there was emergent support for legislative reform of the Comstock laws. Quietly, *Family Limitation* continued to be distributed throughout the country. It was now sought after by women who had learned about it from a friend or at a meeting or in the newspaper. Elizabeth Gurley Flynn wrote to Sanger about a Chicago activist who reported that "the women in the Stockyard district kissed her hands, when she distributed them." At the end of William Sanger's trial, the FSL announced that $1,000 had been raised to publish another edition of the notorious pamphlet.[35]

MARGARET SANGER'S RETURN

A few days before William Sanger's release from prison in early October 1915, Margaret Sanger returned to New York, after an absence of nearly a year, with the intention of fighting the *Woman Rebel* charges and with vague plans to open a birth control clinic modeled after the ones in Amsterdam. Her friends had kept her informed of the grass-roots support for birth control generated by *Family Limitation* and her husband's arrest and trial. But Sanger could not have been prepared for the chilly welcome she received from the more moderate reformers who had filled a leadership void in her absence. With Mary Ware Dennett at the helm, the NBCL had tried to distance itself from Sanger and her outlaw status. And although the League utilized Sanger's *Woman Rebel* mailing list and rallied around the Sanger name, it eschewed her direct-action approach. As Sanger later remembered, the NBCL made it clear in its first meeting with her that it "disagreed with my methods, my tactics, with everything I had done. Such an organization as theirs, the function of which was primarily to change the laws in an orderly and proper manner, could not logically

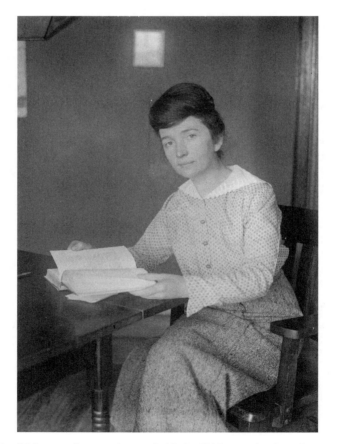

Photograph of Margaret Sanger taken probably in 1915 near the time she returned from her European exile. (Courtesy of the George Grantham Bain Collection, Library of Congress.)

sanction anyone who had broken those laws." She was also disappointed that the birth control agitation had been focused on the middle class. Aside from efforts by some radicals to distribute *Family Limitation*, there had been no attempts to reach working-class women. With no backing from the NBCL and uncertain legal advice from the FSL—her advisors argued over whether or not she should plead guilty— Sanger contacted the assistant district attorney in her case to arrange a meeting and review her options.

However, on November 6, a family tragedy intervened and added a new complication to Sanger's defense. The Sangers' youngest child, five-year-old Peggy, died from pneumonia. Her death sent Margaret Sanger into a state of depression and forced the federal prosecution in her case to consider the new public relations challenge of how to force a mourning mother into court. Guilt-ridden and physically weakened by the loss, Sanger secured a delay of her trial.[36]

THE BOLLINGER BABY

But it was the death of another child that had both a more immediate and lasting impact on the birth control cause. Just two weeks after Peggy Sanger's death, a five-day-old baby boy, born with multiple physical deformities, brain damage, and partial paralysis, died in the German-American Hospital in Chicago. The hospital's chief of staff, Dr. Harry Haiselden, had advised the parents, Anna and Allen Bollinger, to forego surgical intervention that would probably have saved the baby's life. The story unfolded over several weeks in the press, competing with war news on the front pages. "When Dr. H. J. Haiselden allowed nature to take her course in deciding the fate of the Bollinger baby in Chicago, he started the nation talking," ran the editorial in the *Salt Lake Telegram*. "No other event in recent months has been so widely discussed in the newspapers, in the pulpits, in meetings of scientific societies and in the homes of the people." The Illinois commissioner of health and others had tried to pressure Haiselden into performing an operation to correct bowel defects that would have allowed the baby to survive. A Catholic woman even attempted to kidnap the baby and take him to another surgeon. But Haiselden stated publicly that "there was no chance that life would bring this child anything better than an animal existence and imbecility. I had no right to condemn it to that." He said he believed he had done the human race "a favor." Many prominent Americans agreed, including the pioneer of the juvenile court system, Judge Ben Lindsey, civil rights attorney Clarence Darrow, historian Charles Beard, nurse and social worker Lillian Wald, and, surprisingly, Catholic Cardinal James Gibbons of Baltimore, who put forth that Haiselden was "not obliged" to take "extraordinary means" to prolong life.

The death of Baby Bollinger aroused a storm of protest from other clergy of all denominations, as well as many doctors, social workers, and health and children's advocates. The pacifist and settlement house movement founder Jane Addams said, "Under no circumstances has any human being the right to pass judgment of death for unfitness on any other human being." Dr. Ira Wile, an outspoken birth control supporter, thought that physicians should never refuse to save a life, and that Haiselden should have consulted with other doctors at the very least, something he admitted he had not done. Several who spoke out against the doctor referred to Helen Keller as an example of a person who triumphed over her disabilities. "Defectives have reached great heights," noted Bishop Samuel Fallows. Yet Helen Keller herself supported Haiselden's decision in a remarkable letter released to newspapers about 10 days after the baby's death. She wrote that Haiselden "performed a service to society as well as to the hopeless being he spared from a life of misery . . . the world is already flooded with unhappy, unhealthy, mentally unsound persons that should never have been born." She argued that the baby's death was not in vain, for he "has brought us face to face with the many questions of eugenics and control of the birth rate—questions we have been side-stepping because we are afraid of them." Keller used this issue to mount support for the birth control cause, writing, "The case of William Sanger . . . should open the eyes of all intelligent persons to the forces at work against the spread of this new idea." Birth control, she continued, helped "distressed parents to limit the number of their offspring and give a better chance of health and happiness to the children they did have."[37]

Coming on the heels of the William Sanger trial, the Bollinger story kept the issue of birth control alive in the press and provided an opportunity for birth control advocates to appeal to both sides in the debate over infant euthanasia. Several physician advocates of birth control, including Abraham Jacobi, a critic of Haiselden, argued that couples with an inheritable condition should refrain from childbearing. Mary Ware Dennett and Anita Block of the NBCL publicly supported Haiselden's position, and Frederic Robinson, the editor of the *Medical Review of Reviews* and son of William Robinson, used the Bollinger story to try and reignite a legislative campaign to amend the Comstock laws and establish birth control as a necessary component of eugenics. "The Bollinger case," he wrote in a widely printed statement, "has no direct bearing on birth control, for the mother already had had two healthy children. But the publicity which the case has received has at last swept away these barriers of silence which hitherto have kept the subject of child-birth from consideration by our great American public." Around the same time, Robinson also hired a group of poor and ailing men to go out into the streets of New York carrying banners with warnings such as, "I am a burden to myself and the State. Should I be allowed to propagate?" and, "I have no opportunity to educate or feed my children. They may become criminals." Mutual Movies newsreel picked up footage of the pathetic men as did the print press.

In the months that followed, the Bollinger story grew in complexity. Haiselden admitted that he had let many seriously impaired infants die, and that he had not only withheld treatment, but also in some instances had aided the onset of death through the use of narcotics. Other doctors came forward to disclose similar "mercy killings." Newspapers reported on deformed or disabled babies in different parts of the country who had been deprived of medical attention. Haiselden became a supreme self-promoter and propagandist, appearing on the lecture circuit and in newsreels. He went so far as to write and star in a fictionalized movie based on the Bollinger case, *The Black Stork*, which was shown in theaters from 1917 into the 1920s.[38]

THE *WOMAN REBEL* CHARGES

Margaret Sanger was one of the few birth control advocates to remain silent on the Bollinger case. Grieving over her own daughter's death, she refrained from public comment. She was, according to Leonard Abbott, who worked with her on her defense, "in a *very* confused state of mind. She wavers between the attitude prompted by her own weakness, and her desire to be consistently radical and revolutionary." Sanger admitted it was "difficult to get the heart for any thing," and blamed her daughter's death on her exile. Emma Goldman wrote Sanger an impassioned letter in December, telling her that her guilt was unreasonable and that she must collect her strength and take advantage of the "growing interest" in birth control, which has "taken hold of the public as never before." Goldman encouraged Sanger to push through the legal process and plan for a cross-country lecture tour, which would "give the movement an impetus of great force."

Public sympathy for Sanger prompted the district attorney to offer a plea bargain if she promised not to violate the law again. But she refused to plead guilty to publishing obscenity when she believed she had not written anything obscene. Whatever the cost, she wrote in another mass mailing to "Friends and Comrades," the goal was "to raise the entire question of birth control out of the gutter of obscenity and into the light of human understanding." Her legal advisors and concerned friends, like *Masses* editor Max Eastman, thought Sanger was unstable, especially after she decided to forgo counsel as her husband had done. But Sanger recognized that her "personal sorrow" made her story more compelling to the public. She also saw a way to win over additional support by turning the tables on the prosecution. After avoiding trial for more than a year, she now challenged the federal court to try her case as soon as possible. Following several court delays due to scheduling problems, she told reporters in February 1916, "It is not fair to keep me under the shadow of this indictment." She threatened that "if it continues much longer" she might "sue the government for libel."

With public sentiment growing in Sanger's favor, her confrontational strategy succeeded in coalescing support, especially among women. Feminist Alice Carpenter organized a dinner rally of 200 supporters for Sanger in January at the Hotel

Brevoort in New York City. The guests included Abraham Jacobi, who bristled at Sanger's provocative manner and lay status but held firm to his support for changing the laws; writers and friends John Reed and Walter Lippmann, whose opinions carried considerable weight among liberals; and Mary Ware Dennett, who announced that the NBCL stood behind Sanger and her defense (Sanger attributed her support to an attempt to boost membership and raise money for the NBCL). A number of prominent women signed a petition calling for the judge in Sanger's trial to impanel a jury equally represented by women. An impressive group of society women, feminists, radicals, FSL attorneys, and activist physicians accompanied Sanger to her court dates in January and February, only to have the proceedings postponed. The judge assigned to the case received dozens of letters and telegrams each day calling for a dismissal of charges. Resolutions passed by liberal organizations, unions, schools, and women's groups from across the nation declaring support for Sanger were sent to President Woodrow Wilson, the judge, and local newspapers.[39]

Finally, on February 18, 1916, the U.S. Attorney for New York entered a nolle prossequi, and all charges against Sanger were dismissed. The District Attorney did not want to "make a martyr" of Sanger anymore than he already had, and he disliked the constant agitation from her supporters. "They are the queerest lot of cranks," he wrote, "that we have had around here for a long time." Although the dismissal of the case was anticlimactic, Sanger accepted it as a clear victory and cited publicity as the deciding factor and the catalyst for the movement. At a celebration rally she said, "I thank the grand jury for indicting me. I thank the Federal authorities for fanning the flame, and I thank the dear newspapers for publicity. They have done wonders to arouse interest in birth control." Emma Goldman's arrest in New York on February 11 for discussing birth control and the lead-up to her trial had prompted additional articles, updates, and editorials on the subject.

The government's inconsistent attempts to curtail speech starting with the *Woman Rebel* charges had created a mainstream news event that in effect sanitized birth control and made it an acceptable issue of public discussion. Not only did newspapers and radical journals cover the topic, cultural and political commentary magazines such as *Harper's* and the *New Republic*, social hygiene and medical publications including *The Survey, Physical Culture, Medical Times,* and Robinson's *Critic and Guide,* also followed news of the movement and contributed to the debate. Most noteworthy, the *Pictorial Review,* the middle-class women's magazine with a circulation of over 1 million in 1916, published a three-part series on birth control in October 1915 and February and March 1916. "What Shall We Do about Birth-Control?" featured a "for and against" letter-writing contest. The March 1916 issue included the winning letters from men and women, including a male physician, a clergyman, and a woman welfare worker. She wrote: "All normal women want children, but they want them when *they* want them—not just as it may happen."

The esteemed lawyer and constitutional expert Samuel Untermyer, a legal big gun who had been brought in to advise Sanger in December 1915, told her, in recommending that she take the plea bargain, "You cannot even get publicity in these days when the papers are crowded with international news and the big things of history are happening." He was wrong. The newspapers covered every court delay and protest rally. As Sanger, Goldman, and an increasing number of their followers already sensed, the grassroots birth control campaign was well on its way to becoming one of those "big things of history."[40]

SANGER'S EMERGENCE AS MOVEMENT LEADER

As soon as the *Woman Rebel* charges were dismissed—and with them Sanger's public platform of a trial—Sanger finalized her plans for a speaking tour. She seemed eager to get out of town, both to try and put the death of her daughter behind her and to disengage from a birth control turf war that had erupted with Emma Goldman. Goldman's *Mother Earth* had criticized Sanger for letting an important legal challenge slip from her control. Sanger left on a national lecture tour in mid-April 1916, following the trail blazed by Goldman before her. Meanwhile, Goldman rallied the growing number of birth control supporters to her side in several large meetings in New York following her February arrest. At Carnegie Hall on March 1, Goldman whipped up the crowd, assailing the Comstock law and attacking the "narrow-minded bigots" who enforced it. Sanger, suffering from the flu, was noticeably absent from the Carnegie Hall rally, which took place before she left town, as she was from other events surrounding Goldman's trial, sentencing, and 15 days in The Tombs. Most of the FSL crowd and the anarchist contingent that had dutifully escorted Sanger to her rallies now tagged along after Goldman, including William Sanger, who joined the group that gathered at The Tombs on April 20 to protest Goldman's imprisonment. Margaret Sanger bristled over Goldman's headline-grabbing activities that spring and thereafter worked to discount Goldman's influence on the movement.

Ben Reitman's arrest in Manhattan in late April for distributing contractive literature, and his 60-day prison sentence, set off another round of protest meetings and inspired other activists to step forward and risk arrest. Rose Pastor Stokes, a wealthy socialist and feminist activist, feminist lawyers Ida Rauh and Jessie Ashley, along with Leonard Abbott and Bolton Hall, the prominent single-tax advocate, made the news that spring for handing out contraceptive recipes and birth control pamphlets at a Carnegie Hall meeting. They did the same at a Union Square rally that disintegrated into a mad scramble, with both women and men pushing and lunging to grab contraceptive circulars as if they were dollar bills. Rauh, Ashley, and Hall were later arrested.[41]

Yet none of these vocal proponents for birth control expressed interest in dedicating their efforts to this single cause or in taking a strong leadership position in the emerging movement. In these heady days before America's entry into the war in the spring of 1917, most of the New York radicals were passionate but capricious free-agent activists who moved from one cause to another and were beginning to gravitate toward antiwar protest. Goldman understood that her marquee name drew significant radical interest to the cause, but she had no intention of focusing solely on birth control work nor did she wish to risk another arrest. She publically announced in May 1916 that she would open a "birth control headquarters"—essentially an information clinic—on 17th Street in New York but not much came of it. By the summer, Goldman was caught up in labor conflicts in California. Although Mary Ware Dennett continued to lead the tentative NBCL, she turned to pacifist causes and completing her sex education tract, *The Sex Side of Life*, after failed attempts to jostle New York State legislators into reconsidering the obscenity laws. William Robinson and the other physicians who had taken a courageous public stand in favor of legalizing birth control were more comfortable behind the scenes and would not flaunt the law in protest. Only Sanger was both resolute in challenging the law and resistant to being pulled in another direction.[42]

SANGER'S CROSS-COUNTRY TOUR

Sanger's historic 1916 speaking tour not only clearly established her leadership of the movement, it also went a long way toward making her name nearly synonymous with birth control. Sanger started with an April 15 speech in New Rochelle, New York, and moved on to appearances in Pittsburgh and Washington, D.C., before traveling into the Midwest and on to the West Coast, concluding with a July 14 banquet in her honor in Cleveland. Sanger lectured over 30 times in 20 cities that had either started a birth control group or maintained an active free speech contingent. She also gave countless newspaper interviews, which might have done more to gain acceptance for the cause than the lectures. Sanger's speeches (she alternated between two versions on the tour) could be captivating but were choppy. She often blunted emotional appeals for a woman's right to control her own body and obligation to oversee her family's health with prosaic passages on the evolution of family limitation in Europe and self-conscious attempts to establish her expertise. In interviews she tended to be more plain-spoken and to the point. "Birth control," she told a wire reporter, "does not necessarily make for either larger or smaller families; it simply insures, through the mother's knowledge, a square deal and fair chance for whatever children are born . . . it is the logical and sensible and humane thing to do, law or no law." The newspaper profiles and interviews, almost without exception, portrayed Sanger as appealing, soft-spoken, and earnest—a diminutive club woman come for tea. She hardly looked or sounded the part of a woman rebel. A Denver reporter, after meeting Sanger in a hotel room, described her as "looking like a picture of a demure, ultra-feminine gentlewoman more interested in darning socks than defying the government." "I am merely the mother of three children with a message to mothers," Sanger described herself after a talk in Detroit. Through extensive local newspaper coverage, Sanger's message reached a much larger audience than has been depicted in scholarly treatments of her early activism, which have focused on the limited readership of the radical press and the union-fed crowds who came to hear her speak.* Her appearance, manner, and approach helped to elevate discourse and put people at ease with a sensitive subject.[43]

A number of the communities Sanger passed through had been primed by Goldman and Reitman. They had recently agitated both sides in the debate: labor leaders and other radical organizers who booked halls and handled publicity and the guardians of public morality, including local politicians, church leaders, and police, who tried in several cities to interfere with Sanger's public events and, in a few instances, silence her speech. Inevitable confrontations and attempts to muzzle Sanger during the tour only increased her press coverage and won her broader support.

In St. Louis, an attorney for the local branch of the Federation of Catholic Societies, Edward V. P. Schneiderhahn, a self-appointed censor, worked feverishly in the days leading up to Sanger's arrival. He urged Catholic leaders and businessmen to threaten a boycott of the Victoria Theater, which Sanger supporters had booked for an evening lecture on May 22. Caving to pressure, the theater's manager cancelled the booking that morning and refused Sanger's appeals to reconsider. Sanger called it "arrogant Catholic coercion" and threatened to sue. But instead of spreading word of the cancellation, she and her St. Louis organizers stayed mum and showed up just before her scheduled lecture to find many of the 1,800 ticket-holders milling about the street in front of the theater. With a dramatic flourish, Sanger shook and pounded the locked doors, inciting the crowd to cheer and wave their hats in the air. She then returned to the open-top car she had arrived in, where Frank O'Hare, the socialist agitator and editor, was standing on the driver's side, shouting out about suppression and injustice. Sanger spoke briefly, and the other passengers in her entourage, including the political cartoonist Robert Minor, passed out forms for people to sign in support of birth control. They then moved on to the nearby Odeon Theater where Sanger tried those doors in vain, knowing they too would be locked. Police kept the situation from overheating by convincing O'Hare and Sanger to move on or face arrest for blocking traffic. The street theater served its purpose; as one paper wrote, the incident "advertised [Sanger's] propaganda, piqued public curiosity, aroused

---

* See, for instance, Dolores Falmino, "The Birth of a Nation: Media Coverage of Contraception, 1915–1917," *Journalism and Mass Communication Quarterly* 75 (Autumn 1998): 560–71, which looks only at national publications with circumscribed audiences.

popular interest, and gained public support from many who otherwise might be indifferent." Sitting in the back of the car, witness to the entire scene, was a young Roger Baldwin of the St. Louis Civic League who would later found and lead the American Civil Liberties Union (ACLU). Baldwin cited this episode as his baptism into First Amendment activism.[44]

In Portland, Oregon, still stirring from the arrests of Goldman and Reitman in 1915, Sanger ran up against a local government that had grown weary of birth control advocates. An active birth control league had kept the issue in the public eye. Local newspapers had closely followed the events in New York since Sanger's return from Europe, and even city churches had debated birth control in Sunday sermons. The pastor of the Methodist Episcopal Church preached "The Right of Children to be Well Born" in response to a Roman Catholic priest's excoriation of birth control supporters, setting off a clerical letters-to-the-editor debate in the press. When Sanger arrived in mid-June, there were anxious expectations on both sides. The Portland Birth Control League had advertised heavily for Sanger's lectures, seeding the city with propaganda materials. Conservative city leaders spread the word that Sanger would try to open a clinic in Portland, a possibility she had hinted at in interviews. An overflow crowd came to hear her, without disruption, at the Heilig Theater on June 19. However, following Sanger's speech, three union men were arrested, probably on orders of Portland mayor Harry Albee, for selling copies of a newly printed edition of *Family Limitation*, revised by the Portland physician and openly lesbian-feminist Marie Equi. Sanger tried to take responsibility for the charges but had to leave Portland to deliver scheduled speeches in Washington State. In her absence, the Portland City Council unanimously passed an emergency ordinance banning *Family Limitation* as an obscene publication. Sanger returned to the city later in the month to support the three arrested men and protest the new law.

Sanger spoke at an impromptu June 29 protest meeting at Portland's Baker Theater. Afterward, she, Equi, and two other women sold copies of *Family Limitation* in open disregard for the law. All four were arrested, igniting what one paper called a "wild demonstration" that resulted in a swarm of angry birth control supporters running after the patrol wagon that transported the women to the city jail. Sanger, Equi, and one of the other women refused bail and spent the night behind bars. The four women were tried together with the three union men on July 1. The judge expressed concern that *Family Limitation* would be a corrupting influence if it dropped into the hands of an adolescent girl, but he also listened closely to Sanger, who was given an opportunity to speak to the court at length and to the lawyers on both sides. Pro bono attorneys Isaac Swett and Colonel C. E. S. Wood, a prominent author and leading civil libertarian on the West Coast, underscored the court's dilemma as they offered definitions of obscenity that could apply to innumerable medical texts as well as books in the public library. The judge decided to postpone his ruling and released the defendants. The delay led to a lively debate in the press, with the *Portland Morning Oregonian* concluding that *Family Limitation* was "dangerous" because the activists who sold it had little control over who read it. The *Evening Telegram* agreed, calling the pamphlet "vicious." But the *Portland News* mocked the city government, as did many letter writers, who thought their city had overreacted. The wait for a verdict also created some suspense, which made the story more interesting fare for wire services and newspapers throughout the country. Finally, on July 7, Municipal Judge Arthur Langguth found the defendants guilty for distributing obscene material, noting that the pamphlet contained several references to copulation. He fined them each $10 and then suspended their sentences—an acknowledgment that he did not object to birth control per se but had to abide by the law. Sanger called the decision "cowardly . . . it's practically the same old story, that knowledge, if it's hidden away on the musty bookshelves or in the narrow confines of the medical profession, is moral; but as soon as it is distributed among the working people the same book becomes obscene."[45]

That was the concern of the Chicago Women's Club, which publicly turned down Sanger's offer to address the group on birth control after deciding that *Family Limitation* was "too brutally plainspoken for us." The Women's Club's prudish rejection generated plenty of publicity and encouraged other conservative women's organizations in neighboring cities to raise doubts about the appropriateness of Sanger's message. The Women's Council of Akron, Ohio, protested Sanger's scheduled appearance there and successfully pressured a music hall owner to break his contract with her. She left the city after having failed to find another public space. But the publicity generated by these skirmishes gave Sanger all the promotion she needed. In Chicago, Sanger's base as she toured the Midwest, the Women's Club hubbub opened up other venues and stoked the press's interest in highlighting a birth control debate. Sanger spoke at several large public meetings, pointing out the irony of the Women's Club conservatives "enjoying the benefits of birth control for themselves but unwilling to endorse it for the less fortunate of their sex." She also held discussions about opening a free clinic in the Chicago stockyards to reach the working women most in need of contraceptive advice. The city's newspapers not only reported on her speeches, but they also covered a government investigation of Sanger started by the U.S. District Attorney for Chicago, her back and forth in the press with Theodore Roosevelt over race suicide, her proposal for a city-funded clinic, and her suggestion that accessible birth control may have prevented the recent senseless murder in Chicago of a pregnant teenage girl by her boyfriend. The ubiquity of birth control stories in the press struck one anti-birth control citizen as absurd. In a letter to the editor he asked what have been "the big views, the lofty patriotism, the high spots of our national spirit the past three months?" with the United States on the brink of joining the world war "at any hour." He went on to list the top stories: Sanger "preaching publicly nation-wide abortion"; Sanger talking about Sadie Sachs, the young woman who died from a botched abortion; Rose Pastor Stokes handing out "free recipes to pregnant women"; and "sex," the "predominating human interest feature of all news, all theaters, all reform movements."

Acutely aware of all of the attention that she received and the perception in certain quarters that she was passing on impure thoughts and facilitating promiscuity (a Catholic publication in San Francisco referred to "the barnyard morality of the Sanger woman"), Sanger took care to present birth control on a high plane, as a "great social principle," a "new social awakening," and an advancement in eugenic thinking. She argued for its moral legitimacy, rejecting the reasoning that classed her arguments with immorality "while Mr. Roosevelt can go up and down the length of the land shouting and urging this class of women to have large families and is neither arrested nor molested, but considered by all society as highly moral." In turn, she questioned the morality of sexual and economic oppression, of birthing children into poverty, and of relying on dangerous abortion procedures as a birth control measure. And though she had been silent on the Baby Bollinger controversy, she added stronger eugenic language to her public speech in 1916, warning about the burdens posed to society by unfit children born to defective parents. She refrained from publicly discussing how birth control changes the sexual dynamic between men and women, and she would not give out contraceptive information from the podium. She refused to give her critics ammunition to indict her as a dissolute free love radical, and she did not want to jeopardize the tour or her plans to open a clinic with an arrest and prison sentence. However, Sanger did distribute *Family Limitation* in every city she visited, over 20,000 copies by her estimate, somehow avoiding arrest everywhere but Portland. She answered hundreds of letters that were passed or sent to her from women seeking contraceptive information. And she met with people individually: "Women came to me in the hotels with babies in their arms; men ready for work, carrying their lunch baskets, came early to get a little private advice before I left."[46]

BIRTH CONTROL LEAGUES

It is impossible to estimate how many people Sanger reached with her arguments for birth control and with the practical contraceptive information contained in *Family Limitation* or related by Sanger herself in brief consultations. More significant in terms of the growth of the movement were the organizations that cropped up in her wake that produced educational and propaganda materials during the World War I years before any clinics were in operation. Sanger's meetings and lectures brought together like-minded activists, social workers, society women, and other progressive reformers who established birth control leagues in a number of cities. Organizations formed soon after Sanger's visits in Pittsburgh; Washington, D.C.; Cleveland; Spokane; Detroit; St. Paul, Minneapolis; and Indianapolis. Leagues that had formed earlier in 1916, or in 1915 in some of the larger cities such as Chicago, Seattle, Los Angeles, and San Francisco, grew in size and scope following Sanger's tour. With several exceptions, notably on the West Coast, where labor, antiwar, and feminist interests radicalized the new birth control leagues, the local organizations launched in these years generally aimed to apply birth control as a panacea for social ills and to promote it as a matter of good public health, not unlike campaigns to reduce tuberculosis or improve sanitation. They disseminated literature, but were cautious when it came to *Family Limitation* and specific information on methods. Though many of these leagues dissolved within a few years, a number of Planned Parenthood affiliates today had their beginnings in the spring and summer of 1916.

The Cleveland-based Birth Control League of Ohio is one of the organizations that formed after a successful Sanger appearance. The League held its first meeting on June 23, 1916, two months after Sanger gave two well-received speeches to overflowing crowds on Easter Sunday. After a series of informal gatherings of supporters that spring, Socialist agitator Frederick Blossom organized a league with broad-based support. The organization brought together physicians, religious leaders, social workers, and influential businessmen and their wives who were attracted to the potential for birth control to help solve big, underlying social problems that were seen as the cause of much suffering and that thwarted many creative, Progressive Era efforts to achieve meaningful health reform. The League stated that one of its objectives was to extend family limitation practices "as a means of reducing poverty, immorality, crime, physical and mental defectiveness, and other human ills." Upper- and middle-class do-gooders mixed with left-leaning social workers and socialist radicals and found common ground in advocating a modification of the obscenity laws (although Ohio physicians could legally prescribe contraception) and in implementing "a vigorous campaign of oral and printed propaganda to carry the gospel of birth control to every section of the city."

But there was a decidedly conservative caste to the Ohio league. League leaders condemned "the general distribution of printed matter describing methods of preventing conception," advocated using only medical channels to distribute birth control, and refused to assist any activist who violated the law. The League's public statements avoided feminist rationales for family limitation, saying, for example, "Birth control means . . . happier homes and stronger family ties." The organization's short-lived *Birth Control News*, the first movement periodical in the United States, emphasized eugenic improvement—birthing better babies—and offered several medical validations and a vigorous religious defense of birth control. "Because animals reproduce in ignorance and blind obedience to the laws of nature," wrote the Rev. A. T. Wooley, "is no reason why man should abdicate his intelligence and descend to their level." Apart from a few excerpts from Sanger's letters and speeches, nothing in the publication tied the group to the radical roots of the movement. Nor was there any mention of a contraceptive method.

Frederick Blossom (1878–1974), who became the president of the Ohio league, operated as a kind of backroom negotiator, impresario, and educator (he had a Ph.D. in romance languages). As the business manager of Cleveland's Associated Charities, he had learned how to tone down radical rhetoric and reach out to the wealthy. For the new League, he won the support of a few prominent Cleveland society women who helped attract others of high social standing, building a membership of over 400 by the end of the summer of 1916. Sanger was immediately impressed with Blossom, who also arranged her speech before a large social worker's conference in Indianapolis in May. She called him "polished, educated, and clever" and noted that some of his success came from "never waving a red flag in front of anybody's nose as I did; my flaming Feminism speeches had scared some of my supporters out of their wits." In fact, in the years to come Sanger would emulate, on a larger scale, Blossom's leadership of this small, regional group, muting her own radical speech, attracting wealthy society women to fund the movement and make it more acceptable to the middle class. She also surrounded herself with a core group of activists and feminists who did the hard, behind-the-scenes organizational work. Sanger heartily endorsed the Ohio league, finding its program "the most constructive" of the existing organizations. A short time later she talked Blossom into following her to New York to help her start a national publication.[47]

BIRTH CONTROL IN BOSTON

Although Sanger's exhausting trip came to an end in mid-July of 1916, she was back in New York City only a few days before a call from Boston extended her busy summer. Twenty-two-year-old Van Kleeck Allison, co-editor of *The Flame*, a monthly Boston radical paper in the same vein as Alexander Berkman's *The Blast* and Sanger's *The Woman Rebel*, was arrested on July 10 for distributing "obscene" literature. He had handed a copy of Reitman's and Goldman's *Why and How the Poor Should Not Have Many Children* to an undercover detective and published in *The Flame* an article on contraception by William Robinson. Irish Catholics dominated Boston's government, which was headed by the flamboyant Mayor James Michael Curley. His reputation as a censor led to the commonplace phrase, "banned in Boston." The superintendent of police and the municipal judge, both Catholics, came down hard on the youthful Allison, a scion of an upper-crust New York City family who had just arrived in Boston after attending Columbia University. Bail was set at a hefty $1,500. District Attorney Joseph C. Pelletier, a national officer in the Knights of Columbus, the Catholic fraternal organization, personally conducted the prosecution, even though it was a lower court case, typically handled by an assistant.

Boston did not welcome the birth control advocates who came to Allison's defense. Despite the threatening environment, a number of liberal groups passed resolutions protesting the arrest, and members of settlement houses, several Boston-area Protestant churches, and even the YMCA came to rallies in Allison's support. A few activists courageously spoke out for birth control and used the opportunity to organize an advocacy group, even though they were not enamored with Allison. Cerise Carman Jack, the wife of a Harvard professor, paid Allison's bail and declared at his trial, "I shall stand by him to the end." But she later remarked, "Our martyr was certainly not of our choosing—very young, irresponsible, although well-meaning, and, unfortunately, a man." Dr. Antoinette Konikow, a Russian-born, American-trained physician and a founder of the Socialist Party, came forward as the lone local doctor to publicly back birth control. Like William Robinson in New York, Konikow pressed for acceptance of birth control within the medical profession and wrote about sex education for *The Call* and other publications. Elizabeth Glendower Evans, a Beacon Hill society woman, suffrage leader, and labor activist, whose views carried weight with liberal women, made sure to greet Allison in front of reporters at his trial and assure him of her assistance.

The trial, before a jammed courtroom, was a dramatic event that carried the Boston news headlines for several days. The judge allowed District Attorney Pelletier to rant and scold. At one point Pelletier questioned the presence of female spectators at a "dirty sex" case. Another time he demanded that Allison turn over the names of any married women with whom he had discussed birth control. Allison hesitated, but after a recess, 16 women came forward of their own volition to say they were in favor of family limitation and stated their names for the court. In trying to underscore the indecency of Allison's actions, Pelletier asked the defendant if he would discuss such a despicable topic with his own sisters. Allison replied that he had written to one sister, and she was in favor of it. In his closing argument, Pelletier called the case "one of the most far-reaching . . . that has ever been brought into a criminal court in the Commonwealth" because it considered the actions "of a man of education and intelligence, no boy, no drunkard, no criminal, not from the slums and the low type of man," but someone who willingly and deliberately decided he would "violate the law of God and man." The defense attorney focused on the trumped-up charges against Allison (the prosecution also accused him of giving birth control leaflets to young factory girls, though the evidence was weak) and stated that it "is not indecent or immoral to talk of the human body and its natural functions." Judge Michael J. Murray could not restrain his own venom. He called the pamphlet in question "obscene, indecent, impure, vile and unchaste" and without delay sentenced Allison to an imposing three years. Allison was composed on leaving the court room, telling reporters, "I am not sorry now that this happened, for I shall affirm my belief in the doctrines of birth control on every occasion, as I believe them just and sound and right. And there are hundreds of other serious and intelligent members of the community who think as I do, and who are going to make this fight theirs as much as my own."

The Allison Birth Control Defense League, formed by Cerise Carman Jack; Charles Zueblin, the sociologist and writer; Stuart Chase, an accountant better known for his forays into Fabian socialism; and several others, circulated petitions and arranged a mass meeting to which they invited Margaret Sanger. On July 31, Sanger joined a number of other speakers in defending Allison's actions before an estimated crowd of 2,500 in the Majestic Theatre in Boston. A heavy police presence ensured that the speakers stayed focused on the social and economic benefits of birth control but did not attempt to circulate information on methods. Sanger, who later called it "one of the greatest meetings I ever attended," received nearly five minutes of applause before giving her standard speech, well-honed from her tour. She injected a feminist view that had been lacking thus far in the comments of other activists, concluding that birth control "is interlocked with the new social and spiritual movement which says men and women must be free and equal in the joy of living. . . ." Allison, out on bail awaiting an appeal, ended the meeting by reading a few of the thousands of letters that he said he had received since his arrest, "all of them asking for birth control information and telling heart-rending tales of poverty, ill-health, and unwanted motherhood."

Allison later had his sentence reduced to two months by changing his plea to guilty. He served his time and quickly faded from the cause, but not before his case gave rise to the first birth control organization in the Commonwealth. In September 1916, the Allison Defense Committee became the Massachusetts Birth Control League, which opened a downtown office, distributed its own informational pamphlet, and set its sights on pursuing a legislative remedy to the state Comstock laws. The Allison case also agitated those opposed to birth control, mainly Catholic groups. On August 13, the Knights of Columbus organized a protest rally of their own at the Majestic Theatre, drawing over 2,000 to hear David Goldstein, a national lecturer for the organization and a Jewish convert to Catholicism. Goldstein accused Sanger, "immoral rich women," and "the women of the street" of violating the "sacred law of the Bible" and promulgating "detestable acts." In what would become a standard argument used to counter birth control advocates' call for smaller families and quality over quantity, Goldstein pointed to the many great men who came from large families, including George Washington and Ben Franklin. For birth controllers, it was an uphill climb in Boston. This earliest incarnation of a league could not survive a more powerful and better organized, government-backed and police-enforced opposition led by the Catholic Church. The League was gone before the end of World War I.[48]

THE NEXT STEP

In the midst of the Allison episode and still recovering from the hardships of travel, Sanger wrote to an English friend that the country was finally emerging from "its Rip

Van Winkle slumber of Puritanism." Never one to underestimate her achievements, Sanger later claimed that her cross-country campaign "had created a national public opinion in favor of birth control . . . won the press to discuss the subject . . . inspired the organizations of leagues" and "aroused the nation to a realization of its great moral duty toward womanhood." Despite her encouragement, no clinics opened as a result of her tour, with the possible exception of an informal informational office in St. Paul, Minnesota. Nor was there any indication that any of the birth control leagues would take on the risky proposition (though in some states a doctor-directed clinic would have been legal). It is not clear whether Sanger had convinced the activists who started birth control leagues and spread the propaganda that clinics were necessary.

Sanger's own *Family Limitation*, which had come to represent the free dissemination of birth control, undermined her argument for clinic-based contraception. Clinics required women to forfeit a significant degree of privacy and place their trust in a medical provider. They raised issues of control over access and cost, and they challenged the notion of reproductive self-determination. In her speeches, Sanger explained and advocated the network of Dutch contraceptive clinics, emphasizing the need to increase contraceptive effectiveness and bring down infant and maternal mortality rates. But Americans had always been suspicious of European models of health care. And there were indications that poor and working-class women, the group Sanger most wanted to reach, would not come to clinics whether because of fear, exhaustion, family responsibilities, or lack of money. The Danish IWW organizer Caroline Nelson, a founder of the San Francisco Birth Control League, told Sanger that the only way she saw to get contraceptive information to women in the working areas was to send out a trained field nurse "who speaks the language of the district." But based in part on the remarks of many women who wrote to Sanger and pulled her aside after speeches, Sanger remained confident that a woman-run clinic would draw poor, immigrant, and working women. Her next challenge was to prove it.[49]

THREE

BIRTH CONTROL CLINICS

This movement has assumed national proportions, and now it is a question of whether the people shall have access to the knowledge they demand or whether the authorities will continue to execute a law that has generally fallen into disrepute. The end is not hard to foresee. In this case as in numerous others, history will repeat itself. The law will be ignored and defied with increasing frequency till general sentiment will compel its repeal. What is a crime today will be an accepted and approved fact tomorrow.[1]

—Alexander Berkman, July 1, 1916

In the summer of 1915, as Margaret Sanger monitored from England the emergence of sustained birth control activism on the U.S. coasts, she recognized that the cause had in some ways already moved beyond the fight for free speech, although First Amendment rights would always be at the heart of the birth control campaign. The self-replicating *Family Limitation* had blasted through the antiquated traps set by Comstock and his cohorts to expurgate obscenity. And the press, responding to public interest, had shelved its tacit ban on covering issues related to human sexuality. Birth control in all its permutations, as it related to eugenics, health concerns, population control, and women, had become legitimate news and an issue worthy of public debate, even if the open discussion of contraceptive methods continued to be off limits.

While still in England, Sanger had decided that after she returned to the United States and resolved the *Woman Rebel* charges she would "establish a free clinic in New York's Lower East Side," modeled after the Dutch clinics. Her brief practicum in Amsterdam convinced her that the occlusive vaginal diaphragm used in tandem with a spermicidal cream or jelly was the best choice for most women. To be consistently effective, the diaphragm had to be fitted, preferably by a trained medical professional, and inserted properly, which required some basic instruction. Follow-up examinations and adjustments were also necessary to ensure comfort and effectiveness. Thus clinics were needed to reach women who could not afford a private doctor or find one willing to prescribe contraception and to serve those who did not want to consult their own physicians for privacy reasons. Not only would women receive effective contraception, clinics, as Sanger envisioned them, could offer advice on sexual matters and hygiene and give out referrals for therapeutic abortions (many states allowed medical abortion if the woman's life was endangered).[2]

THE DIAPHRAGM: FEMINIST BIRTH CONTROL

Sanger and others who recommended the diaphragm likely were relying on their own experience, feedback from friends, and recommendations from medical professionals. There were no statistical studies on the success rates of the diaphragm until the 1920s. It had its drawbacks: it was cumbersome and more expensive than most other methods; it interfered with spontaneity; it required proper cleaning and care to avoid infection and to preserve the rubber; and it could be difficult for some women to insert, especially those who were squeamish about touching their bodies. But when sized and inserted correctly, the diaphragm was extremely trustworthy. Its flexibility—the combination of rubber and a coated watch-spring rim—allowed it to be folded on insertion and to regain its shape when put in place, completely covering the cervix and vaginal wall, creating a more expansive and stable barrier than the smaller cervical cap. Paired with a spermicide, the diaphragm presented a seamless rubber curtain lethal to sperm.

The major selling point of the Mensinga diaphragm, the type used widely in Europe and that Sanger recommended, was how it shone in contrast with other methods. It was far more comfortable and safer than the early intrauterine devices used by a small percentage of women at the turn of the century. These rubber or wire IUDs (often called permanent pessaries) were extremely uncomfortable for many women and more likely to cause inflammation and infection. Douching, which had been popular in the late 19th century, had become even more widely used in the 1910s because of *Family Limitation* and other publications that recommended regular cleansing of the vagina. This generated the growth of an entire industry of solutions and syringes that were marketed for hygiene purposes. But the douche was an extremely ineffective contraceptive; it was often administered too late and could actually assist in transporting sperm to their destination rather than washing them away. A number of questionable douching solutions caused irritation, burns, and other painful reactions; the caustic disinfectant Lysol remained among the most popular. Suppositories, such as boric acid bound with cocoa butter, which Sanger recommended in *Family Limitation*, also came up short in terms of effectiveness. Some of the active ingredients turned out to be compatible with sperm, and, caught up in the moment, women often did not give the suppository enough time to melt and spread prior to intercourse. Condoms varied in quality but were a reliable contraceptive if used with some care. However, they still carried the stigma of being associated with prostitution and venereal disease. Many men and women disliked condoms because of discomfort and loss of sensitivity, but they were relatively easy to acquire, being sold as prophylactics. Other barrier methods used with spermicides, such as the sponge, medicated tampon, and cotton plug, all worked to varying degrees but not as reliably as the diaphragm.

Withdrawal, which probably remained the most common birth control practice, was extremely unreliable and, according to sexologists of the day, dangerous for women. Sanger and her British counterpart, Marie Stopes, echoed the accepted medical belief that coitus interruptus caused nervous disorders and frigidity in women. Many experts also claimed that it denied women the beneficial vitamins and hormones absorbed from semen in the vaginal canal (this belief was another strike against the condom as well). The shaky science obscured a core feminist argument that a woman's climax is as necessary as a man's for sexual health and overall well-being, and withdrawal is more likely to frustrate female orgasm than any other form of birth control. Women birth controllers attacked abstinence for similar reasons. Sanger also rejected the rhythm or safe period method, not only because it did not work very well and experts could not agree on when a woman was most fertile, but also because it compelled women to have intercourse during the days of their cycle when, according to Sanger, they were least likely to be in the mood. Increasingly, birth control leaders and women physicians in the movement viewed the diaphragm and other female barrier methods as feminist birth control, since these means gave women more control over the scheduling of sex and a better opportunity to achieve orgasm.[3]

THE RATIONALE FOR MEDICAL OVERSIGHT

Despite Sanger's contempt for doctors and her feminist assault against the medical profession, which she blamed, along with the government and the Catholic Church, for maintaining women's inferior status, her experience as a nurse and the hundreds of desperate appeals for help she had received each week since her tour ended underscored for her the importance of providing women with birth control under medical supervision. Although women lost a degree of independence under medically supervised birth control, Sanger thought that the benefits far outweighed any inconvenience and sacrifice. It was the only way she knew to ensure contraceptive safety and effectiveness. She did not trust the unregulated practitioners, healers, and quacks who peddled devices and medicines. And she feared the lucrative underground abortion trade that endangered women's lives. Nor did Sanger feel confident that women, especially the uneducated, would make the right decisions about reproductive control without medical consultation. Anecdotal evidence suggested that women gravitated toward the easiest-to-use methods, not necessarily the most reliable. And though Sanger was bent on breaking the law again by opening a clinic, her planned defiance was the calculation of a moderate reformer seeking acceptance for her cause. She had decided to treat each woman individually and begin the long process of reining in the amorphous contraceptive trade. She sought to establish reasonable guidelines for contraceptive care. And she intended to provide a countermeasure to abortionists. Sanger had observed the way community leaders, including police officials, politicians, judges, doctors, and clergy—even many who endorsed family limitation—became alarmed at the thought of young, unmarried women gaining access to contraceptive publications. The fear that such information led to promiscuity kept many Americans from approving easier access to birth control, even if they used it themselves. Taking contraception off the street and giving it a medical context in a clinical setting had the potential to alleviate at least some of the concerns stemming from America's continuing anxiety over uncontrolled sexuality—and sex in general.

Although Sanger had not yet completely committed to a clinic model for contraceptive distribution, her resolve to open a clinic in 1916 represented a startling about-face, moving from grassroots, do-it-yourself contraception to birth control under medical supervision. Only two years previously she had taken ownership of the anarchist, IWW slogan, "No Gods, No Masters," and printed it on the masthead of *The Woman Rebel*. Though not immediately apparent, Sanger's emphasis on clinic creation redefined the terms of the debate over reproductive rights and women's sexual freedom as it eroded the ideological foundation of the early birth control movement, with its anarchist roots and strong allegiance to individual autonomy.

THE BROWNSVILLE CLINIC

In mid-July 1916, at the conclusion of her cross-country tour, Sanger returned to New York and, trying to keep up the momentum, told reporters a few days later that she would open a clinic in the poor and mostly Italian and Jewish immigrant neighborhood of Brownsville, Brooklyn, in the early fall. Papers from as far away as Kansas City reported that Sanger planned to have nurses instruct the poor in birth control practices in the same way that they instruct new mothers about "infant feeding"—as if to say that contraception was a most natural and necessary component of health care. The Brownsville site was a serendipitous find; Sanger had been home only a few days when a group of Brownsville women tracked her down at her hotel in Manhattan and asked for contraceptive advice. Although Sanger later claimed that she explored the five boroughs of the city and studied health statistics to find the right location, she simply chose the first opportunity that presented itself. And, like today, rents were cheaper in Brooklyn. In most respects it did not matter to Sanger where she set up shop, as long as it was in a working-class neighborhood. Her writings and correspondence offer nothing to suggest that she had any intent at this point of operating a clinic for a sustained period. Her goal was to break ground with a simple model that could be approximated elsewhere and to challenge the law.[4]

In 1915, both the National Birth Control League (NBCL) and William Robinson's fleeting Committee on Birth Control had tested the waters for a legislative approach to legalizing contraceptives in New York State but found Albany lawmakers unwilling to tackle the issue. Sanger never entirely dismissed the possibility of a legislative remedy and would concentrate on lobbying efforts in years to come, but reasoned that it would be "a slow and tortuous method of making clinics legal." As she explained a few years later, the law in America was "sacred" and extremely difficult to amend without the public will to do so. The movement would have to win wide public acceptance before politicians would be willing to shoulder the political risk that came with endorsing birth control legalization. As the legal scholar, C. Thomas Dienes, put it, "legal revision itself would have to grow out of a refashioning of the social environment." Sanger's activist training with the IWW in direct action and confrontation taught her to "agitate, educate, organize" before you can "legislate." She told an audience in 1921, "Agitation through violation of the law was the key to the public which would ultimately make the other three tactics workable."

While the federal Comstock Law prohibited the circulation of contraceptives and related information through the mails and did not directly apply to the activities of a clinic, the relevant sections of the New York State Penal Code (most likely drafted by Comstock) made it a misdemeanor to sell or exhibit contraceptives or impart contraceptive information. The Code did provide an exception for doctors to prescribe contraception to prevent disease, which everyone understood, with a wink, to mean condoms to protect men from syphilis and gonorrhea. Sanger looked to broaden that exception by forcing a test case that would consider women's health as an indication for contraceptives. However, to strengthen a potential legal challenge, she needed to establish medical oversight of the clinic, a difficult task that nearly upended her plans. She tried to secure a doctor (preferably a woman), but none of the physicians she knew was willing to risk a license suspension or prison time. Desperate for help, Sanger contacted William Robinson who, though he would not offer his own services, told her that as long as she gave "hygienic advice" and did not attempt to dispense contraceptives, she would probably avoid interference from local and national medical organizations or federal authorities. The federal law would not come into play unless Sanger used the mails. Sanger's goal of fitting diaphragms would have to wait, however. As a whole, the medical profession continued to keep its distance from public birth control discussions and blocked efforts to instruct medical students in contraceptive techniques. Doctors remained, generally, either opposed to or indifferent toward birth control and often lacked the practical knowledge to overcome professional constraints. According to Robinson, Sanger needed to fear the vice societies and state authorities. He warned her not to give information to unmarried women or even to imply that such a thing was feasible, or "you will have the law down on you at once." "The whole thing," he wrote, "is to conduct it [the clinic] in such a way as to avoid unnecessary antagonism." He concluded, "If you do as I say and if you don't charge the people for anything . . . they would have great difficulty in doing anything to you, and this Birth Control Clinic might become the germ of thousands of similar clinics."[5]

Not only did Sanger have trouble finding a doctor to associate with the clinic, she also encountered an indecisive radical community that continued to support free speech agitation but was disconnected from practical efforts to distribute contraceptive devices and information. As Linda Gordon has written, "the American Left had had little experience with the provision of services through counterinstitutions such as birth control clinics." Their uncertainty, combined with a fear of prosecution and the distraction of the war, held back organizers in Boston, Cleveland, and some West Coast cities from advancing the cause to the logical next phase of actually providing contraception.

Failing to find a willing physician, Sanger engaged her sister, Ethel Byrne, a registered nurse. For administrative help she hired Fania Mindell, a Jewish immigrant who was fluent in several languages, including Yiddish, which was widely spoken among the many first-generation Jews in Brownsville. A Chicago-based activist, Mindell had helped Sanger organize meetings that spring. Sanger also added social worker Elizabeth Stuyvesant to help with recordkeeping and supplies, and Frederick Blossom, the charismatic, multitasking Cleveland organizer to manage her new "birth control headquarters," a small office on Fifth Avenue not far from Union Square. Blossom did not want to be connected with the clinic but agreed to help with publicity, develop a monthly journal devoted to the movement, and start a new organization, the Birth Control League of New York (BCLNY), to compete with the NBCL, which often disagreed with Sanger's tactics.[6]

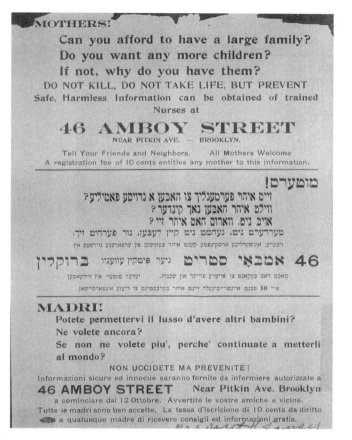

Flyer for the Brownsville Clinic, 1916, written in English, Yiddish, and Italian. (Courtesy of the Sophia Smith Collection, Smith College.)

In early October, Sanger and Mindell rented a suitable storefront at 46 Amboy Street in Brownsville, cleaned it up, and turned it into a makeshift clinic. Furnishings included a portable examination table with a rubber mat, desks, a few chairs, a couple of metal stands with jars of cotton balls and water basins on top, some scrub brushes and soap. Contraceptive articles for demonstration included condoms, Mizpah pessaries, cervical caps, suppositories, and probably douching syringes. Most of these devices were available locally in pharmacies and sold for medical or hygienic uses, while the preferred Mensinga diaphragm was difficult to obtain. The first month's rent of $50 was paid by Kate Crane Gartz, an heiress to a steel fortune, who had met Sanger in Los Angeles that summer. Gartz was one of the first society women to hand Sanger (who otherwise relied on meager pamphlet sales and lecture fees) a check; she helped open a productive tap of wealthy women, a tap that Sanger never closed. For several days, Sanger and her small crew canvassed the area, circulating flyers printed in English, Italian, and Yiddish that announced:

MOTHERS:

Can you afford to have a large family?
Do you want any more children?
If not, why do you have them?
DO NOT KILL, DO NOT TAKE LIFE, BUT PREVENT
Safe, Harmless Information can be obtained of trained
Nurses at
46 AMBOY STREET
NEAR PITKIN AVE.—BROOKLYN.
Tell Your Friends and Neighbors. All Mothers Welcome.
A registration fee of 10 cents entitles any mother to this information.

On October 16, they opened the doors to the nation's first birth control clinic. Over 100 women came that first day, in small groups or alone, many pushing baby carriages. There were Russian, Polish, Hungarian, and Italian women; Jews, Catholics, and Protestants. The majority were working mothers—scrubwomen, chambermaids, and sweatshop workers. A few were sent to Sanger by their physicians. One woman pointed out, "It is so much easier to talk to a woman than to a man, that is why I never tell my doctor." For the 10-cent fee each woman received brief instruction in how to use each of the contraceptives and where to find them in a drugstore. Some were given pamphlets, though this act was more clearly unlawful than simply transmitting information orally. Women were invited to return if they needed help inserting or fitting a cervical cap. The staff recorded information on file cards about each woman's reproductive history. It is not clear if the examination table was ever used, though possibly some women were checked for signs that they might be pregnant.

For many clients, the clinic served as a kind of confessional where they could unburden themselves of the guilt of an abortion or complain about health problems, difficult husbands, sickly children, and other ills associated with poverty. "They all tell the same sort of story," Sanger told a reporter. "Some fear their husbands might object; sometimes the husbands come with them. 'We can't feed any more mouths,' is the burden of their message." She added that they were all "so pathetically grateful." A Russian woman told Sanger that first week, "God must have sent you to us. We are too poor to pay a doctor to tell us what you have told us. If the police fight you, they must fight us too." One woman told a local reporter,

This is the kind of place that we have been wanting all the time. I have had seven children, two are dead, and my husband is a sick man. Do you know how I got bread for them? By getting down on my hands and knees and scrubbing floors for the baker; that's what I did when we couldn't pay the bill. Seven children, that's enough for any woman.

There were incredible stories of excessive childbearing: one woman had 15 children by the age of 36; another mother had seven surviving children out of 11 and claimed to have self-aborted 28 times. The "most pitiful," according to Elizabeth Stuyvesant, were the pregnant women seeking abortions who had "a desperate determination to risk all" but had to be sent away.[7]

After four days, a steady stream of women, and no clear sign from the police as to their intentions, Sanger issued several statements hailing the clinic's success. She described her "national plan," which was little more than a boast about how quickly she could snap supporters into action and how rapidly birth control would transform society. "The poor, century-behind-the-times public officials of this country might just as well forget their moss-grown statutes and accept birth control as an established fact," she told reporters gathered at her Manhattan hotel. She said that four more clinics would be running in New York within days, followed by clinics in over a dozen other cities. "Within two years every man and woman in this country will know how many children they can afford to have. And when they know that, I predict that two generations of birth control will wipe out all the slums, eliminate the birth of mental defectives, minimize the number of humans in insane asylums, and automatically put a stop to child labor and prostitution." The press coverage advertised the clinic to the wider world. In its second week, women came from all five boroughs, Long Island, New Jersey, and from as far away as Philadelphia and New England.

Newspapers around the country picked up Sanger's comments as well as wire service reports that police were combing Brownsville in search of the clinic. In reality, beat police had already visited and affably moved on. Sanger had also written to the Brooklyn District Attorney to ensure that her law-breaking would not be ignored. It was not. On October 20, Margaret Whitehurst, an undercover police woman, entered the clinic posing as a new mother. Wearing "an old shawl thrown over a stylish suit" and "looking very well fed and comfortable," she did not fool anyone. Nevertheless, she was treated like any other client except that she was allowed to purchase a cervical cap at cost. Sanger pinned the two-dollar bill to the wall and wrote on it "spy money." Whitehurst reappeared in uniform on October 26 with three other officers and arrested Sanger and Mindell, the only staff in the clinic at the time. On being arrested Sanger reportedly screamed at Whitehurst, "You dirty thing! You're not a woman! You're a dog!" The police confiscated about two dozen Mizpah pessaries, condoms, suppositories, copies of pamphlets, including *Family Limitation*, and all of the patient records. Refusing to walk to the police station, Sanger and Mindell were forcibly dragged out of the clinic and into a patrol wagon. Ethel Byrne was arrested

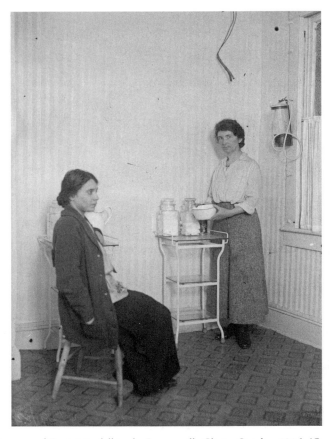

Margaret Sanger and Fania Mindell in the Brownsville Clinic, October 1916. (Courtesy of the George Grantham Bain Collection, Library of Congress.)

at her home that evening. All three were released the next day on bail, arraigned on November 6, and scheduled for trial in the Court of Special Sessions.[8]

OTHER ACTIVISTS AND ADVOCATES

The clamor surrounding the Brownsville clinic was not all that was going on with birth control activism. On October 20, Emma Goldman was arrested yet again for circulating birth control information, after she confessed the crime as a defense witness in Bolton Hall's trial, stemming from his June arrest for handing out pamphlets in Union Square. She was bailed out the same day as Sanger, Byrne, and Mindell. On October 23, Dr. Abraham Jacobi and 10 women physicians attempted to get the

New York County Medical Society to vote in favor of a recommendation to change the New York penal law to allow a licensed physician to give contraceptive advice. They lost narrowly, 77 to 69. Nonetheless it was an encouraging sign for advocates that many doctors thought that the law should not encroach on their private conversations with patients. On October 30, the same court and panel of judges slated to hear the Brownsville case convicted and fined Jessie Ashley for distributing contraceptive literature that past spring. Two other less prominent New York activists, Stephen Kerr and Peter Marmer, were also found guilty of the same charges. The well-connected Ashley, an NBCL founder with strong ties to suffrage leaders and free speech advocates, garnered extensive press coverage and proved instrumental in helping to rally wealthy liberals to the cause.

The event that heartened birth control advocates the most came from an unlikely source. On October 12, Judge William H. Wadhams of the Court of General Sessions of New York stunned observers when he suspended the sentence of Rebecca Schnur, a petty thief, and publicly endorsed the legalization of contraception under certain conditions. Schnur was a domestic, the mother of six children and wife of a garment worker with tuberculosis who had been forced to leave his job by a city health inspector. Desperate to care for her family, she stole money from an employer's home. "I stole," she told the court, "because my six children must have something to eat." She had been convicted previously on a similar charge. Judge Wadhams said he was troubled over the fact that the law prohibited the tubercular husband from working with others, "Nevertheless he goes on becoming the father of children who have very little chance under the conditions to be anything else but tubercular, and . . . to repeat the process with society. There is no law against that." Yet, the judge noted that those who attempt to give out birth control information, to help precisely people such as the Schnurs, are arrested and brought to his court. He pointed to Europe's success with "birth regulation" and questioned America's "common sense." "I believe," he wrote in his decision, "we are living in an age of ignorance, which at some future time will be looked upon aghast." Birth control advocates publicly applauded Wadhams's decision, and a picture of the harried mother and her children appeared in newspapers alongside wire service reports of the story. A judge in Des Moines issued a similar ruling that fall, and a number of other judges spoke out in sympathy with these decisions.[9]

Such constant birth control agitation magnified the attention focused on Sanger following the clinic arrests. After laying low for two weeks, Sanger met with reporters on November 12 to announce that she would reopen the Brownsville clinic. In the 10 days it functioned, over 500 women had received contraceptive advice, and now countless more had heard about the clinic and wanted it to resume. To the press, Sanger emphasized that the clinic was not a radical venture; "even very conservative thinkers agree that a clinic is the best method for spreading the information about family limitation to the people whom each additional child means an additional burden." She reopened it on November 13 and was arrested the next day for maintaining a public nuisance. Out on bail again, she attempted to keep the clinic running, but police forced the building's landlord to evict his tenants, and the clinic closed for good.

Despite Sanger's predictions of dozens of clinics cropping up in other states, there is only limited evidence of informal birth control offices in St. Paul, Minnesota, and Ann Arbor, Michigan, and possibly advice rooms in Los Angeles and San Francisco. They all may have given out information but probably not contraceptives. A number of doctors, such as Sanger's two physicians in New York, Drs. Morris Kahn and Mary Halton, maintained private clinics that resembled public dispensaries, in that the costs were low and the consultations brief. But they reached relatively few women, mostly middle-class. Remarkably, no birth control dispensary clinic opened until Sanger established the Clinical Research Bureau in New York City seven years later.[10]

THE BROWNSVILLE TRIALS AND THE COMMITTEE OF ONE HUNDRED

There was much legal wrangling in the fall of 1916 over various motions, including unsuccessful attempts by the Brownsville defendants to secure a jury trial or be tried together. Sanger and her pro-bono attorney, Jonah J. Goldstein, who was representing all three women and also became Sanger's lover around this time, did succeed in forcing Judge James McInerney, one of the three judges in the Court of Special Sessions in Brooklyn assigned to the case, to recuse himself. McInerney had presided over both the William Sanger and Jessie Ashley cases and made no secret of his belief that birth control was ungodly and its users "selfish."

Ethel Byrne, charged with selling articles prohibited under Section 1142 of the New York Penal Code, came up first on the docket on January 4, 1917, before the three-justice court. Attorney Goldstein, only 31 years old but already a player in city politics and fully cognizant of the potential magnitude of this case, opted not to challenge the evidence or police procedure, or claim his defendant had not acted as charged. Guilt was predetermined. Instead he argued that the law was arbitrary and unconstitutional, and he approached the case as a stepping stone to an appeal process and clarification of the law from higher courts. He held that contraception must be legally available to women as a matter of health and because women have a fundamental right to control their fertility. "This is nothing more," he stated, "than having the court determine once and for all the present standing of women in our modern society." In a preliminary hearing in December, Goldstein put forth that the law was "an infringement" on a woman's "free exercise of conscience and pursuit of happiness" because it denied "her absolute right of enjoyment of intercourse. . . ." The judge had rejected this line of reasoning outright, ridiculing Goldstein's assertion of a sexual right and adding that fear of pregnancy acted as an important deterrence to fornication. Fearing another public acknowledgment of a women's right to sexual pleasure, the judges in the Byrne hearing tried to contain Goldstein, limiting his argument on the unconstitutionality of Section 1142 to 15 minutes and refusing to admit expert testimony by Dr. Morris Kahn, who regularly dispensed birth control out of his private practice.

Byrne admitted to violating the law but repudiated the prosecution's additional allegations that the clinic was out to make a profit and was attempting to do away with Jews.* After only one full day of hearings, the court found Byrne guilty. She was sentenced on January 22 to 30 days in the workhouse and hauled off to the local jail, then to Blackwell's Island prison. "I shall go on a hunger strike at once," she announced, planning to emulate the well-publicized tactic of imprisoned British suffragettes. She also refused to be bathed or to work. To further goad prison officials, Byrne said she was giving out contraceptive information to other inmates. Her hunger strike succeeded in drawing national press attention, including daily wire service updates on her weakened condition. To placate reporters the Commissioner of Corrections released a daily bulletin on Byrne's health: January 25: "Pulse–Normal; Temperature–Practically Normal; Respiration–Normal; General Physical Condition–Fair . . . Walked to bathroom and returned twice in order to wash some handkerchiefs." After five days with no food and little water, Byrne collapsed in her cell and was forcibly fed by the prison physician and attendants. In a state of lethargy, she offered little resistance. Forced feedings of eggnog (milk, eggs, and brandy) continued over the next few days, leading up to the start of Sanger and Mindell's trials.[11]

The courtroom on January 29 was packed with supporters, as it was during Byrne's trial. About 50 Brownsville women, "shawled and tired-faced slum mothers," had been subpoenaed by the prosecution or represented the Mothers' League of Brownsville. They sat alongside a smartly-dressed contingent of society types—the "women of furs and autos," as one newspaper called them. The line of limousines outside the court, the glitz and hobnobbing inside, enveloped Sanger with the light of celebrity. The *Tribune* described these trials as looking more like receptions "with Mrs. Sanger as the guest of honor." But these buttoned-up club women were not there for show only; many of them belonged to the Committee of One Hundred, the group organized by Gertrude Minturn Pinchot on November 28, 1916, to aid Sanger's legal fight and help with educational and propaganda work for the movement. As of mid-January 1917, the Committee was 37 short of 100, but its members included a number of prominent and powerful women. Sanger described Pinchot, the well-born wife

---

* Though completely unfounded, the conspiracy theory that the birth control movement had genocidal intentions has never gone away, only refocused on African Americans.

of progressive political leader, Amos Pinchot, as "Aristocratic of bearing, autocratic by position," adding that, "she was one to command and be obeyed, and was easily a leading personality in the philanthropic smart set of New York." Another recognizable figure was Florence Jaffray Harriman, the well-known suffragist, founder of New York's exclusive Colony Club for women, and widow of banker J. Borden Harriman. There were several other Committee members who, like Harriman, shuttled between Fifth Avenue splendor and palatial Newport, Rhode Island, mansions, or who were well situated in New York's financial and political power base—names such as Cabot, Tiffany, Creel, Belmont, Delafield, and Havemeyer.[12]

Two other important Committee members, both born in 1875, were among the more eccentric women of their generation and attached to enormous Midwest manufacturing fortunes. Juliet Barrett Rublee, a restless and adventurous heir to a Chicago roofing company fortune and wife of attorney and Washington insider George Rublee, drafted the Committee's statement of purpose. Within a couple of years she became Sanger's best friend and most significant financial backer. In the days before Sanger's trial, Rublee went to Washington to lean on her connections in hopes of setting up a meeting between Committee of One Hundred members and President Wilson. A mercurial personality, Rublee was sometimes outlandish in her pursuits—she directed her own feature film in Mexico, a fiasco that drained her bank account, and she led an expedition to test a newly-invented deep-sea diving cylinder off the coast of Italy that resulted in her kidnapping. Hence she could not always be relied on within the movement. Another Committee member, who kept a low profile during these tumultuous early years of the movement, was Katharine Dexter McCormick, one of the first women graduates of the Massachusetts Institute of Technology. She had married Stanley McCormick, the heir to the International Harvester Corporation. Shortly after their marriage, Stanley was institutionalized for schizophrenia. His illness and Katharine's forced independence spurred her interest in legalizing birth control in order for women to achieve sexual autonomy and to keep from passing on inheritable diseases. McCormick stood out not only because she was often the smartest person in the room but also because her dress and comportment harked back to Victorian times, while her outlook and opinions were thoroughly modern. Her work in support of women's causes eventually led to a long career in medical philanthropy, and she joined with Sanger in the 1950s, funding and overseeing the research that led to the birth control pill.

Also part of the Committee was a core group of Greenwich Village radicals who had come from wealth and had remained loyal to the cause since Sanger's *Woman Rebel* indictments, including the feminist lawyer Jessie Ashley and anthropologist Elsie Clews Parsons. The ever-present Rose Pastor Stokes, the Russian-born cigar maker and writer who married into a sizable fortune, was often in the first row of every birth control trial and took a leading role in organizing Committee functions.

Mary Ware Dennett and several other NBCL stalwarts rounded out the Committee of One Hundred's impressive membership list.

There is no underestimating the significance of this group in putting the movement on firm ground. Not only did these Committee women bankroll Sanger, the NBCL, and the *Birth Control Review (BCR)*, but they also provided influential legal, political, and press contacts that proved invaluable to the movement over the next decade. In addition, Committee members bridged feminist camps within the birth control and women's suffrage movements, although many suffrage leaders continued to avoid the birth control question and its inherent controversies, fearing a side show to their central aim of voting rights. These women's high standing in society, their limousine flash, and big-hat visibility made an emphatic statement that one could be in favor of birth control without fearing an association with free-lovers and anarchists. The Committee of One Hundred helped to reframe the movement as a progressive solution to social problems, enabling Sanger to distance the cause from its radical beginnings and expand her base of support. "Formerly," Sanger wrote, "a few women of wealth but of liberal tendencies had been actively concerned in the movement, but now some who were prominent socially were coming to believe on principle that birth control should not be denied to the masses. The subject was in the process of ceasing to be tagged as radical and revolutionary, and becoming admittedly humanitarian."[13]

With so many birth control supporters and a largely sympathetic press presence in the courtroom, the three judges of the Court of Special Sessions tried to avoid making Sanger into a martyr as her sister had become. They called first on Fania Mindell, who was charged with selling an obscene publication, Sanger's *What Every Girl Should Know*, which was widely distributed in New York and did not contain contraceptive information. Her trial on the morning of January 29 was brief, as the judges decided they would need to read the pamphlet at a later time. Sanger, charged with conducting a clinic to disseminate contraceptive information and a separate violation of maintaining a public nuisance, watched a curious turn of events unfold as her trial began. Presiding Judge John J. Freschi questioned the prosecution's assumption that the contraceptive articles entered into evidence were for illegal purposes only; might there not be legal intent, he asked, since these articles were available in drugstores and the Penal Code allowed for contraception to prevent disease? The prosecution failed to adequately address this question and opened the way for an interpretation that could extend the use of birth control for health reasons. Put on the defensive, the prosecution stumbled further when, in a comic moment, they called a Mrs. Alice Cohen to the stand to testify as a clinic patient only to find out that they had subpoenaed the wrong Mrs. Cohen. Nevertheless, the prosecution called a number of other Brownsville mothers who admitted they had received contraceptive information from Sanger. Rather than challenging the mothers' testimony, since

Sanger's guilt was never in question, defense attorney Goldstein encouraged them to describe their predicaments and list the reasons they sought birth control. After hearing many accounts of multiple miscarriages, infant deaths, exhaustion and illness, paltry earnings and the burdens of poverty, Judge Freschi said he could not stand to hear any more and adjourned the court for several days so that the attorneys could prepare briefs on the meaning of birth control and its function in preventing disease.* The Brownsville women had made the case for birth control more effectively than any activist.

That night, Sanger appeared before a crowd of 3,000 as the guest of honor at a Carnegie Hall rally organized by the Committee of One Hundred and the BCLNY. The new league, a smaller and more radical rival to the NBCL, though there was some overlap in membership, principally existed to raise funds to cover legal fees and other expenses related to the clinic cases, and release publicity materials. League president Frederick Blossom used the occasion of the Carnegie Hall rally to distribute the first issue of the *BCR*, which quickly became Sanger's mouthpiece and the chief source of information on the movement and educational material on birth control. In a speech that hit several histrionic highs, Sanger told the mostly female crowd, "I come not from the stake of Salem, where women were burned for blasphemy, but from the shadow of Blackwell's Island, where women are tortured for obscenity."

Even with Sanger on trial, the focus remained on her sister, Ethel Byrne, still imprisoned and weak but in fair condition. The nation's newspapers would not let go of the story, reporting every detail of Byrne's health and forced diet. Her tube feedings continued on a regular schedule and now included "malted milk and beef juice," along with eggs and coffee. As Edward Mylius wrote at the time, "The whole country seemed to stand still and anxiously watch this lone woman's fight against an iniquitous law and against the authorities who were mercilessly enforcing it." Photographs of Byrne's solemn face appeared next to the updates that newspapers ran each day of her hunger strike, from the *Daily Herald* in Biloxi, to the Spanish-language *La Prensa* in San Antonio, to the *Daily Alaska Dispatch* in Juneau. The scope of publicity compared to that of the Bollinger baby case, despite the fact that this story competed with America's approach to entering the war. And the coverage extended from the front page to the editorial page, where there continued to be much consternation over the spread of birth control propaganda. The *San Jose Mercury News* called Sanger and Byrne

---

* The defendant's briefs, along with later appellant statements and supplementary briefs, were edited by Sanger and published as *The Case for Birth Control* in May, 1917. The book amounted to a compilation of historical analysis, contemporary articles, statistical information and excerpts from medical and scientific works on the benefits of birth control. For many years it stood as the most complete socioeconomic, eugenic, and medical justification of birth control.

"ill-balanced women" that were part of an "ignoble cult," "dangerous to the country's future and of no interest to the clean American home." Nevertheless, they believed it was a passing fad: "A few more arrests and the propaganda of birth-control will vanish as quickly as it appeared." On the other side, the *New York Evening Post* ran an editorial questioning the enforcement of a law that was being broken by people every day.

Prison officials refused to let Sanger or attorney Goldstein visit Byrne, further escalating fears of her demise. Sanger then called for her sister's release on humanitarian grounds. Failing to get help from the mayor's office, Sanger joined a delegation of five Committee of One Hundred members who traveled up to Albany on January 31 to lobby the governor to support birth control legislation. With Gertrude Pinchot, a close friend of Governor Charles Whitman, at her side, Sanger convinced the governor to grant Byrne a conditional pardon, with the understanding that she would not repeat her offense. Whitman also agreed to appoint a commission to study the state laws governing the dissemination of contraception. Sanger and Pinchot went to pick up Byrne on February 1 and found her emaciated and unable to walk. Kept awake with smelling salts and wrapped in Pinchot's fur coat, Byrne was carried out in dramatic fashion on a stretcher and taken by ambulance to Sanger's Manhattan apartment. The Commissioner of Corrections called the whole episode a "farce" and said Byrne was in better shape going out than coming in. The Committee of One Hundred immediately declared Byrne's hunger strike a victory. Attention turned to the resumption of Sanger's trial and the expectation that if found guilty she, too, would go on a hunger strike.

But the judges had leniency in mind. Bound to the law, they had little choice on February 2 but to find Sanger guilty as charged. However, at a sentencing hearing three days later, they offered her clemency if she promised to observe the law in her continuation of the birth control campaign. She responded, "I cannot respect the law as it stands to-day," but planned to obey the law pending appeal to the higher court, "This is a test case," she told the judges. Sanger was then sentenced to 30 days in prison. "As far as I am concerned," she told reporters, "I have accomplished as much as is possible at this time. We have aroused public opinion and created an agitation which will bear fruit." Therefore, she saw no reason to starve herself or refuse to cooperate with police or prison officials. The same day Fania Mindell was found guilty and fined $50. Goldstein appealed the Mindell and Sanger convictions (a writ of prohibition in the Byrne case was denied following her pardon), and Sanger spent her time in the Queens County Penitentiary without incident.[14]

THE BENEFITS OF MATYRDOM

With the publicity blitz from the clinic cases, the movement lunged ahead in the spring of 1917. New birth control leagues and societies cropped up and older ones expanded; by the end of the year there were more than 30 organizations spread across the country, including in Elizabeth City, North Carolina; Harrisburg and Johnstown, Pennsylvania; New Orleans, and several cities in New Jersey. Sanger and Blossom had trouble keeping up with all the incoming regional reports to the *BCR* and news of legislative initiatives in several states. As one newspaper editorial made clear, "The folly of making a martyr of Mrs. Sanger . . . by imprisonment and persecution, is bearing fruit throughout the country. Instead of squelching the doctrine preached by her, public sentiment is being strongly aroused in its favor in many localities."

The efforts by Sanger and others to address the socioeconomic and eugenic benefits of birth control paid off, attracting more moderates and helping to shield the movement from the criticism that it was an extreme radical pursuit. The subject began to win endorsements in sermons in Protestant churches and synagogues. Positive articles on birth control appeared with greater frequency in scientific journals. Increasingly, settlement house personnel and social workers, nurses and midwives were taking a stand in favor of birth control in professional societies, at conferences, and in their daily work. Margaret Lynch, a visiting nurse working for the Baby Milk Supply in conservative Lexington, Kentucky, and known throughout the area as the "babies' woman," had the courage during "Baby Week" to speak out for "legalized birth control and prohibition," after which "the problem of caring for the undernourished and sick babies of this community will be solved."

Even the intransigent medical profession was gradually moving toward a grudging acceptance of birth control, at least in cases that warranted the protection of women's health. On the whole, doctors remained opposed to a socioeconomic justification for contraception, and the profession continued to lash out at the birth control movement. Physicians suggested a link between abortionists and birth control activists, cast doubt on the safety of diaphragms and other methods, and completely rejected lay efforts to distribute contraceptive information. Medical sanction of legalized birth control was still a pipe dream for movement leaders. However, the prominent physician proponents of birth control, including William Robinson, Abraham Jacobi, and tuberculosis expert S. Adolphus Knopf, had been doggedly educating their colleagues and providing the public with professional substantiation of the movement's propaganda. Public health physician Ira S. Wile and Mount Sinai surgeon A. L. Goldwater went a step further and confronted their profession with accusations of hypocrisy. Wile publicly charged that many of the doctors in his own medical society in New York regularly performed abortions and at the same time opposed birth control legalization. Wile's colleagues hissed at his accusations. Goldwater raised a ruckus after his informal 1916 survey of physicians in New York found that those who favored preserving the anti-birth control provisions in the law had, on average, less than two children. Most physicians, he argued "not only *believe* in the doctrine of Birth Control, but most generally *practice* it." The Brooklyn-based gynecologist Robert Latou

Dickinson declared at a Chicago Medical Society meeting in February 1916 that he was a "confessed criminal," in that he furnished contraceptive information to his patients. Dickinson wanted the profession to "take hold of this matter and not let it go to the radicals, and not let it receive harm by being pushed in any undignified or improper manner." Over the next two decades he would become one of the key players in trying to bridge the gap between the medicos and the lay activists.[15]

SANGER'S STAR POWER

In the aftermath of the clinic trials, Margaret Sanger sought to assert her preeminence as movement leader and remain the focal point of publicity. She was jealous of her sister's hunger strike fame and determined to keep Ethel Byrne a footnote to the movement (years later she went so far as to have their prison roles reversed in a Hollywood film script for a bio-pic that was never made). She had misgivings about Frederick Blossom, who had counseled her against opening the clinic but seemed keen to share some of the ensuing limelight, and she tried to contain his growing influence among birth control supporters. She even looked to separate somewhat from the society women who had become her key supporters, telling reporters in Chicago, where she went to lecture in April 1917, that these women who came out for birth control had made it into a "pink tea movement." Sanger elaborated, "The people naturally do not want it to be placed in the hands of women with lorgnettes, who will make it [birth control] an affair of class and will ask so many questions before they are willing to give out the information that it will be too late to do any good." Her comment might have been prompted by the news that the same Chicago Women's Club that refused to host her lecture in April 1916, looked into establishing a clinic that spring, a remarkable turnaround in only a year's time.

Sanger was still struggling with the rapid transformation of the movement from a working-class, radical identification to a "first citizens" (as the socialist Blossom called them) campaign of society women and liberal professionals who treated the Brownsville trials and imprisonments as a cause célèbre and entry point for their own brand of highly-organized and well-funded group activism. Sanger needed the support of these wealthy and powerful women but resented their increasing influence and visibility in the press, not to mention their loosely veiled disapproval of her one-woman leadership. Virginia Heidelberg, an NBCL officer, complained in March, in a letter to Mary Dennett, "Sanger . . . is herself so uncertain about policy. No movement ever succe[ed]ed that was a one person movement." Dennett and other emerging leaders, like Massachusetts suffragist and blue-blooded Republican Blanche Ames Ames, the new president of the Birth Control League of Massachusetts, were well-positioned to lure in birth control proponents who had no stomach for Sanger's direct action tactics. Yet none of the other leading advocates could match Sanger's charisma or flare for publicity. Nor did they exhibit that elusive combination of fervor, daring, and equanimity that attracts followers and projects leadership.[16]

BIRTH CONTROL ON THE BIG SCREEN

Sanger looked to market her compelling personal story, reach a wider audience with her message, and further solidify her hold over the movement by making and starring in a propaganda film in the spring of 1917. *Birth Control*, co-written by Sanger and Blossom the previous fall and filmed around Sanger's trial and imprisonment, followed a series of silent films that took on the issue of birth control in the middle part of the decade, contributing to the phenomenal media hype over the subject since 1915. These included the antiabortion *Miracle of Life* (1915), which "lays bare the fallacies of race suicide;" Haiselden's *The Black Stork* (1917), which implicitly advocates birth control; the anti-birth control film, *The Unborn* (1916), which moralizes against "the greatest evil of the day"; and *Where Are My Children?* (1916). This last film starred Tyrone Power Sr. as a district attorney who, while prosecuting a case

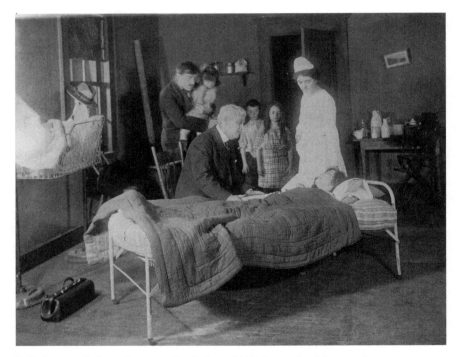

Still photograph from the movie *Birth Control* (1917), starring Margaret Sanger as a nurse. (Courtesy of the Sophia Smith Collection, Smith College.)

against an abortion doctor, discovers his wife's name on the nefarious doctor's client list. There were a few birth control plays as well, such as *The Home without Children*, about a childless marriage that is transformed by the birth of a bastard nephew. (When the frustrated would-be father tells his wife to listen to Theodore Roosevelt on race suicide, she shrieks in response: "I'd rather know what his wife thinks!") None of the productions that ostensibly advocated family limitation presented a clear cut endorsement of birth control. They offered contraception preferable to abortion, something worth defending but not necessarily promoting, or one element in a eugenic approach to bearing healthy children.

Birth Control, however, unabashedly affirms the moral necessity of family limitation. Produced by the Message Photo-Play Corporation, the film depicts the highlights of Sanger's brief career to date, from nurse to activist, in dramatic scenes intended to educate the masses and galvanize new support. In a somber tone, the "five reel photodrama" underscores the disparity between large, poor families and small, wealthy ones, then heralds the beginning of a new era where working-class women could secure contraception. The movie brings the story of the movement right up to date, covering Sanger's trial and imprisonment, and concluding with the subtitle: "No matter what happens, the work must go on." *Variety* thought that filmgoers would be "electrified with the intense convictions of the propagandist," and noted that "facts are given that if not making everyone who sees the picture a convert to her cause will certainly make everyone think twice before denouncing the movement." The National Board of Review found the film commendable, leading the producers to advertise to wary theaters, "We'll Guarantee You It's Law Proof and Censor Proof." In late March, Sanger announced that she would tour with the film, which was scheduled to premier at the Park Theatre in New York City on May 6. But just prior to its first public showing, the movie was suppressed.

George H. Bell, the Commissioner of Licenses for New York, had not seen the film but had heard from others, including representatives from the Catholic Theatre Movement, that *Birth Control* was unsuitable. Bell told the Park Theatre management that the film was "immoral, indecent, and directly contrary to public welfare" and threatened to revoke the theater's license if they screened it. He may have been influenced by the Brooklyn branch of the Motion Pictures Exhibitor's League's earlier vote against its exhibition. Within hours, Jonah Goldstein, representing Message Photo-Play, sought a court injunction to bar the commissioner's action and instigated a lawsuit to collect on damages due to a loss of receipts. Meanwhile, Sanger set up a private screening for the press and other invitees to demonstrate that the film was, as the *Tribune* reported, "clean and the performance unobjectionable." In early June, New York Supreme Court justice Nathan Bijur found that Bell had violated the filmmakers' free speech rights and enjoined Bell from interfering with its presentation. He stated that "there is nothing in it which can reasonably be viewed as against morality, decency, or public welfare." However, in July, the State Supreme Court's Appellate Division reversed Bijur's decision and upheld the ban, citing Bell's argument "that the film would have a tendency to arouse class hatred, as it tends to show that the rich have small families and favor the poor having large families."* Another film, *The Hand That Rocks the Cradle*, which opened several weeks after *Birth Control* was suppressed, met the same fate. It also depicted Sanger's arrest and imprisonment, as well as Byrne's hunger strike, though fictional names were used and Sanger had no involvement in its production.[17]

GOVERNMENT SUPPRESSION, RELIGIOUS OPPOSITION, AND THE FEAR OF RACE SUICIDE

The threat of government suppression loomed over the birth control movement during the later World War I years, but officials at both the state and federal level were much more concerned with antiwar propagandists than with birth control advocates. There were isolated incidents apart from Sanger's run-ins with the law, such as the arrest of a clubwoman in Cleveland, a Mrs. Ralph D. Mitchell, for distributing pamphlets by Sanger, and Emma Goldman from her home. Ben Reitman was arrested twice in December 1916, in Cleveland and in Rochester, for distributing birth control pamphlets. His two trials, in January and February of 1917, attended by a colorful assortment of radicals, garnered headlines in the local press. He was acquitted in Rochester but convicted in Cleveland and given a six-month prison sentence.

Some state legislatures were active in the spring of 1917 in tightening antiobscenity laws and fending off attempts to legalize contraception: the Pennsylvania House of Representatives passed a bill forbidding the dissemination of birth control literature; the state legislature in Boston tabled a bill that would have authorized medical schools in the Commonwealth to provide contraceptive instruction to students; and the Assembly of Codes Committee of the New York State legislature killed two birth control bills instigated by the NBCL and Committee of One Hundred. The movement had learned to leverage government interference to increase publicity, but antagonism toward birth control from other quarters was growing and becoming less predictable.

Opposition from the Catholic Church had increased in 1916 and 1917. More priests lashed out against birth control in sermons, and some regional Catholic groups, such as the Catholic Theatre Movement and several Catholic women's organizations, issued statements condemning "this unnatural and utterly anti-Christian propaganda." In March 1917, Pope Benedict XV reacted to the birth control agitation

---

* The few copies of the film disappeared and have never been found.

in the United States by instructing the international Sacred Heart League to pray for "large and holy families" during that month. Several Catholic publications made scurrilous remarks about Sanger. One went so far as to call for the imprisonment of all birth control activists, prompting Sanger, in the summer of 1918, to pronounce the Church "the bigoted, relentless enemy of birth control." The Church also clarified and defended its teachings on marriage and reproduction, and made more of an effort to confront penitents. Catholic prelates were nervously aware that a growing number of Catholics practiced some form of family limitation. But American Catholic Church leaders did not yet mount a concerted opposition campaign perhaps remaining too uncomfortable with the subject.[18]

One of the most publicized attacks on birth control at this time, though fleeting, came from the hyperbolic evangelist, Billy Sunday. Speaking to a woman-only meeting in New York, Sunday rasped that he "despised the women who shrink from maternity because they love ease and fashion. Their hands are stained with the blood of their unborn children, and they are murderers just the same as if they put their hands on the throats of their 12-year-old children and choked them to death." Sunday did not dwell on birth control; he spent more time attacking other liberal movements, as well as divorce, various forms of debauchery, and especially drink—becoming one of the leading proponents of prohibition. But he tapped into the country's ongoing fears about race suicide, made more acute by rising numbers of immigrants from Eastern and Southern Europe, black migration to northern cities, and deaths of American soldiers overseas.

Eugenicists were raising a panic during the later years of the war about the differential birth rate between rich and poor, white and black, native and immigrant, educated and uneducated. As the sterilization advocate Paul Popenoe wrote in 1917, "The superior parts of the population are limiting their families so much that they are not even reproducing their own numbers, while the increase of inferior families is checked only by the death-rate, because they do not practice effective methods of birth control." This fear was felt across the country by "old stock" populations who expressed concern that the United States would lose its distinctive ingenuity, drive, and idealism if newcomers and nonwhites proliferated at an increasing rate while the so-called native white population remained stagnant. And more than government suppression or opposition from the Catholic Church or evangelists, the fear of race suicide posed the most insidious threat to the birth control movement because it pushed many individuals who had no clear moral objections to birth control into conflict with it. Popular and quickly spreading movements for eugenics and human betterment, determined to preserve racial hierarchies and reduce foreign-born populations, were not always opposed to contraception. However, eugenicists endeavored to replace birth control and the concept of individual reproductive autonomy with the notion of birth regulation and the imposition of fertility standards based on class, race, and ethnicity. The eugenics movement posed a particularly vexing challenge to the reproductive rights movement's feminist goal of woman-controlled fertility, and Sanger would spend much of the next decade trying to figure out how to align the two movements' objectives while upholding her commitment to voluntary mother-hood.[19]

RADICAL RIFT

During this period of limbo, with wartime pressures on leftist movements and as birth control activists awaited a decision on the appeal of Sanger's Brownsville conviction, the movement also faced heated internal squabbles, with Frederick Blossom at the epicenter. The fundamental disagreement between the NBCL and BCLNY over the degree of birth control deregulation in proposed New York legislative bills spilled over into disputes about funding sources and shared responsibilities. Sanger accused the NBCL of holding on to contributions meant for her and resented the support given to the NBCL by the Committee of One Hundred. The NBCL made no secret that it lacked confidence in Sanger's leadership and found Blossom, who resigned from the League's board in December 1916, disagreeable and untrustworthy. Sanger defended Blossom against outside attacks until the two had a falling out sometime that spring.

An argument over the war and Blossom's refusal to run a pacifist piece by Sanger in the *BCR* spiraled into accusations of mismanagement and embezzlement. He accused Sanger of profiting from the movement and using donations to live high on the town. She questioned Blossom's bookkeeping and demanded a full accounting, prompting him to resign as editor of the *Review* and depart with the cash on hand and even some of the office furniture. The rift resulted in the suspension of the *Review* after the June 1917 issue. The war of words escalated to the point where Sanger hired attorney Goldstein to threaten charges of slander and fraud against Blossom, a move that angered the socialist community which thought the dispute should be settled in house, among "comrades." A number of radicals held a recent grudge against Sanger for keeping mum on Ben Reitman's arrests and trials earlier in the year instead of rallying support for him; Emma Goldman called it an "inexcusable breach of solidarity." Sanger backed away from legal threats when the BCLNY appointed a committee of three socialists to investigate Blossom. The committee found no wrongdoing and scolded Sanger for taking actions "contrary to the fundamental principles of radicalism." The investigation was a fait accompli, for the committee had no intention of impugning Blossom or releasing information that would disgrace the BCLNY.

For Sanger, who had distanced herself from New York's radicals since returning from her exile, the Blossom episode sealed her split from the Socialist Party and further identified her with the wealthy progressive set. It did not, as some scholars have suggested, result in a complete break with the radical community, as Sanger continued to hire seasoned radical activists. Within a year of Blossom's departure from the *BCR*, she brought in William (Billy) Williams, a socialist journalist from Kansas City, and Agnes Smedley, the socialist political activist and writer, to do editorial work and writing for the *Review*. She also kept many of her friendships with leading radical figures, such as Eugene Debs and Carlo Tresca. Sanger's battle with Blossom resulted in a public announcement of her ouster from the BCLNY in July 1918, which Sanger shrugged off, as she had never formally been a member. The BCLNY briefly split into two factions, for and against Sanger, before dissolving later in 1918.[20]

THE *BIRTH CONTROL REVIEW*

Sanger turned her attention to resuscitating the *BCR* in late 1917. In October she was rebuffed, once again, by the NBCL when she approached them for money for the periodical. She briefly considered handing the magazine over to William Robinson to run, but Jessie Ashley, who would shortly become one of the *Review's* literary editors, Gertrude Pinchot, and Juliet Rublee donated enough money to clear debts and enable Sanger to return to a monthly publishing schedule starting in December 1917. In January 1918, Ashley and Helen Todd, a social worker and member of the Committee of One Hundred, devised the formation of a holding company as a long-term financing solution. The New York Women's Publishing Company (NYWPC) was created in February 1918 and sold enough shares of stock to Committee of One Hundred members to put the *Review* on stable footing. The board of directors of the new company included Sanger, Rublee, Ashley, Cerise Carman Jack from the Massachusetts League, other Committee of One Hundred women, and NBCL executive secretary Mary Ware Dennett, giving the League a greater presence in the *Review*. The *BCR* had a modest subscription base but fairly high street sales. It gained wide visibility, publishing articles by a number of notable writers, including in its first year Havelock Ellis, the eugenicists Paul Popenoe and Roswell Johnson, and the well-known South African feminist author, Olive Schreiner. That it served as a clearinghouse for movement news made it indispensable to activists across the country. And with the demise of the BCLNY, the *Review* became Sanger's organizational base and the only other national presence along with the NBCL.

One reason that the *Review* was able to restart during a difficult wartime economy and a key to its success over the next decade was the intrepid street hawking of Kitty Marion (1873–1944), who sold 1,000 copies of the December 1917 issue. For many New Yorkers, Marion became the face of birth control. With a satchel of *Reviews* hanging in front of her and one in each hand, she stood for hours each day in Herald Square, Times Square, Grand Central Station, the Coney Island boardwalk, and other pedestrian hotspots and called out "*Birth Control Review*, twenty cents a copy." The German-born Marion, who had moved to England in her teens, was a veteran of the English Women's suffrage movement, where she had built a reputation for confrontational behavior and sometimes violent protests. She had been imprisoned a number of times for various destructive acts in Britain, such as breaking windows of government buildings and setting homes on fire. In one prison she set her cell on fire by burning a bible. One of the figures most closely associated with the suffragette hunger strikes in Britain, Marion claimed to have been forcibly fed over 200 times. She was deported at the beginning of the war and made her way to New York.

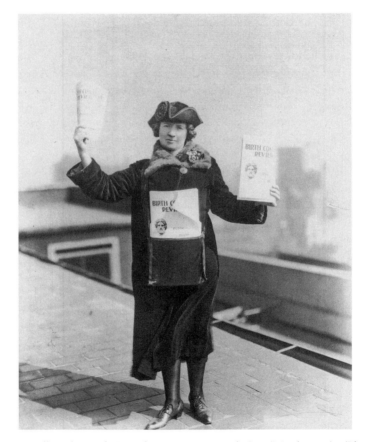

Kitty Marion selling the *Birth Control Review* in New York City (March 1925). (Photograph by Underwood & Underwood. Courtesy of the Sophia Smith Collection, Smith College.)

She attended the Carnegie Hall rally for Sanger in January 1917 and soon after joined the small staff of the *Review*. Sanger immediately set her to work on street corners selling the *Review* and handing out flyers, a job that Sanger admitted, after trying it herself, was "torture." Marion endured death threats, heckling, spitting, physical abuse, and police obstruction. Many passers-by prayed for her or crossed themselves indignantly. In August of 1918 Marion was arrested by an undercover agent for the New York Society for the Suppression of Vice, Comstock's old organization, which continued to hound birth control advocates. For imparting contraceptive information to an undercover officer, she was sentenced to 30 days in The Tombs. Yet even behind bars, Marion relentlessly pitched birth control, holding small meetings with other inmates. Agnes Smedley, who was also in The Tombs in the fall of 1918 on charges of distributing contraceptive information and an unrelated charge under the Espionage Act, said, "Kitty is turning the place into a birth control branch." Smedley remembered that Marion "came clattering down the stone corridors every morning with her scrub pail in hand. 'Three cheers for birth control,' she greeted the prisoners and matrons. And 'three cheers for birth control,' the prisoners answered back." Over the next 10 years, Marion was arrested eight more times for her birth control work. She called the trouble she faced nothing more than "water on a duck's back."[21]

THE BROWNSVILLE APPEAL: CLEARING THE WAY FOR CLINICS

It took nearly a year for the appeal of Sanger's Brownsville conviction to travel through the courts. Jonah Goldstein won a small victory in November 1917 when the Court of Appeals overturned Fania Mindell's conviction for selling Sanger's *What Every Girl Should Know*. He argued the Sanger case a final time in December 1917 before the Court of Appeals in Albany. As he had in Sanger's first trial, he challenged the constitutionality of Section 1142 of the New York State Penal Code that prohibited any sale or distribution of contraception. He argued that the law violated the Fourteenth Amendment in that it deprived married women of the right to individual liberty by, in effect, forcing conception on them. Although the state does not compel marriage, he submitted, the prohibition on birth control made motherhood compulsory for women who were required by the marriage contract to engage in intercourse with their husbands or face marriage annulment. Goldstein emphasized that the law "precludes physicians from giving any information even where conception would make pregnancy dangerous or fatal." As Sanger wrote in the *Review*, "no more tyrannous infringement of personal liberty could be imagined." Goldstein also submitted briefs on which he, Sanger, and others had worked in 1917, which included extensive data, much of it taken from foreign studies, linking excessive childbearing to poverty, disease, mental deficiency, and high rates of maternal and infant mortality.

Although the breadth of sociological and medical information in the defendant's briefs was impressive, the court found it irrelevant to the particulars of the case and applicable to legislative consideration only. By unanimous decision the court upheld the constitutionality of Section 1142 and affirmed Sanger's conviction, noting that because she was neither a doctor nor a person claiming to be affected by the law, she had no right to challenge the law on a constitutional basis. However, Judge Frederick Crane, the author of the opinion, offered a backdoor approach to attaining some degree of latitude. He highlighted Section 1145 of the Penal Code that contained a medical exemption to the inflexible wording of the state Comstock provision. It stated "An article or instrument, used or applied by physicians law-fully practicing, or by their direction or prescription, for the cure or prevention of disease, is not an article of indecent or immoral nature or use, within this article. The supplying of such articles to such physicians or by their direction or prescription, is not an offense under this article." This law, referred to earlier, had been enacted as a public health measure to allow for the legal use of prophylactics to control venereal disease. Crane then established a fairly broad understanding of the term *disease*, relying on this dictionary definition: "an alteration in the state of the body, or of some of its organs, interrupt-ing or disturbing the performance of the vital functions, and causing or threatening pain and sickness; illness; sickness; disorder." He added, "This exception in behalf of physicians," while it did not permit "promiscuous advice to patients irrespective of their condition" was "broad enough to protect the physician who in good faith gives such help or advice to a married person to cure or prevent disease." He then extended this protection to pharmacists and vendors acting on the physician's orders. Judge Crane's intent was clear: to offer greater access to contraception to satisfy the reason-able health needs of married women and families while respecting the underlying intent of the law as a check on immoral sexual behavior. Crane's decision established that there was a legitimate public health interest in birth control apart from venereal disease prevention. It afforded doctors significant leeway in determining the medical indications for prescriptive contraception.

The loss of the appeal was reported in the press as a defeat for the movement, but Goldstein and Sanger viewed it as a victory, though not necessarily clear and deci-sive. The court had not accepted Goldstein's argument that the law was an infringe-ment on individual liberty, thereby denying any claim to a legal right of reproductive choice. Sanger cynically noted that the ruling put contraception on an even legal ground with abortion, which the law permitted for physician-determined therapeutic health reasons. But the decision did help begin a process of legitimization, treating contraception in a medical context as a public health issue. More importantly for the movement, the decision validated Sanger's plan to place contraception under medical supervision; in fact, the Crane decision ensured that this was the only way to proceed in New York, barring a legislative remedy. The decision put in place the framework for opening a legal clinic, though a considerable educational challenge remained. "We can no longer say that the Doctors can not give this information to [tubercular] women & those suffering with other ailments," Sanger wrote to Juliet Rublee. "Now we must let the Doctors know this decision, & get the women to ask them for it."[22]

The Crane decision had no bearing outside of New York, and coming out of the war, none of the other state or regional birth control organizations across the country had the financial, legal, or political support to open clinics. Sanger did not seem in a hurry to test the law again and thought it prudent to wait while Goldstein appealed the New York Appellate Court's ruling to the Supreme Court. She also anticipated that hospitals would be first in line to pivot off the Crane decision and offer contraceptive advice. As Cathy Moran Hajo noted in her recent study of birth control clinics, "Hospital-based obstetrical care was one of the fastest growing services," as fewer and fewer women bore children at home. To advocates, hospitals seemed ideal sites for contraceptive instruction. However, conservative hospital boards and a circumspect obstetrical profession were not ready to associate with a cause that continued to be identified with feminism and radicals. Furthermore, most hospitals preferred to leave preventive care and health education to social service organizations. In 1919, Sanger's personal physician, Dr. Mary Halton, formed a committee under NYWPC auspices and surveyed over two dozen New York City hospitals to see if they would offer contraceptive advice to a woman with tuberculosis and a woman with syphilis who wished to avoid pregnancy. "Each hospital," Halton wrote in the final report, "refused to allow the patients to come, and each hospital said that under the present law it could not give such information to any such patients" out of fear of charter revocations and arrest. Because of the urgency of these patients' health problems, several hospital superintendents recommended staff doctors who "might be willing to break the law in their private offices." Remarkably, if the women had been pregnant, the severity of their illnesses would have warranted a legal therapeutic abortion at the same hospitals that denied them contraception. It would take a number of years before a few hospitals began incorporating contraceptive services.[23]

Ever since her imprisonment, Sanger had conducted an occasional and informal clinic out of the *BCR* office on Fifth Avenue. She called it her "little room" and received funding from Juliet Rublee to keep it supplied. A dozen or more women came each week to receive contraceptive information. Kitty Marion and other *BCR* staffers referred women while always on the lookout for undercover police. Donations from Gertrude Pinchot enabled Sanger to print additional copies of *Family Limitation* to hand to clients and to translate the pamphlet into Polish and Lithuanian and keep it circulating in working-class neighborhoods. By 1918 there were also Yiddish, Hungarian, and Russian editions; and by the early 1920s it had been translated into half a dozen other languages. Now in its sixth edition, the pamphlet continued to be the most effective means of reaching thousands of women in all economic classes. The censors had largely given up trying to curtail its spread, though a Pittsburgh woman was arrested in the summer of 1918 for handing out copies to mine workers.[24]

DENNETT ASSERTS HER LEADERSHIP

The Crane decision coincided with the reemergence of Mary Ware Dennett as a leading voice in the movement. Dennett had devoted most of her time during the war to work with various peace and civil liberties groups. In January 1918, she accepted the position of executive secretary of the NBCL and pledged to kick start an organization that lacked a strong agenda and had become wholly reactive to Sanger. Although the NBCL had doubled its membership in 1917, it lacked funds and had failed to take advantage of its affiliation with birth control leagues across the country. Dennett sought new ways to nationalize the movement and better position it to lobby for a birth control amendment to the federal Comstock Law. She analyzed the laws affecting birth control in all states, noting which had strict prohibitions and which were free of restrictions (there were only five), and arranged petition drives to urge the amendment of specific state laws as well as the federal penal code. In May 1918, Dennett organized the two-day Eastern States Conference on Birth Control in New York, which included delegates from Boston; Philadelphia; Syracuse; Buffalo; Washington, D.C.; Indianapolis; and Chicago. These advocates discussed strategy, shared information, and argued for the importance of birth control during wartime. "It lowers the birth rate," Dennett later wrote, "but lowers the death rate and infant mortality rate still more. Fewer people are born but more survive" to contribute to the war effort. "In other words," she told readers of the *BCR*, "birth control is the highest, most far-reaching kind of patriotism." Dennett also took to the road in 1918, speaking to women's, civic, and medical groups in upstate New York, where she established several new NBCL committees. Her infusion of energy and well-honed organizational skills paid off impressively in 1918. She increased the membership of the League tenfold, raised close to $5,000, and put out over 100,000 flyers and pamphlets.

Dennett viewed her role in the movement as educational and remedial. In effect, she believed she was cleaning up after Sanger's "atmosphere of violence." Politicians and doctors, the two key constituents for changing the laws, she argued, were "repelled by the racket of the birth control movement" and its ties to "revolutionary 'radicalism.'" Dennett aimed to cleanse the movement of the strident tones of anarchists like Goldman and Berkman and elevate it above Sanger's brand of street theater and unlawfulness. Dennett went so far as to refuse to send women who wrote to her any practical contraceptive information out of respect for the law; in fact she asked for their assistance in supporting a legislative amendment. "The League," she wrote one advice seeker, "cannot be in the business of breaking laws it is working to change."

Dennett also emphasized the need for education on both sexuality and birth control to rescue these subjects from the taint of obscenity. To this end she looked to publish an essay, *The Sex Side of Life*, that she had written in 1915 to educate her two sons. In February 1918, Frederic Robinson printed the essay in the *Medical Review of Reviews*, where it received positive attention. It was republished in June in *The Modern School* magazine and then privately by Dennett in 1919 in pamphlet form. Like some of Sanger's early sex-education writing, *The Sex Side of Life* placed human sexuality in the context of Mother Nature while celebrating the distinctively human ability through sex to merge instinct and emotion, mind and soul. "It is *not* a nasty subject," she insisted. "It should mean everything that is highest and best and happiest in human life. . . ." Her prose is devoid of sentimentality and her explanations clear and precise. The pamphlet, not unlike *Family Limitation*, took on a life of its own and was circulated widely in 1919 and the early 1920s, turning Dennett into a recognized sex expert. A number of educational institutions distributed it to students, and it received widespread medical and clerical endorsements. Even the YMCA, which had first sponsored Comstock's vice crusades, sold the pamphlet through its bookstores. In 1922 the U.S. Post Office declared the pamphlet obscene and unmailable under the Comstock Law, setting the stage for a later court battle that became one of the pivotal censorship cases in the 20th century.

"The task before me seems so colossal to undertake alone," Sanger wrote to Juliet Rublee in December 1917, which is why, in part, she decided to invite Dennett to serve on the NYWPC board and give her a page each month in the *Review* to update NBCL members. Despite Sanger's differences with Dennett, she found her to be "a good promoter and experienced campaigner" and appreciated her "shrewdness." However awkward, Sanger's reaching out to Dennett was also a matter of survival, for neither group had deep pockets. Cooperation, though it fell short of consolidation, helped both the *BCR* and the NBCL gain larger audiences for their publications and more subscriptions and membership fees. Following the Blossom troubles and in the midst of government intimidation of leftist movements, it made good sense to rally the movement together.[25]

SUPPRESSION OF DISSENT AND THE RED SCARE

There were warning signs in August 1918 that the birth control movement might become one more target of the government in its crackdown of radical organizations following the passage of the 1917 Espionage Act and the 1918 Sedition Act. Kitty Marion's arrest by an undercover agent that month and the Post Office's confiscation of the August issue of the *BCR* for running a review of a banned book, Marie Stopes's *Married Love*, portended more severe acts of suppression. Moreover, Sanger still was considered a dangerous radical with ties to individuals and groups that had been accused by the government of treason.

The new laws made it a crime to express antiwar sentiment or opposition to conscription, and could be construed to prohibit any criticism of the government. The public had largely supported—and the press egged on—the vicious and often extralegal government brutality, suspension of civil rights, and acts of vigilantism occurring across the country against German Americans and other immigrant groups, socialists, anarchists, and so-called "red" organizations of any kind—especially after the October 1917 Bolshevik Revolution in Russia. Labor groups and the radical press were the main targets of the government's campaign of repression, which included mass arrests of radicals and violent raids of radical organizations. The government went all out to destroy the IWW, which had not agitated against the war but had conducted a series of wartime strikes that affected industries vital to the war effort. By 1918, most of the leaders of the Wobblies were in prison or had been forced to leave the organization, including the early birth control supporters Bill Haywood, Elizabeth Gurley Flynn, and Carlo Tresca. Emma Goldman and Alexander Berkman were arrested in June 1917 for obstructing the draft. They had formed the No-Conscription League in May 1917 and had been holding rallies in New York. News coverage of the No-Conscription League and the League for Amnesty of Political Prisoners, organized in 1918 by Goldman from her prison cell in Missouri, mentioned that radicals prominent in "birth control circles," including Leonard Abbott, were among the draft obstructionists. Goldman and Berkman were deported in 1919. Other radical friends of the movement and close Sanger supporters, Roger Baldwin, Eugene Debs, and Scott Nearing, most prominent among them, were arrested for sedition.

The birth control movement was also linked to several suppressed leftist publications, such as the *The Masses*, whose staff, including Max Eastman, Floyd Dell, John Reed, and the political cartoonist Art Young—all friends of Sanger's and early backers of the cause—was indicted for publishing antiwar material. The socialist paper *The Call*, still one of the most vocal champions of birth control, was declared unmailable over 20 times in the first half of 1918 and had its mailing permit suspended for expressions of dissent and pro-Bolshevik sentiment. Although *The Call* limped along for a few more years, scores of radical publications dissolved, including *The Masses, Mother Earth,* and Berkman's *The Blast,* all of which had provided space to Sanger and other birth controllers, and had been among the most steadfast supporters of the movement.[26]

Sanger grew more cautious after the U.S. entry into the war in the spring of 1917. By the end of that year, the content of the *Review* had become less overtly political and defiant, and more focused on socioeconomic and health issues. Yet she could not refrain from asserting her deep-rooted belief that overpopulation led to war, and she published several articles calling on women to protest the war and cease childbearing. "She must deny the right of the State or Kingdom," Sanger wrote in "Woman and War," "to make her a victim of unwilling motherhood, and the handmaiden of militarism." The case could be made that these words were every bit as seditious as those of many other authors and activists charged with conspiracy to interfere with the war effort. Sanger also used the pages of the *Review* to protest government suppression and the round-up of radicals; her article calling for support of the arrested IWW leaders was printed in the issue deemed unmailable by postal authorities. Yet she escaped any serious trouble apart from a December 1918 arrest, along with Kitty Marion, for selling an issue of the *Review* that contained an article on birth control and abortion. The charges were dismissed two weeks later. The *Review* otherwise remained unscathed and continued to publish.

While the antiradical hysteria shattered the left and drove many radicals underground, Sanger acknowledged that the war had halted the progress of the cause only "temporarily." How the movement escaped more severe damage is something of a mystery. Sanger's fallout with socialists over the Blossom affair and the gradual drift of the movement away from its antiauthoritarian beginnings may have insulated it against the radical purges of 1917 to 1919. Unlike many other organizations on the left, it does not appear that Sanger, the *BCR* or NBCL came under FBI scrutiny until the early 1920s. The Lusk Committee of the New York State Legislature, empowered to investigate subversive activities, created a file on Sanger in 1919 but never took any action. Possibly the Committee of One Hundred members' powerful connections safeguarded the movement. In particular, Juliet Rublee's husband, George, had served in several positions in President Wilson's administration and may have put in a word to leave the birth control women alone. More likely, government officials reasoned that as long as there were no egregious violations of the law, it was better to do nothing; a forced legal entanglement would give the movement yet another propaganda opportunity. Federal and state authorities had observed the martyrdom of Byrne and Sanger in New York and Van Kleek Allison in Boston, and it appears they had learned their lesson, at least for a time.

CONDOMS AND THE WAR AGAINST VENEREAL DISEASE

The government's efforts to combat venereal disease (VD) in World War I also complicated its dealings with the birth control movement. Following Sanger's arrest with Kitty Marion in December 1918, Sanger and Jonah Goldstein made an effective argument that quickly led to the dismissal of their case and shielded them from further obscenity charges. Goldstein pointed out in court, and Sanger in the *Review*, that the War Department, the Navy, and the U.S. Public Health Service had printed and distributed a number of pamphlets on VD that were more explicit than the *BCR* article that led to their arrest. In fact, it appeared that passages from Sanger's *What Every Girl Should Know* had been lifted nearly verbatim and used in army publications on VD—an irony Sanger relished.[27]

The government's newfound interest in sex education literature as part of its anti–VD "Fit to Fight" campaign and the more than 4 million men who returned from military service with an unprecedented education in sex had a profound and lasting effect on the birth control movement far beyond censorship issues. Before the war, men with venereal disease had been rejected for service. But with infection rates in many areas over 10 percent among new enlistees and demand for manpower high, the surgeon general had little choice but to lift the ban. Shortly after the United States entered the war, the War Department created the Commission on Training Camp Activities (CTCA) to stem the tide of venereal infection before recruits were sent overseas. The CTCA undertook a sophisticated education campaign that, historian Allan Brandt has written, "combined elements of uplift and distraction, coercion and repression in its efforts to make the military venereal-free." The CTCA fell under pressure from progressive sex reformers, purity advocates, and moralists of different stripes, both within and outside the government, to create and preserve a moral environment in the military. As a result, the Commission focused almost exclusively on behavior. It closed down red light districts, provided recreational outlets, and emphasized abstinence. Disease rates fluctuated but remained high, so the CTCA took its message to the public, blurring the line between private morality and public health. The move brought the government into the public dialogue on sexuality that had been cultivated most effectively thus far by the birth control movement. "The war is doing one good thing," said William Zinsser, chair of a Council of National Defense subcommittee charged with gathering public support for the campaign. "It is making people speak out loud about a subject that before was either ignored or dealt with in whispers." Ultimately, however, the military had to depend on chemical prophylaxis rather than moral suasion. Soldiers were ordered to report to prophylactic stations after sexual activity to be injected with a chemical solution that was effective against chancroid, gonorrhea, and syphilis if taken within the proper time frame and under appropriate conditions.

At no time did the military and the various public health agencies condone the use of condoms, which were still technically illegal to distribute. During World War I the United States was the only Allied country to send its troops into battle lacking this one crucial piece of armor. The concern that condoms encouraged prostitution and indiscriminate sex overrode the practical consideration of disease prevention. The no-condom policy frustrated military doctors who had to cope with the repercussions of rampant VD. One exasperated surgeon, Dr. Louis Schwartz of the U.S. Public Health Service, writing in the journal *Military Surgeon* in May 1918, was convinced that "the free distribution of [the condom], together with the teaching of its proper use to our soldiers and sailors, would at one stroke not only wipe out venereal disease from the military forces, but would prevent its spread amongst the civil population." He noted the main objection to handing out condoms, that men will "indulge" their sexual desires "more freely," was unreasonable since other attempts to curb military men's sexual appetites had failed. Even the "fear of infection rarely prevents the gratification of sexual desire." Schwartz concluded, "Let us not shut our eyes against the truth, just because the truth is not nice to see."

Despite such common sense arguments, the military did not reverse its policy on condoms until the next war. Yet not surprisingly, American soldiers and sailors regularly used condoms during the war years. Inexpensive rubbers were relatively easy to obtain near urban centers in the United States and plentiful in Europe, where many doughboys first learned about them from prostitutes or fellow servicemen. After they settled back into civilian life, many veterans continued to use condoms as a method of marital birth control. "Every soldier in the World War was told to use them," Sanger wrote some years later, "and they have not forgotten." One well-regarded study found that couples married before 1912 used condoms about 20 percent of time, preferring withdrawal as their main source of birth control, while couples married after 1921 used condoms more than 40 percent of the time, an increase attributed in large part to the war.[28]

World War I benefitted American condom manufacturers, who sold their goods in England to supplement the European market, which had previously relied on German brands. A few companies leveraged their wartime success to become dominant players in the lucrative postwar condom market, including Youngs Rubber (maker of the Trojan brand) and manufacturer Julius Schmid (Ramses brand), who had been arrested by Comstock in 1890. His company supplied the U.S. military with condoms during World War II. Better manufacturing techniques and the Crane decision, which effectively decriminalized the prophylactic condom, cleared the way for condoms to become the most visible form of birth control in America. In many circles, however, they were still viewed as a crude tool of the prostitute. Birth controllers continued to malign them as untrustworthy and uncomfortable. Boston physician and contraceptive activist Antoinette Konikow liked to quote a German expert who quipped, "From the point of view of prevention a condom is as thin as cobweb, but from the point of view of the joy of the sexual act it is as thick as the wall of a fortress." Some of the first studies on contraceptive effectiveness, released in the 1920s, found a condom failure rate between 50 and 70 percent due to improper use and breakage, as well as a high dissatisfaction rate.

Not only did World War I lead to a greater acceptance and use of condoms for both disease prevention and birth control, it also marked a turning point in the U.S. government's handling of a sexual issue. Never before had the government instigated and participated in an open and sustained public discussion of a sexual matter or allowed health and medical concerns to encroach on established standards of morality. As Andrea Tone has persuasively written, "The VD crisis freed Americans to reclassify sex as a legitimate subject of scientific and social research and made sexual behavior a matter of public welfare. Most important, it established a credible justi-fication for contraception—public health—that placed the birth control debate on less incendiary grounds."[29]

BIRTH CONTROL FOR BETTER HEALTH

In her speeches and writings since her cross-country tour in 1916, Sanger had been guiding the movement toward a greater emphasis on birth control for better health. Her trial defense in 1917 yielded compelling data on the potential for birth control to: reduce maternal and infant mortality; reduce abortion deaths and the myriad problems associated with abortion, including sepsis, tetanus, and sterility; reduce the incidence of birth defects and childhood disabilities due to syphilis and congenital diseases; and reduce many of the illnesses and harmful social behaviors associated disproportionately with large families living in poverty. Relying on statis-tics taken from the U.S. Children's Bureau and other government agencies, sources in England, the Netherlands and elsewhere in Europe, and personal stories from the thousands of women who wrote to her, Sanger authored a series of articles in the *BCR* between 1917 and 1919 that focused on birth control and health. Together they read as not only a plea for legalization, but also an appeal for a public health plan for birth control. Is it not, she wrote, "the right of an individual to demand, yes, *demand* of sci-ence, of the medical profession and of the State, the benefit of the knowledge society has accumulated on the subject?"

In lieu of the kind of government public health guidelines she sought and that were ubiquitous in the government's anti-VD campaign, Sanger issued her own. In November 1918 she published her recommendations for when a woman should avoid childbirth. She established a minimum childbearing age of 22 and a preferred age of at least 25 (when "she has attained a ripe physical and mental development"). Sanger advocated waiting two to three years between pregnancies ("the mother requires at least this much time to regain her normal strength"). She advised against having chil-dren when either parent had any number of diseases ("tuberculosis, gonorrhea, syphi-lis, cancer, epilepsy, insanity, drunkenness, or mental disorders" and "In the case of the mother, heart disease, kidney trouble, and pelvic deformities"). She also discour-aged having additional children after the birth of a "physically or mentally defective" child and ruled out bearing children "whenever the conditions of life and the uncer-tainty of livelihood make it improbable that children can be given proper care. . . ." Sanger's efforts to underscore the health benefits of and biological arguments for birth control shifted the movement into a better position to gain credibility from within the medical and eugenic communities and take advantage of both official and public interest in sexual science.[30]

POSTWAR PROBLEMS

In the short term, the upheavals brought by war and the Red Scare, which did not begin to recede until more than a year after armistice, inhibited the growth of the birth control movement. The two national organizations, the NBCL and *BCR*, remained New York-centric. The Committee of One Hundred existed in name but had been largely subsumed by the NBCL. The Committee of One Thousand, another support group that cropped up in 1917 under the direction of Dr. Ira Wile, does not appear to have conducted any meaningful work. Regional groups had declined in numbers—about 10 fewer in 1919 than 1917—and scope of activities. Most significantly, by 1919 the leadership of the movement was in disarray.

Sanger, suffering from a flare-up of tubercular lymph nodes, exhaustion, and financial worry, went west to spend the winter of 1919 in southern California to regain her strength and begin a book that set out to merge feminist arguments for birth control with theories of eugenic improvement. Her health declined again that fall, and she turned inward. Immersed in morbid thoughts, she wrote impulsive farewell letters to her estranged husband and several former lovers, and temporarily handed the editing duties of the *Review* over to Mary Knoblauch, a NYWPC board member. Sanger ended the year in a sanitarium in Staten Island, New York. When the Supreme Court dismissed the Brownsville appeal in November 1919, leaving the Crane decision intact, Sanger could not offer her followers any clear indication of what came next. Her long absences from New York and failure to devise a clear postwar agenda created an opportunity for Mary Dennett to assert her strengths as an organizer.[31]

THE VOLUNTARY PARENTHOOD LEAGUE AND THE BATTLE OF THE BILLS

Dennett, frustrated with the inability of the NBCL to establish state legislative campaigns and stay solvent, decided to start over with a new national organization, launched in May of 1919. The Voluntary Parenthood League (VPL), she announced, would engage in an educational and lobbying campaign in Washington to repeal the federal Comstock laws. Dennett lured a number of NBCL members and well-known birth control supporters to join her, including William Robinson, the Reverend John Haynes Holmes, and Katharine Dexter McCormick, immediately lending the group some prestige. The NBCL could not survive the shakeup and disbanded several months later, with many members signing on to the VPL. Dennett extended an invitation to Sanger to serve on the VPL executive committee, but Sanger passed, still smarting from Dennett's earlier calculated snubs. By the summer of 1919, Dennett

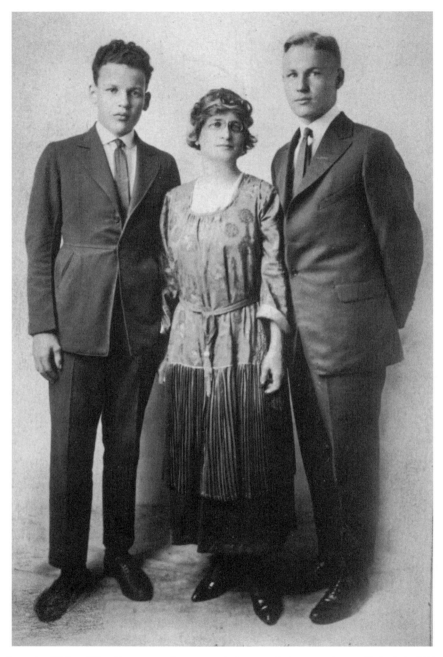

Portrait of Mary Ware Dennett and sons in 1919, around the time she established the Voluntary Parenthood League. (Courtesy of the Schlesinger Library, Radcliffe Institute, Harvard University.)

had shifted into full gear with the VPL legislative program and had begun preliminary interviews with prospective bill sponsors in Washington.

Sanger reacted to Dennett's legislative initiative defensively, using the *BCR* to
criticize the VPL's proposed bill and highlight her alternative one. Sanger had previously expressed minimal interest in pressing for federal legislative change, believing it
to be unattainable in the near term, though she did hold out slightly more hope for
state reforms. Both Dennett and Sanger resurrected competing bills drafted by the
NBCL and BCLNY in 1916 to amend the New York State Penal Code. Though they
both believed that contraceptive information was of legitimate scientific importance
and had been erroneously labeled by the Comstock laws as obscene, they differed
over whether it should be available without restriction to married couples. Dennett
advocated a complete repeal of the law that would strike out the words "prevention
of conception" in five separate sections of the Federal Criminal Code. Also called
the "unlimited" or "open bill," if passed it would have enabled lay people to impart
contraceptive information, send materials through the mails, and distribute contraception without medical oversight. Alternatively, Sanger backed a "doctors-only" bill
that sought to exempt physicians, nurses, and midwives from the prohibition and to
remove (in most incarnations of the bill) any association between birth control and
indecency.[32]

Sanger's commitment to forging a clinic-based contraceptive delivery system neces-
sitated practical considerations that hinged on medical regulation. She framed the
issue around her preferred method, the diaphragm, which required individual fitting.
If "everyone is permitted to impart information," she wrote in the summer of 1919,
"those who receive it have no guaranty that it is correct or suitable to the individual's physical requirements." Medical control would increase effectiveness, and, most
important, ensure better standards of safety. In an unregulated environment, Sanger
argued, women would be deluged with harmful quack remedies and inferior products, and the line between contraception and abortion would be too easily blurred.
In theory, a doctors-only bill provided at least some assurance that "the important
factors of health, physiological structure, temperament, and economic condition can
be considered and their requirements accurately met." She added:

> A system of disseminating information which depends largely upon neighbors, friends,
> and kindly relatives is not likely to give the best results. Neither is it likely to improve
> present methods and develop more desirable ones. I do not believe it to be more advis-
> able to have an amateur instructor in contraceptives than to rely upon an amateur
> dentist or surgeon.

Dennett was incensed by Sanger's sudden interest in federal legislation, just weeks
after Dennett launched the VPL. She viewed Sanger's public disapproval of an open

bill as petty and obstructionist. She roiled at the hypocrisy of Sanger's doctors-only endorsement, knowing that Sanger, a laywoman, persisted in handing out *Family Limitation* and meeting with women in her office. Added to that, Sanger continued to champion birth control for the poor, yet her proposed bill would favor the middle- and upper-classes, which had better access to medical care. How can one "account," Dennett later wrote, "for Mrs. Sanger's extraordinary swing of the pendulum from revolutionary defiance of all law to advocacy of special-privilege class legislation. . . ." Dennett feared that the doctors-only bill "would create a medical monopoly of the dispensing of information." She dismissed Sanger's concerns that an open bill would unleash unreliable and dangerous information, arguing that such spurious publications would not be able to compete with authoritative guides.

Both reformers were somewhat disingenuous in their rhetoric. Dennett was unwilling to admit that returning to the free market system in the contraceptive trade that operated prior to the Comstock laws would expose women to harmful and ineffective products; it remained a huge problem even under the Comstock restrictions. But she was a stickler for the letter of the law and could not fathom continuing her birth control activism in an environment—either under the Comstock Law or a doctors-only amended version—in which violation of the law was the rule and doctor-supplied birth control the exception. "A legal house-cleaning," she wrote, "seems the only hope for putting this country on either a self-respecting or a democratic basis, so far as this subject is concerned." For her part, Sanger downplayed her deep distrust of the medical profession and failed to address the fact that very few doctors and nurses received training in this area or were in any better position to inform women than, for instance, many social workers. Sanger's advocacy of the doctors-only bill had, at this stage, more to do with frustrating Dennett's push for power than achieving sensible legislative change. She made it abundantly clear that a legislative fight was not her first priority: "The most important thing in the movement is not to change the law, but to relieve the suffering of overburdened women, law or no law. Meanwhile, however, it becomes desirable incidentally, to seek to change the statute. . . ."[33]

In the short term, the VPL bill had greater appeal to birth controllers, many of whom stood for complete repeal on principle and sought a unified movement. As longtime birth control activist and open bill supporter James F. Morton wrote in the *BCR*, "we are suddenly faced with a division in our ranks" which he believed opponents would exploit to their advantage. However, the open bill showed little prospect for Congressional sponsorship, let alone passage, and Dennett's limited medical support gradually pulled away. Sanger's legislative approach showed much more political savvy and pragmatism. The doctors-only bill complemented the Crane decision and anticipated future cooperation and compromise with physicians. It also promised, on the surface at least, to be more palatable to legislators aghast at the thought of contraceptive free will.

Less immediately apparent, the doctors-only bill was yet another manifestation of Sanger's evolving strategy to lift birth control to a higher plane, to a respected field of scientific endeavor. "The scientist," she bragged in 1920, "is giving it reverent and profound attention." Along with emphasizing public health, Sanger had, since the war, increasingly worked to define the cause as something weightier than pregnancy and disease prevention—as "a high mission of freedom and regeneration," nothing less than "a working social philosophy." She spoke in these years of birth control as a social, biological, and economic force that must be subject to scientific scrutiny in a carefully managed environment. The doctors-only bill continued the movement on this trajectory. Medical oversight would facilitate controlled research studies, lead to better contraceptive devices and advance a more thorough understanding of the long-term health and economic benefits of birth control. Sanger saw unfettered access to contraception as threatening to hinder the movement's scientific progress by thwarting the establishment of guidelines and professional standards that could only exist in a medically-directed setting.[34]

RIVAL LEADERS

The sparring over legislative strategy energized both Dennett and Sanger and created two distinct camps in the movement that pulled further apart heading into the new decade. The resumption of their rivalry seemed to break Sanger out of her funk, and her more sanguine disposition returned after a restorative trip to England in the spring of 1920. Before Sanger left town, Dennett resigned from the NYWPC in January 1920, ostensibly over a Sanger editorial in the *BCR* that called on women to go on a five-year "birth strike" to alleviate demands on a limited postwar food supply. Dennett said her federal lobbying work was "seriously menaced" by the article because it was "injecting into the situation a militantly feministic policy. . . ." Sanger seemed relieved to have her out of her way. And Dennett, encamped in Washington much of the time, could now declare she was no longer associated with the more radical wing of the movement.

The jostling for leadership was relatively short-lived. Dennett had trouble finding and keeping a sponsor for her bill and was again running low on money. She no longer had a space in the *BCR* to air her views, and her cautious maneuvering and avoidance of controversy kept her and the VPL out of the newspapers, with no significant public or media leverage to pressure congressional votes. Meanwhile Sanger, who returned from England and a tour of war-torn Germany in the fall of 1920, was sought after by women's and civic groups for her international perspective. In terms of public exposure and leadership identification, it was no match: Sanger remained the face and voice of birth control. Even so, over the next two years, Sanger rather cunningly took steps to isolate Dennett and her cohorts—leaving them off of invitations, keeping VPL letters and articles out of the *BCR*, and attacking Dennett's character behind her back.[35]

WOMAN AND THE NEW RACE AND THE MOTHERS' LETTERS

Sanger received a new round of press attention following the October 1920 publication of *Woman and the New Race*, her first original book apart from the early pamphlet series. Havelock Ellis supplied an introduction and the socialist writer Billy Williams reworked Sanger's disjointed prose into a fluid—and at times florid—style. She did not intend for the book to educate the working class but rather targeted feminists and social-control progressives who were working to find government solutions to social problems and who had not yet made a place for birth control in public health endeavors. Many feminists and women's rights groups had been wary of birth control because they believed it was too focused on women's sexuality—still a discomforting topic in feminist circles—and could be perceived as being disparaging of motherhood and chaste living. The well-known suffragist Carrie Chapman Catt wrote to Sanger, "Your reform is too narrow to appeal to me and too sordid." In the book, Sanger tried to change both of these perceptions, presenting birth control as a broad social reform, a "fundamental remedy" for "child slavery, prostitution, feeble-mindedness, physical deterioration, hunger, oppression, and war," and a means of attaining sexual fulfillment "through knowledge and the cultivation of a higher, happier attitude toward sex. Sex life must be stripped of its fear. This is one of the great functions of contraceptives."

As Sanger biographer Ellen Chesler explained, *Woman and the New Race* "was written in the extreme, exhortatory style characteristic of the radicals," replete with affirmations, admonishments, and evangelizing. It was more forceful than most feminist tracts and, contradictions and false assumptions notwithstanding, made a clear argument that a woman finally had the tools to emerge from reproductive bondage and "assume her responsibility" to create a better human race. Coming just after the enactment of women's suffrage and in the midst of the birth control movement's internal arguments over medical control of contraception, Sanger chose an opportune time to reassert that the movement stood for a "woman's *basic* freedom" that women, individually and as a group, must fight to secure. "No woman can call herself free who does not own and control her body," Sanger wrote midway in the book, in what has become a familiar aphorism for the reproductive rights movement. "No woman can call herself free until she can choose consciously whether she will or will not be a mother."[36]

More than any other birth control publication, *Woman and the New Race* generated an unprecedented response from women seeking contraceptive advice. Published by the New York bookseller, Brentano's, the book sold out three editions in a little over a year, due in no small part to deceptive advertisements that erroneously suggested it contained actual contraceptive advice. The closest the author came to practicalities was a brief description of the birth control clinics in the Netherlands. Thousands of women, sometimes several hundred a week, wrote to Sanger in reference to the book and in need of birth control information, sexual and relationship advice, or simply someone to hear their story. Sanger had been receiving these "mothers' letters," as they became known, since *The Woman Rebel*. She regularly published a selection of them in the *BCR* and included excerpts in *Woman and the New Race*. Other activists had been deluged in the past with similar letters, including Rose Pastor Stokes in 1916 to 1917 when her name was often in the news, and William Robinson following the publication of his books. But no one received anywhere near the number of letters as Sanger. She eventually had to hire staff to answer them. Though she claimed to have responded to thousands of such letters, it is unclear how many women received useful replies, as few of Sanger's responses survive. To some women she did send the name of a nearby sympathetic doctor, an address of a contraceptive manufacturer, and/or a copy of *Family Limitation*.

The majority of extant letters are from the rural poor, those who had limited choice in doctors, were distant from urban centers, and who had few places to turn to for help.* These letters share a remarkably similar sensibility. They often include affirmations of motherhood, faith in God, and love for family, along with both veiled and direct criticisms of the medical and social practices that placed men in control of fertility. Husbands, as depicted in the letters, carried on a tradition of sexual self-fulfillment. The letters generally portrayed male doctors as mum on birth control even though they increasingly influenced all aspects of childbearing, reversing a long history in America of women asserting nearly complete control over their most sacred and empowering domain. Over and over again, women who complained of constant work, few pleasures, and indifferent husbands wrote to Sanger that they just wanted to do the "right thing," to be the "right" kind of mother or wife. They feared that they were letting others down because their bodies and temperaments did not recover from incessant pregnancies. "Mrs. Sanger I have always been a decent girl & I am still a decent Woman," wrote a mother from Galatia, Illinois, after reading *Woman and the New Race*. "I am a believer in the God above & I want to lead a Christian life but

---

* Most of the mothers' letters have not been found. They were treated as confidential client records and probably destroyed. Several hundred letters are interspersed in Sanger's papers in the Library of Congress and the Sophia Smith Collection, Smith College, and a book-length selection of transcribed letters was published by Sanger in 1928 under the title *Motherhood in Bondage*.

it is awful, awful hard to live it & give birth & carry babies & care for them & suffer & nearly die with misery & pain & do what is right." A frequent refrain appears in many of the letters, "I would rather die than have another baby."[37]

More often than not these women felt compelled to chronicle their reproductive histories as justification for their request. "Married at 20 to a laboring man," wrote a woman from Nevada, "in eleven years I had 5 living children, 1 still born, and 5 miscarriages. Left a widow at 35 with no means of support and 3 children at school." Another from Florida told Sanger, "My parents rushed me into marriage at 16 yrs. In 5 yrs time I had 4 living babies, but one of them died with pneumonia." From Minnesota, a woman wrote:

> Dear Mrs. Sanger:
>   Your book of "Woman and the New Race" received. But did not get what I most needed in it is some very important help. Now I would like to ask you to help me as soon as you can. I am a mother of 11 children, 10 living. Green, that is what I am, only 34 years old and am 3 months in a family way again. I have a man that thinks it's my fault because we have children. I do confess it is.

The letters became an anecdotal source of the health consequences arising from too frequent childbirth and too many children born into poverty. Later in the decade, one of Sanger's assistants, Mary Sumner Boyd, tabulated the ailments and diseases mentioned in a random sample of 5,000 letters sent to Sanger over many years. At least 100 specified illness or injury among children, including rickets, tuberculosis, dropsy (edema), blindness, deafness, abscesses, convulsions, VD, kidney disease, eczema, and various unknown ailments. Eight hundred fifty letters in the sample reported serious maternal health problems related to pregnancy and parturition. Women attributed asthma, epilepsy, influenza, tuberculosis, goiter, heart, bladder and kidney trouble to pregnancy, as well as "intolerable itching," St. Vitus's dance (chorea), back problems, partial paralysis, piles (hemorrhoids), rupture, constipation, liver and stomach complications, severe varicose veins, dizziness, numbness, deafness, blindness, and insanity. Many of the same conditions were given as a consequence of childbirth, along with infections, puerperal fever, lacerations, adherent placenta, hemorrhages, fistula, prolapsed or retroverted uterus, blood poisoning, abnormal weakness, lameness, and breast abnormalities. The analysis claimed that nearly 10 percent of the women were invalids, but gave no criteria for the finding.[38]

The mothers' letters demonstrate as well as any source the prevalence of abortion in the early 20th century. Roughly a third mention abortion or describe a means of family limitation or experience of miscarriage that could be construed as a reference to abortion. Though it is impossible to estimate the percentage of terminated pregnancies at this time, the abortion expert Frederick Taussig came up with a widely accepted formula that pegged one abortion to every 2.5 births in urban areas and one to every five births in rural districts. Progressive Era antiabortion campaigns, which had mostly dissolved after the war, had done little to stem the tide of abortions or reduce the number of abortionists, although they did make it more difficult and anxiety-ridden in regions that aggressively enforced the law. Many women freely admitted to Sanger that they regularly resorted to abortifacients or visited abortion doctors. Some were not clear about the difference between contraception and abortion. A number of the letter writers held back this information because of the stigma and legal implications. Quite a few of the mothers divided their births into "live" and "dead," and grouped together abortions, miscarriages, and stillbirths. Some of the indirect references to abortion include "getting rid" of a baby, "taking drugs," or the "awful thing." One typical letter writer asked Sanger "if you could help me in some way to have me miscarry this third baby of mine . . . for I just dread the kind of life that I am leading." Sanger relied on these letters to remind supporters and opponents alike that abortion remained an all too conventional form of family limitation because of limited access to contraception. "Family limitation will always be practiced as it is now being practiced—either by birth control or by abortion. We know that," she wrote in *Woman and the New Race*. "The one means health and happiness—a stronger, better race. The other means disease, suffering, death."[39]

The movement employed the mothers' letters nearly every step of the way. Dennett, who also received hundreds of letters from women in reproductive distress, sent out a small selection to members of congress during her VPL lobbying campaign in the early 1920s. She was inspired to do so by stories of Comstock's success when he circulated in Congress examples of pornography and sex toys that provoked Congressmen into passing his obscenity bill. In 1921, Sanger and Juliet Rublee assembled about a dozen letters written by mothers in response to *Woman and the New Race* and published them as *Appeals from American Mothers*, which the NYWPC used for fundraising and propaganda needs. At key moments in Sanger's oration and in her writings, she dispensed with statistics and expert opinion and drove home her point with excerpts from the mothers' letters. The movement relied on these desperate calls for help much like abortion rights groups in the late 1960s used speak-outs to publicize individual women's stories about illegal abortion. These types of emotional propaganda tactics embolden movement workers and knock opponents off their talking points. Mary Sumner Boyd told an interviewer, "They get you. You cannot read them without something happening to you inside, which you do not get over."[40]

PROMOTION AND EXPANSION

By the end of 1920 the *BCR* group was having trouble keeping up with the response to *Woman and the New Race*, increased demands on Sanger's schedule, and several new undertakings. The NYWPC had enlisted Mary Halton to explore the possibility of opening a clinic in New York City, and Sanger began looking for physicians to sponsor such an endeavor. Sanger also formed, in December 1920, a legislative committee to lobby for a doctors-only bill in the New York State legislature that would reinforce the Crane decision and clarify the legal foundation for a clinic. She kicked off the new campaign with a luncheon of 500 prominent women in New York, another effort to expand the movement's base of society women.

Between November 1920 and April 1921, Sanger made 46 appearances to speak or debate on birth control, including a speech before the National Women's Party convention in Washington in February. There she unsuccessfully attempted to convince the women's rights organization that it should endorse birth control as part of

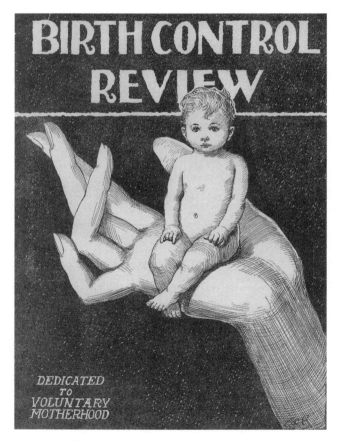

Cover of the *Birth Control Review*, February 1921. (Courtesy of the Sophia Smith Collection, Smith College.)

its post–Nineteenth Amendment agenda. Party head Alice Paul believed issues such as birth control and black women's voting rights confused the organization's focused efforts on pursuing equal rights legislation for women.

In the spring of 1921 Sanger sent out 200 queries to prominent professionals across the country who supported birth control, including physicians, eugenicists, sociologists, and economists, asking their opinion about holding a national birth control conference in the fall of 1921. The positive response convinced her to forge ahead with conference plans. Heading into the summer of 1921, it was readily apparent that the *BCR* staff and the NYWPC board were too small to handle Sanger's ambitious plans.

Several factors, including the need for a larger staff, pushed Sanger grudgingly toward the formation of a new and broader organization. Operating much of the time as a free agent, she had avoided joining the NBCL, the BCLNY, and the VPL, citing the tendency of such groups to be "rigid, lifeless, and soulless." Yet she lacked the prestige that an organization could give her, prestige that a publication could not offer. More importantly, Sanger needed a more conventional organization to attract the broad support from the professional class and scientific community that she believed was crucial to changing the law and building a network of clinics. By late 1920 Sanger had already begun making moves toward this goal, bringing in Anne Kennedy, an experienced club organizer from California, to begin to systematize the often chaotic *BCR* office and take over Sanger's schedule. In the spring of 1921 Kennedy helped Sanger establish a conference committee and the rudiments of a new league, which Sanger announced would be formed at the close of the "First American Birth Control Conference" to be held in New York City in mid-November.[41]

THE FIRST AMERICAN BIRTH CONTROL CONFERENCE

The conference, Sanger's largest organizational undertaking to date, was deliberately scheduled to follow the Second International Congress of Eugenics, held at the Natural History Museum in New York, and to coincide with the American Public Health Association's semi-centennial convention and "Health Fortnight" in midtown Manhattan. The Washington Naval Conference and disarmament talks began the same week, and Sanger hoped to draw international attention from the many reporters and dignitaries arriving in the United States to cover the negotiations. The form letters and flyers that went out, and the announcements in the *BCR* promoted the conference as "recognition of Birth Control as the Science of Population"; an "open discussion" by "men and women of international importance"; "A New Approach" and "A New Diagnosis"; "a fundamental step toward National and Racial Health. The Abolition of Poverty. Disarmament and World Peace." Invitations were specifically tailored to eugenicists and public health workers. The conference committee included many of the same old names from the Committee of One Hundred and other groups, but with the addition of several prominent eugenicists and social scientists, including Lothrop Stoddard, the most popular eugenics writer of the time, the well-known economist Irving Fisher, and the Harvard biologist and eugenicist, Edward M. East. There was a noticeable absence of references to women in the promotional materials and proposed conference agenda.[42]

Through the conference and the creation of a new national league, Sanger aspired to "reach into every state in the Union" and pull the disparate elements of the movement together. She invited birth control leagues and women's organizations from across the country to the pioneering event. However, she did not inform the VPL or invite Mary Dennett to participate. The animosity between the two rivals had deepened earlier in the year when the New York Academy of Medicine rejected the VPL's legislative program, but its Health Committee endorsed Sanger's more physician-friendly state bill. Then Sanger used a *BCR* editorial to urge all birth control supporters to abandon the VPL-sponsored open bill, prompting a remonstrative letter-to-the-editor from Dennett that Sanger refused to publish. Nor would Sanger give publicity to Dennett's fledgling journal, the *Birth Control Herald*.

As soon as Dennett got her hands on a conference brochure she wrote to the *BCR* board to ask that the VPL be given time to present. Additionally, she wanted the delegates to vote on whether to create a new organization or enlarge the VPL, "the only existing national organization." In a personal letter to Sanger, Dennett called for a joining of forces now that Sanger had again "fluctuated" and decided to adopt an organizational as well as a legislative approach. Dennett further irked Sanger by disclosing that she intended to open "some special independent *demonstration* clinics in a few big cities," an idea that appeared to contradict Dennett's efforts to respect the law. Reluctantly, Sanger sent a tardy invitation to Dennett, requesting that she submit a report on the VPL to be read at the conference. Their rancor intensified in the lead-up to the conference when Dennett invited Marie Stopes, who opened England's first birth control clinic in March, to speak in New York in late October under the auspices of the VPL. Sanger had worked closely with Stopes and helped promote her books in the United States, and she cautioned Stopes that Dennett was "outside the pale of honesty & decency" and that the VPL had brought "disintegration to the cause." Stopes, who claimed to support both American leaders, nevertheless shared Sanger's letters with Dennett who then threatened Sanger with charges of libel and slander. The tension reached a violent breaking point at the close of the conference.[43]

The conference went smoothly right up to the last day. Over 300 delegates attended the three-day event at the Plaza Hotel, including more than 100 from the American Public Health Association. At the opening session, conference organizers urged the delegates to send telegrams to the concurrent disarmament conference and to the

U.S. Congress calling for commissions to study the role of birth control in relation to world peace. The maneuver, part of a clever promotional effort started by press release a month before the conference, generated news headlines across the nation linking birth control with lower population rates, the potential for increased food supplies, and a cessation of world hostilities.* This was followed by a session on "Overpopulation and War" on day two. Other sessions focused on health, social problems, and legal aspects of birth control, with a disproportionate number of speakers from medicine and academia rather than from activist causes and social services. In comparison to past discussions, there was a definite shift in emphasis from free speech rights and issues related to women's sexual emancipation, to societal and scientific concerns about the quality of human life, articulated in the new nomenclature of eugenics.

The first day of the conference also included a closed-door (its legality was questionable) medical meeting on contraception that exhibited a disconcerting lack of consensus among medical practitioners who regularly dispensed contraception. Not one of the major methods was found to be without serious flaws, and two male physicians regarded common types of pessaries (cervical caps and diaphragms) as injurious to most women. Sanger, who had attended the International Congress on Contraceptives in Amsterdam in August, and who probably had more experience with occlusive pessaries than anyone else in the meeting hall, reviewed the widespread success experienced in Holland and elsewhere with the Mizpah pessary. The renegade Boston physician and socialist Antoinette Konikow, and Sanger's own doctor, Mary Halton, concurred with Sanger's findings, and the women battled to defend the ease of use and effectiveness of the Mizpah and similar models against methods, such as the condom and suppositories, that limited women's control or interfered with sexual pleasure. The group discussed a number of other methods, including a new contraceptive jelly from Germany and a controversial x-ray sterilization technique that had shown positive results in temporarily sterilizing both men and women. Dr. Edward W. Lee, a gynecologist, advocated vasectomy as a simple and safe sterilization procedure for men. His interest failed to impress the others who, like most in the medical establishment, thought it wise to preserve a man's ability to father a second brood later in life, even if it meant greater hassle and hardship for women.

Sanger also shared some of the data that she had collected from one of the few surveys of contraceptive use to date. The *BCR* staff had sent out a questionnaire on contraception to 31,000 names taken from various subscription and mailing lists. They ended up with 1,250 complete responses, which showed that roughly a third of

---

* See, for instance, "Birth Control May Be Argued at Arm Parley," *Tulsa Daily World*, October 13, 1921; "Family Limitation Seen as War Cure," *Washington Post*, November 5, 1921; "Birth Control Urged to Bring World Peace," Ft. Wayne, Indiana, *News Sentinel*, November 11, 1921.

the sample relied on condoms and a third on some form of pessary. The remaining couples that reported regular birth control use listed suppositories and coitus interruptus, followed by the sponge, the "safe period," and cotton plugs. Douches were widely used but mostly in combination with another method. Most striking were the number (the survey identified at least 16) of douching solutions, including Lysol (by far the most popular), salt, vinegar, cream of tartar, soap suds, Listerine, iodine, and borax. There was one vasectomy and two female sterilizations listed.[44]

Sanger waited until a formal dinner the second night of the conference to announce that the first legal birth control clinic would be opened the following week in the Lower East Side of Manhattan, where she used to work as a visiting nurse. Prior to the conference, Sanger and Mary Halton had secured the support of several New York physicians. Among them was the eminent pediatrician, L. Emmett Holt, the Dr. Spock of his day, known for his bestselling childcare bible, *The Care and Feeding of Infants*. His name lured other doctors, but none of them wanted to actually run the clinic. Finally, Sanger got a commitment from the gynecologist Lydia Allen DeVilbiss, part of William Robinson's fleeting Committee of Birth Control in 1915 and a fearless and experienced public health doctor. She had joined the staff of St. Mark's Hospital in New York earlier in 1921 and had started a small contraceptive dispensary clinic that she later claimed was the first in the nation, though a number of other doctors had quietly done the same. Sanger claimed to have lined up 40 other physicians to be associated with the clinic, 30 in regular attendance. The clinic would operate strictly within the confines of the law, explained Anne Kennedy, and "afford an opportunity to women suffering from a disease, such as tuberculosis, to inform themselves." A hat was passed and about $1,200 collected. There was talk of clinics opening in other cities, starting with Baltimore. The news made for a resounding conclusion to the main program of the conference, but it was immediately overshadowed by the events that interrupted the final meeting.[45]

THE TOWN HALL RAID

The concluding public meeting on Sunday evening at the Town Hall theater was widely advertised in the press as a way to "Get the facts about Birth Control." Sanger was scheduled to give a closing address and introduce keynote speaker Harold Cox, the editor of the *Edinburgh Review* and a former Member of Parliament, who had become part of Sanger's social group in England. The theme of the night was the morality of birth control. But before Sanger and Cox arrived, police had raided the hall and locked the doors, keeping out hundreds who waited outside and locking in nearly a thousand who had already taken their seats. When the police announced that the meeting would not be permitted and opened the doors to escort the crowd out, a rush of new people pushed in, carrying Sanger and Cox along with them.

Sanger was lifted onto the stage to the chant, "Defy them! Defy them!" She quieted the crowd and cried out, "This meeting is not suspended. It is a legal meeting, legally announced. We have a right to hold it under the Constitution. . . . Let them club us if they want to."

Two officers seized her arms, but she pulled away to the front of the stage and began her prepared remarks to a crowd that was yelling taunts and hissing at the police. A sergeant told her to stop speaking and again grabbed her arms, as scores of people climbed up on the stage in a show of support, including Juliet Rublee, Lydia DeVilbiss, and Sanger's publisher, Lowell Brentano. Near pandemonium broke out with several women trying to speak to the crowd about birth control, another group huddling around Sanger and several others calling for an uprising against the police. Captain Thomas Donohue, the officer in charge (who coincidentally had been the precinct commander in Brownsville during the clinic arrests in 1916) backed by a force of nearly 100 men, ordered Sanger to leave the stage. She refused and was arrested for disorderly conduct, along with Mary Winsor, a veteran suffragist and conference committee member, who would not quiet down. Police then escorted the two women out of the hall as the crowd broke into "My Country 'Tis of Thee." Out on the street, Sanger and Winsor resisted getting into the police wagon and instead were led on foot the several blocks to the precinct station, followed by a crowd of over 1,000 and a procession of cars and limousines. The women were booked on public disorder charges, taken to night court, and released to counsel. Wire reports relayed the news of the raid and arrests across the country, casting the phrase *birth control* again in bold headlines.

Amid the chaos that ensued in the police station, Mary Dennett made her way in and approached reporters with the intent of giving a statement of support for Sanger on free speech grounds. According to Dennett, as she waited to speak to a reporter, Juliet Rublee turned and struck her, "with a backward swing of her arm, saying 'This is our affair, we don't want you in it.'" Dennett wrote to Rublee later that night seeking an apology and attributing Rublee's behavior to the "emotional stress" of the evening, but neither Rublee nor Sanger would acknowledge any wrongdoing on Rublee's part. They countered Dennett's allegation with one of their own—that Dennett had informed New York detectives that Sanger had been sending illegal pamphlets through the mails. When VPL members wrote to Sanger to express their outrage over Rublee's aggressive act, Sanger replied that Dennett was not of sound mind. The incident furthered the divide between Sanger's supporters and the VPL and pushed Dennett farther to the fringe of the movement.[46]

The Town Hall raid turned into tabloid sensation in New York when reporters learned the following day that Catholic Archbishop Patrick J. Hayes had directed his secretary, Monsignor Joseph P. Dineen, to pressure police to shut the meeting down. Dineen had called police brass and met with Captain Donohue at Town Hall prior to Sanger's arrival. He had pointed out four children in the audience and demanded that Donohue take immediate action. "Decent and clean-minded people," he told the press, "would not discuss a subject such as birth control in public before children or at all." His remarks made for alarming news and were echoed and exaggerated in editorial reaction. The *Tulsa Daily World*, for instance, decried the "number of young boys and girls" in the Town hall audience. The four children, it turned out, were Barnard College students with bobbed hair, attending the meeting as a class assignment. The birth control contingent demanded an investigation to discover who authorized the raid. An indignant press accused the police of intimidation and persecution—"a clear violation of recognized civil rights," wrote the editor of the *New York Tribune*. However, the more conservative *New York Times* scolded the activists for failing to obey the police, comparing them to "a crowd of anarchists."

The next morning, a magistrate dismissed the charges against Sanger and Winsor for lack of evidence. On leaving court, Sanger explained that she had sent a personal invitation to attend the Town Hall meeting to Father John Ryan, who directed the Social Action Department of the National Catholic Welfare Council, the Catholic group most actively engaged in opposing birth control legislation. The Council had been working assiduously against both Dennett's open bill in Washington and Sanger efforts in 1921 to get a doctors-only bill passed in Albany. The invitation may have egged on the Catholic hierarchy in New York. Sanger added that she had rescheduled the closing conference meeting and sent an invitation to Archbishop Hayes "to present the Catholic Church's side of birth control." He had not responded.

The imbroglio with the police and Church obscured news of an event that did not happen as planned—the clinic opening. Sanger had not been able to obtain a dispensary license from the State Board of Charities, and Lydia DeVilbiss refused to risk her medical license on an unsanctioned clinic. It did not help that the Public Health Committee of the New York Academy of Medicine issued a statement that it "emphatically opposed . . . the methods, principles, and program" espoused by Sanger, even though it had earlier offered a tepid endorsement of her doctors-only bill. The much ballyhooed medical support for the clinic may have been exaggerated, judging from the relative silence among pro-birth control physicians after it was announced that the plans had been shelved.

The rescheduled final meeting of the conference took place on November 18 under heavy surveillance but without incident. The publicity had drawn an overflow crowd of several thousand, many of whom had to be turned away. Birth control workers and Paulist fathers competed to sell pamphlets and books outside the theater. The press reported that, since the raid, Sanger had sold about 1,000 copies a day of *Woman and the New Race*. Inside she gave her closing remarks, following an intense panel discussion between three birth control advocates and four opponents. With nearly 2,000 people and a large press contingent in attendance, Sanger questioned the logic of the opposition's prevailing alternative to artificial birth control: abstinence or as many phrased it, "self-control." She said,

> Now I contend that the argument is perfectly absurd because it places man upon the same level as animals. In other words, you use the procreative act only for procreation, and I contend that there is another side, and another use of this relationship. I contend that it is just as sacred and just as beautiful for two people to express their love when they have no intention whatsoever of being parents.

By now this type of frank sentiment brought more blush than controversy; all the same, this simple affirmation of a nonprocreative sexual bond was rarely uttered in a public forum. Bringing the issue back to a very human equation, Sanger's words ended a groundbreaking conference that largely achieved her goal of advancing the movement along scientific lines. As the *Tribune* concluded, "People may differ about the questions raised by the advocates of birth control. The subject is one, however, for serious public discussion."[47]

BIRTH CONTROL VERSUS THE CATHOLIC CHURCH

More wire reports went out two days later when Archbishop Hayes ended his silence and released a statement on birth control. Although he did not specifically comment on the Town Hall raid, he asserted that discussions on birth control should take place only "within the walls of a clinic." At the same time he questioned the legitimacy of the movement:

> The law of God and man, science, public policy, human experience, are all condemnatory of birth control as preached by a few irresponsible individuals, without indorsement or approval . . . of a reputable body of physicians or a medical society, whose province it is to advise the public on such matters.

Despite the public declarations by scores of scientists in favor of family limitation, at both the birth control and eugenics conferences, Hayes insisted that the most respected scientists opposed the tenets of birth control. Curiously, he applauded the eugenics congress for encouraging a "better-born" race and "more children in the families of the well-to-do as a moral duty," revealing an unseemly class bias. He then justified large families by stating that successive children are more likely to succeed and geniuses are often born after the fifth child. The seventh position in the birth line, he claimed, was particularly propitious. As others had before, Hayes noted that Ben Franklin was the fifteenth child in his family, conjecturing that the relative lack of geniuses was because "we are not getting to the ends of families."

Sanger responded in the press the next day, creating an extraordinary public dialogue. She started off by agreeing with the archbishop that "a clinic is the proper place to give information" but clarified that the "theoretical discussion" should be carried out "on the public platform and in the press, as the Archbishop himself has taken the opportunity to do." She then refuted Hayes's theory of the later born genius, cheekily turning to the bible for illustration: "If the Archbishop will recall his Bible history, he will find that some of the most remarkable characters were first children. . . . By the Roman Catholics, Jesus himself is said to be Mary's first as well as her only child."

Hayes thundered back with a doctrinaire condemnation of birth control in the form of a pastoral letter to the Archdiocese. "Children troop down from heaven because God wills it," he stated emphatically. "Woe to those who degrade, pervert, or do violence to the law of nature as fixed by the eternal decree of God Himself!" He called abortion "a horrible crime" and birth control "satanic." He warned, "Keep far from the sanctuary of your Christian homes, as you would an evil spirit, the literature of this unclean abomination." Sanger replied that she had "no objection to the Catholic Church inculcating its doctrines to its own people," but found its attempts to "enforce its opinions and code of morals upon the Protestant members of this country" an "interference with the principles of this democracy."[48]

While Sanger and Hayes locked horns in the press, Sanger's attorney in the Town Hall case, Robert McCurdy Marsh, along with the American Civil Liberties Union, and several physicians and civic leaders, helped initiate an internal police investigation that quickly descended into a farce. Not only did the police inspector grill Sanger on her 1916 conviction, a settled matter, incredibly the investigators arrested Juliet Rublee after she stated she had read the pertinent section of the Penal Code and disagreed with it. "This is nothing but an attempt at intimidation," Rublee told the *New York World*, "but I do not frighten easily." Her arrest made for a new round of headlines and provoked some of New York's most respected leaders, including the financier Paul Warburg and diplomat Henry Mogenthau Sr., to petition the mayor for a formal, city-administered investigation of the police. In late-December 1921, the mayor directed the Commissioner of Accounts to undertake a thorough inquiry into the Town Hall raid and Rublee's arrest. Accusations flew back and forth in the press for several months before the police finally admitted that there were no grounds for shutting down Town Hall or arresting Sanger, Winsor, or Rublee. Captain Donohue was made a scapegoat for his superiors, who denied ordering the raid, and the Commissioner downplayed the influence of the Church. A frustrated Sanger wrote of the outcome: "exactly nothing happened."

The movement's victory, however, was won in the press. In what was clearly becoming a pattern, the suppression and bullying of birth control activists paid incalculable dividends in publicity. In this case in particular, the opposition's disregard for First Amendment rights and its mishandling of investigations created a sense of outrage and exasperation on the part of many in the ruling and professional classes—especially the younger generations—who had not previously come out for birth control but who now came forward in support. The young businessman Robert Lovett, later the Secretary of Defense under President Truman, was among them, as was Evelyn Marshall Field, wife of the heir to the Field department store fortune. She stood in solidarity with the wronged birth control advocates even though she was unsure about the movement, telling a reporter, "I will decide later if I wish to identify myself with it."

The Town Hall episode marked a shift in birth control opposition. In the role of chief antagonist, the government was receding into the background. Sanger, an inveterate Catholic critic, seized the opportunity to publically pull back the curtain on the new enemy. An editorial in the *BCR* stated that Archbishop Hayes' directive to police "has had the invaluable effect of revealing and exposing the source of the opposition to the Birth Control movement in this country . . . the Roman Catholic Church, which attempts—and to a great extent succeeds—to control all questions of public and private morality in these United States." Sanger later wrote, "It was now a battle of a republic against the machinations of the hierarchy of the Roman Catholic Church." She shrewdly tapped into pervasive anti-Catholic bigotry as she looked to score points with Protestant groups and old-line Americans who decried the intrusion of the Catholic Church into secular affairs. Almost overnight, she now attributed to the Church all opposition to the birth control movement, forcing non-Catholic opponents into an uncomfortable association. As historian Leslie Woodcock Tentler has pointed out, by demonizing the Church, Sanger held in check "more conservative Protestant churches, those most likely to oppose contraception," that were "also apt to be the most anti-Catholic. Few of their leaders were eager to make public cause with what Sanger liked to call 'a dictatorship of celibates.'"[49]

THE FORMATION OF THE AMERICAN BIRTH CONTROL LEAGUE

Before the dust of the Town Hall raid had settled, two dozen members of the conference committee and most of the staff of the *BCR* had formally created and joined the American Birth Control League (ABCL). Conference literature hyped the new league as the first truly national organization and predicted a membership of 1 million. Though the league aspired to send out a force of workers to start organizations and clinics in every state, its more modest and immediate mission was to educate the public through outreach efforts such as mailings, conferences, lectures, and exhibits, and to lobby for a New York State amendment. At the ABCL's first annual meeting in January 1922, Sanger was named president and Juliet Rublee, vice-president, along with Charlotte Delafield, a Committee of One Hundred member who was married to a prestigious New York attorney.

The ABCL's "Principles and Aims" codified the movement's scientific make-over and positioned birth control as the keystone to a eugenic program for racial betterment.

> Everywhere we see poverty and large families going hand in hand. Those least fit to carry on the race are increasing most rapidly. People who cannot support their own offspring are encouraged by Church and State to produce large families. Many of the children thus begotten are diseased or feeble-minded; many become criminals. The burden of supporting these unwanted types has to be borne by the healthy elements of the nation. Funds that should be used to raise the standard of our civilization are diverted to the maintenance of those who should never have been born. To create a race of well-born children it is essential that the functions of motherhood should be elevated to a position of dignity, and this is impossible as long as conception remains a matter of chance.

This founding document put a premium on women's health and held that every woman "must possess the power and freedom to prevent conception" and "must be conscious of her responsibility to the race in bringing children into the world." By deftly regarding women's reproductive freedom as a prerequisite to the eugenic improvement of the race, Sanger and the ABCL boldly set out to advance free motherhood as a guiding eugenic principle and unite the two movements, eugenics and birth control, into a "science of population."[50]

BIRTH CONTROL AND EUGENICS

The convergence of eugenics and birth control in the immediate post–World War I period further legitimized the birth control movement and created new opportunities to assess and promote its contributions to social progress. Birth control's acceptance of many eugenic ideas was a natural progression for a movement that had come to focus on the health and medical benefits of contraception and, in an increasingly conservative political climate, needed a new context, removed from radical associations, for its feminist assertions.

The term *eugenics,* meaning the science of human improvement, was conceived in 1883 by the British statistician Sir Francis Galton, who had been influenced by the work of his cousin, Charles Darwin, on evolution by natural selection—the catalyst concept for eugenics. Grounded in biology, eugenics was, nonetheless, a protean field of study in its formative years, enamored of hereditary tendencies but accommodating of diverse—and sometimes contradictory—theories about what caused human behavior, what shaped human intelligence, and what factors ensured the "survival of the fittest"—the Darwinian-sounding phrase introduced by English biologist Herbert Spencer in 1864. The rediscovery of Mendelian genetics (the studies of Gregor

Mendel on hybridized pea plants) at the turn of the century reset eugenics on a more rigid, hereditarian course. Likewise, the advent and immediate popularity of intelligence testing in the pre–World War I years opened the way for an activist agenda to encourage those of better than average intelligence and higher social standing to produce more children (known as positive eugenics) and discourage or prevent the "unfit"—a nebulous category of supposed undesirables, including those who carried a transmissible disease or were of lower intelligence—from having any children (negative eugenics). A number of studies conducted before the war by the American psychologist Henry Goddard, zoologist Charles Davenport, and others in the United States and England advanced the belief that dysgenic groups were breeding excessively, while the strongest and smartest were limiting family size, creating a growing disparity between the fit and the unfit. These pioneering eugenicists specifically targeted the *feebleminded*, another catchall term that lumped together those with certain mental and/or learning disabilities. Their alarming findings added to already well-established fears that traditional white Americans were being overwhelmed in numbers by the poor, by dark-skinned people, and by new immigrants.[51]

Before World War I, eugenics had been widely promoted on lecture circuits and university campuses and had seeped into the popular culture through films, books, and articles in magazines and newspapers. The war magnified concerns about racial health and heightened interest in human betterment initiatives. Public hygiene campaigns were promoted in eugenic terms, postwar eugenic groups proliferated, "fitter family" and "better baby" contests sprang up in middle America, families paid for pedigree analyses, and colleges offered courses in eugenic science alongside of chemistry and biology. The newspapers were filled with stories of eugenic and pronatalist schemes like that of a developer in St. Joseph, Missouri, who would only rent out cottages to childless couples if they agreed to have children within a year. A number of prominent and respected English and American men in the first two decades of the century became associated with and gave credence to the eugenics movement, including Alexander Graham Bell, Theodore Roosevelt, John D. Rockefeller, Charles William Eliot, Winston Churchill, George Bernard Shaw, Havelock Ellis, and H. G. Wells. Eugenics seemed to appeal to conservatives and liberals alike and had few vocal critics, although they were growing in numbers.

The pseudoscientific philosophy was always more show than tell, more of a diagnosis than a treatment. As a remedial force to counter what supporters called the differential birth rate between the top and bottom tiers of society, eugenics had little to offer on a practical scale. Most eugenicists opposed birth control for its shrinking effect (which they often exaggerated) on the middle- and upper-classes and because they did not think the poor and less intelligent would or could effectively use contraception. Instead they urged both voluntary and compulsory sterilization for the unfit, marriage licensing restrictions for those afflicted with VD and other conditions, and education and outreach programs to convince the "better stocks" to have bigger families.[52]

In contrast, the notion that family planning could aid in the eugenic improvement of the human race has always been an underlying factor in the advocacy of birth control in America. Nineteenth-century birth controllers such as Charles Knowlton and later the free lovers Moses Harman and Ezra Heywood advocated child-spacing for health reasons (both the mother's and child's)—a fundamentally eugenic concept. In the early years of the birth control movement, controversy sparked by the Bollinger baby case and Helen Keller's assertion that certain severely disabled persons should never have been born helped link birth control and eugenics for the American public, as did the race suicide debate and Teddy Roosevelt's fatherly entreaties to the middle- and upper-classes to have more children. Physician proponents of birth control, William Robinson and Adolphus Knopf foremost among them, frequently justified the legalization of contraception not to reduce the population but to, in Knopf's words, increase its "vigor by reducing the number [of] physically, mentally, and morally unfit and adding to the number of physically strong, mentally sound, and higher morally developed men and women." Both Emma Goldman and Margaret Sanger warned about the quality of progeny produced by poor women with no access to birth control and resorted to standard eugenic terms such as the *unfit*, the *feebleminded*, and *degenerates*.* In the age of birth control, "Never in the history of the world has woman been so race conscious as she is to-day," Goldman declared. Mary Ware Dennett, though critical of many eugenic assumptions and fear-mongering about the fertility of the poor and nonwhite, recognized after World War I "the possibilities of birth control in connection with racial health . . . and its bearing on eugenics," which because of the loss of manpower "are thus brought to the center of the stage as never before." Many public health programs and hygiene campaigns claimed to be eugenic in the early 1920s. It was fashionable and forward-thinking. The birth control movement asserted in simple terms that it would alleviate social problems and improve the race better than any other social reform.[53]

Sanger was out in front of everyone else in the movement in trying to make birth control relevant to eugenics and to bring well-known eugenicists on board. Her courting of eugenics was an obvious strategic move to position birth control to benefit from the mania over the well-born child. Though she was highly critical of the eugenics movement (and it of her), Sanger marked off their common ground in several articles in the late 1910s, emphasizing that both groups sought to "assist the race toward the elimination of the unfit." She went a step further in *Pivot of*

---

* See, for instance, Sanger's short piece, "The Unfit" in *The Woman Rebel* (April 1914): 10, and Goldman's "The Social Aspects of Birth Control," in *Mother Earth* (April 1916): 468–75.

Civilization in 1922, her follow-up book to *Woman and the New Race* and her most sustained discussion of eugenics, calling the "lack of balance between the birth rate of the 'unfit' and the 'fit' . . . the greatest present menace to civilization." It is important to note that Sanger understood "unfit" to indicate "physical or mental defects." She wrote that "if 'unfit' refers to race or religions, then that is another matter which I frankly deplore."

Pivot was a skillful work of propaganda, designed to "appeal to the scientist for aid, to arouse that interest which will result in widespread research and investigation," rather than target women and the working class. In the book, Sanger goes to great pains to reject Marxism and distance the movement from what she now considered its youthful radical phase. But in trying to win new adherents, she overreached in every way, painting doomsday scenarios of societal parasites and delinquents sucking the world dry, and holding up birth control as "an emergency measure," a panacea for all social ills. Nevertheless, *Pivot* gave the movement something of a road map for finding the intersecting lines of birth control and eugenics.[54]

Sanger's eugenic rationale for birth control borrowed heavily from Havelock Ellis's work on "race regeneration" and his feminist perspective on eugenics. "The breeding of men lies largely in the hands of women," Ellis wrote in 1913. "That is why the question of Eugenics is to a great extent one with the woman question." Ellis found eugenic value in how birth control separated sex for pleasure from the serious business of creating new life. Sanger restated this logical reasoning in more overtly feminist terms, writing, "First: we are convinced that racial regeneration like individual regeneration, must come 'from within.' That is, it must be autonomous, self-directive, and not imposed from without. In other words, every potential parent, and especially every potential mother, must be brought to an acute realization of the primary and central importance of bringing children into this world." If, Sanger believed, women are free to space births, to determine family size, to consider health and economic factors in planning for a child, they will do what is best for their family, which is usually what is best for the community and the human race as a whole.

Like Ellis, Sanger emphasized negative eugenics and sought to discourage parenthood for those who were too poor, too sick, or too unstable to adequately feed, clothe, and shelter a child. She advised that anyone with a hereditary disease or defect should not risk having children. There was broad medical agreement to support this position at the time, even though there were many unknowns when it came to genetic inheritance and much disagreement over which diseases could be considered transmissible. Sanger wrote about the many burdens, financial and otherwise (the "dead weight of human waste") posed by the proliferation of the three established categories of mental retardation: morons, imbeciles, and idiots. This preferred nomenclature, devised by Henry Goddard, corresponded to specific mental ages. Sanger latched onto the popular but specious theory that the feebleminded breed recklessly—each one "a potential source of an endless progeny of defect." She rejected charity, no matter how well-intentioned, because it encouraged "the perpetuation of defectives, delinquents, and dependents." Shortly after witnessing the devastation and misery of war-torn Germany, Sanger told an audience in New York that instead of contributing money to "feed the starving children of Europe," Americans should "send over a quantity of chloroform to put them out of their misery," adding that it would be "the best thing for the children and for the future of the world." It was strong and objectionable rhetoric, then as now. Nevertheless, Sanger's remarks were "enthusiastically applauded." For that postwar audience, she effectively made the point that the temporary alleviation of social problems only postponed greater suffering to come. Birth control offered the only practical solution.[55]

Sanger found that the eugenics movement had served a noble purpose in systematically correlating uncontrolled fertility with increased disease, crime, and poverty. However, she parted ways with most eugenicists in several key areas, most significantly on the question of positive eugenics. She consistently rejected attempts to promote increased childbearing for any group. Holding firm to her belief that every able woman must choose for herself if and when to have a child, Sanger dismissed incentives and pressure tactics aimed at increasing the family size of the educated and elite. She said, "Eugenicists imply or insist that a woman's first duty is to the state; we contend that her duty to herself is her first duty to the state." This was a deal-breaker for many eugenicists who might otherwise have considered giving their support to the ABCL. Neither did it sit well with other birth control advocates in the years to come who positioned family planning programs as a way to build up certain types of families and reduce others. Yet Sanger has been attacked repeatedly for purportedly declaring, "More children from the fit, less from the unfit—that is the chief issue in Birth Control," a statement made in an *American Medicine* editorial in 1919 that was reprinted in the *BCR* with an accompanying rebuttal by Sanger. The statement has been erroneously attributed to her in many biographical and secondary sources and has been widely used as her epitaph.[56]

Sanger also criticized eugenics for minimizing environmental influences while elevating heredity to "the position of an absolute." She thought eugenicists discounted the virtues of "variety" in a population, so intent were they on producing uniformity based on a preferred model of a white, educated northern European descendant. She identified a "distinct middle-class bias" that prejudiced the distinctions made between the fit and the unfit. And she warned that there was insufficient knowledge about genetics to support involuntary sterilization programs, popular among eugenicists. Sanger did back voluntary sterilization for those who were at risk for passing on a disease or defect, and she endorsed compulsory sterilization for the mentally ill and feebleminded "of the hereditary type"—essentially those she thought were incapable of controlling their fertility and were likely to have a disabled child. But she remained cautious about sterilization and questioned its eugenic effectiveness.

Neither Sanger nor the movement as a whole defined fitness in racial terms, as did a number of leading eugenicists who assumed that race and ethnicity determined behavior and then manufactured or modified research results to prove it. Charles Davenport and popular eugenic authors such as Lothrop Stoddard and Madison Grant relied on flawed intelligence tests and dubious "scientific" observations and genetic analyses about specific racial groups to declare certain races, blacks and Jews especially, inferior. Grant's immensely popular *Passing of the Great Race* (1916) helped establish a rubric for Nazi racial policies years later. Harry Laughlin, who with Davenport ran the prestigious Eugenics Records Office at Cold Spring Harbor, New York, and Grant were largely responsible for convincing key members of Congress and much of the American public that immigrants from southern and eastern Europe over bred, underachieved, and accounted for a disproportionate number of patients in insane asylums and inmates in correctional facilities. Metaphors about the bottom of the "melting pot" falling out and horrific visions of the coming "mongrelization" of America stirred up resentment toward new immigrants and black Americans and increased public support for immigration restriction.[57]

Sanger and others in the birth control movement shrugged off the obvious racism inherent in these views and accepted the seemingly well-documented findings by Laughlin and others that fueled immigration restriction, believing that "the slums of Europe dumped their submerged inhabitants in to America." Sanger's concerns centered on the economic status and health conditions of new immigrants and the country's ability to absorb, educate, and employ them, rather than on immigrant's particular ethnicity. However, she certainly lamented the fact that many new immigrants were Catholic and predisposed to oppose birth control. And Sanger quite effortlessly looked the other way when others spouted racist speech. She had no reservations about relying on flawed and overtly racist work to serve her own propaganda needs.

Sanger's wholesale dismissal of the mentally and physically disabled is more troubling from today's vantage point, though her views—echoed throughout the movement—on this segment of society were seen as logical and expedient in the post–World War I era. The near universal ignorance about mental disease, retardation, and many debilitating physical conditions and the institutionalization and segregation of many types of "defective" people—not to mention the labels with which they were saddled—had a dehumanizing effect. Sanger was not alone in seeing the futility of expending money and resources on unproductive segments of society who could not be helped by the limited medical therapies of the day. Her relentless drumbeating about the "over-fertility of the mentally and physically defective," even after the flimsy "science" behind this assumption collapsed years later, suggests that raising this alarm succeeded in winning public support for wider access to birth control. Part of Sanger's success was that she could be ruthless in the promotion of her cause, a trait that we still have trouble accepting in women leaders. Nevertheless, there is a disturbing disconnect between Sanger's clarion call for women's reproductive freedom and her inability to extend rights and liberties to the mentally or physically disabled.[58]

Sanger and the ABCL's commitment to racial improvement persuaded an increasing number of physicians and academics to endorse some aspect of their program but failed to win over many eugenicists. The more orthodox or hard-line hereditarians, like Charles Davenport, Harry Laughlin, California eugenicist Paul Popenoe, and most of the others that came together in the American Eugenics Society, never budged from their belief that birth control exacerbated the disparity in birth rates between the educated and the working class. A conservative lot, many eugenicists disapproved of contraception on moral grounds as well, and associated Sanger and the movement with free love and radical feminism. Lothrop Stoddard, a popular eugenics author and promoter of white supremacism, served for a time on the ABCL national council, an advisory group, and tried to sell Sanger and the movement on his racist theories to no avail. He faded from the picture rather quickly.

There were, however, a group of more moderate and less dogmatic eugenicists who came into the birth control movement in the early 1920s, including Harvard biologist Edward East, sociology pioneer Edward Ross, University of Michigan president Clarence Little, and Raymond Pearl, who ran the Institute of Biomedical Research at Johns Hopkins. These academics emphasized quantitative as much as qualitative problems and looked to birth control as the best means to curtail higher birth rates among the poor and unfit. They became important advocates for birth control in academia, served on ABCL advisory boards, represented the league's interests at scientific conferences, and validated research data on the eugenic value of contraception. In addition, several influential eugenics leaders who had previously shunned the birth control movement issued various levels of endorsement of birth control in direct response to Sanger's efforts to reel them in. Major Leonard Darwin, Charles's son, the president of the British Eugenics Education Society and a towering figure in the eugenics world, had long opposed fertility control and had gone out of his way to avoid discussing the subject. But he gave in to aggressive questioning in New York in 1921, stating, "The birth control movement and eugenics meet in their effort to restrict parenthood among the unfit." Yale economist Irving Fisher, who became an influential voice in the American Eugenics Society, lent his name to the 1921 birth control conference. Fisher said at the 1921 Eugenics Conference, "without question, birth control is today the great new factor affecting the future character of the human race."[59]

Fisher's statement, unexpected from a mainstream eugenicist and all but unthinkable a few years earlier, was one of many indications that control of reproduction was, in Sanger's words, "becoming apparent to the enlightened and the intelligent." The determined effort to rebrand birth control as scientific and eugenic had gained further respectability for the cause and, as historian David Kennedy put it, "underscored the conversion of the birth control movement from a radical program of social disruption to a conservative program of social control." This gradual transformation placed the movement in a better position to lobby for legislative change and secure the medical support needed to open clinics and incorporate contraception into public health programs.

Sanger too had undergone something of a personal makeover parallel with the movement. As president of an organization, she garnered a new level of respect, and her serious intellectual justifications for birth control in *Woman and the New Race* and *Pivot of Civilization* had earned her admiration from a growing number of professionals and academics who had been turned off by her early activism. Sanger's trip around the world from February to September 1922, highlighted by unprecedented speaking tours in Japan and China to warn of the dangers of overpopulation, brought her new recognition as an international figure and gave her a public platform as a population expert. Significantly, the trip ended in London with her marriage to J. Noah Slee (Margaret and William Sanger were divorced in 1921), the millionaire founder and president of the Three-in-One Oil Company, who had been courting Sanger for more than a year. That summer Sanger had written to her close friend and sometime lover, the English writer Hugh de Selincourt, "I shall marry for wealth some day soon. . . ." Two months later she did. The marriage put Sanger on sound financial ground for the first time in her life and gave the movement an insurance policy for the future.[60]

THE CLINICAL RESEARCH BUREAU

When Sanger returned to the United States in the fall of 1922, her immediate aim was to finally get a clinic up and running under the provisions of the Crane decision, which would allow a doctor to prescribe contraception to help cure or prevent disease. No progress had been made in her absence. In fact, the situation looked bleak, as none of the medical men who had initially offered to support a clinic were willing to come on board after Lydia DeVilbiss backed out. Nor had any progress been made on securing a dispensary license, which would have allowed nurses to dispense contraception under the supervision of a licensed physician. The New York State Board of Charities refused to grant such a license to the ABCL because it was not incorporated as a medical organization and did not meet several other requirements. Realizing that it could take years to battle the bureaucracy in Albany, Sanger opted for a stealth approach.

In October 1922, Sanger contacted Dr. Dorothy Bocker, whom she had briefly met in 1921. Bocker directed the Division of Child Hygiene in Georgia but held a New York medical license and had expressed interest in Sanger's campaign. In a letter to Bocker, Sanger outlined her plan to have Bocker open a private practice through which she would dispense birth control to women for specific health reasons, not unlike other doctors had done, including DeVilbiss. Sanger and the ABCL would quietly send clients to Bocker, who would operate initially without any oversight board or medical committee. "To all effects and purposes," Sanger wrote, "it would be a birth control clinic and you would keep clinical records upon which other public clinics would be established in the future." Sanger emphasized that without a dispensary license they would have to call the clinic a "research bureau" and act as if Bocker was engaged in research work only. She warned Bocker that the young doctor might lose her license or even be arrested and face jail time. "On the other hand," Sanger told her, "for one doctor to stand up and assert her right under the legal opinion would give tremendous impetus and encouragement to thousands of other doctors throughout the country to do likewise." Bocker accepted the offer but demanded a large salary, $5,000, because of the risks involved. Sanger had just begun to tap her new husband's money for the movement and rounded up contributions from other sources, including English businessman Clinton Chance, who had befriended Sanger in 1920; the always dependable Katharine Dexter McCormick; and Addie Wolff Kahn, wife of investment banker Otto Kahn.[61]

Sanger gave up the expiring lease on the clinic space she had rented on Tenth Street and set Bocker up in offices across the hall from the ABCL at 104 Fifth Avenue, making little effort to separate the two entities. The doors of the Clinical Research Bureau (CRB) quietly opened on January 2, 1923. Fearing police interference, Sanger did not contact the press or make an announcement in the *BCR*. She did write to selected friends of the movement to inform them "that arrangements have been made to give contraceptive information to those who are entitled to it under the law." The word clinic was never mentioned, and the stated purpose was to collect "scientific data." With no advertising, the clinic depended on word of mouth and referrals from hospitals, private physicians, charitable organizations, and the ABCL.

In the first year Bocker treated over 1,500 women without charge. She filled out a record card for each patient, noting religion, husband's employment, past contraceptive use, and childbearing history, and indicating the health condition for which each patient was being given contraception. There is no record of how many were denied treatment, but the ABCL claimed that the CRB dispensed contraceptives in 1923 to only one-third of the women who sought help. It is doubtful that Bocker turned so many away without giving them information, but clearly both she and Sanger proceeded cautiously. Of course, only married women were admitted, though the clinic made no effort to confirm a patient's marital status. Due to both difficulties in obtaining sufficient quantities of certain contraceptives and questions about effectiveness and patient preference, Bocker prescribed methods in series of 100. For instance, the 100 patients in Series I were given a Mizpah pessary with a Lysol, boric acid douche; Series II, the slightly smaller French pessary with the same douching solution. Other types of diaphragms were paired with suppositories, contraceptive jellies and pastes, and various douching solutions. Although the data were incomplete when Bocker tabulated results in January 1924, none of the 14 series had failure rates above 10 percent, and most were much lower. The Mensinga pessary, made in the Netherlands, and a similar model called Ramses, made in Germany, proved to be the most reliable but were difficult to obtain. However, Bocker's constant fiddling with method combinations and insufficient information on follow-up consultations undermined the validity of her data.

Nevertheless, the CRB was a groundbreaking venture as the first legal clinic in the United States; it remained an independent clinic for 45 years. It quickly grew in size and scope, becoming, within a few years, the leading contraceptive training and research facility in the world. And the CRB served as a model for many of the doctor-staffed clinics that opened across the country in the interwar years. That first year, apart from the State Board of Charities' continuing concern over the true nature of the Bureau—"we have no intention of giving the impression that we are conducting a Birth Control Clinic," Sanger equivocated to a skeptical state inspector—no one tried to interfere with the clinic. When Sanger finally disclosed the CRB to the public at a December 5, 1923, luncheon in New York, the chief of police ordered detectives to pay a visit, but nothing came of the investigation. In fact, the CRB's existence was anticlimactic in every way, covered only briefly in the press and minimized by the ABCL, which did not want to call attention to its questionable, across-the-hall connection. The lack of fanfare and controversy was the clearest sign yet that after 10 years of persistent advocacy and agitation, birth control had become widely accepted by the press and the public.[62]

FOUR

❧

BIRTH CONTROL
AND PUBLIC ACCEPTANCE

We are coming down now, not to a question of principle, but a question of methods.

—Margaret Sanger, January 19, 1934[1]

"The whole of the United States," wrote the suffragist and birth control activist Annie Porritt in 1923, "has . . . become equilibrated to the idea of Birth Control. Even the most conservative and reactionary people now speak the words without self-consciousness, and the words so fully express the idea that they cannot be spoken without their meaning being present in mind." So familiar was that nine-year-old phrase that it began to appear with frequency in popular culture, even in contexts far removed from human procreation. In 1923, a business writer urged "corporation birth control" to cut down on the rapid multiplication of companies in America. In 1920, a housing commissioner in New York called old tenement dwellings converted into studio apartments "birth control houses," because "no one brings a family into them or tries to raise one." *Life Magazine* published "Birth Control of the Seas" in 1923, a satirical poem that read, in part:

The Turbot told it at the Crab's,
    She had it from the Sole –
The very latest thing in thought
    To-day, is birth-control.

Oh, think, Sardine, what this will mean
  To such poor fish as we,
Who give to Commerce, without stint,
  Our countless progeny!

Every type of publication discussed the subject, not just newspapers and news maga-zines. These included women's magazines and religious periodicals; books on mar-riage and childrearing, sociology and eugenics; publications on international relations, economics, and population; and professional journals in science, medicine, and social welfare. One curious example was the *Coast Artillery Journal*, published by the Coast Guard Artillery Training Center, which reviewed Sanger's *Pivot of Civilization*, calling it the "most important" and "most challenging" book of 1922. An early dissertation study of the movement that surveyed hundreds of books and articles pertaining to birth control up until 1927 found that more than two-thirds of the publications presented the subject favorably and that the coverage grew more positive into the 1920s.[2]

SEX AND BIRTH CONTROL USE

At the same time Americans were growing more comfortable with the concept of sex for pleasure and more willing to seek sexual fulfillment. "Sexual expression" in the early 1920s, write D'Emilio and Freedman, "was moving beyond the confines of marriage, not as the deviant behavior of prostitutes and their customers, but as the normative behavior of many Americans." Birth control was the key component in the evolution of a more sexually permissive society but not, by any means, the only determinant of changing sexual behavior. Improved mobility increased opportunities for sexual contact, greater anonymity in urban America created an environment more conducive to casual sex, and (though some historians have overstated it) women's gains in economic and political independence hastened the realization of new sexual freedoms. Contraception was a factor in all of these developments, a common tool for easing the moral encumbrances left over from the Victorian era. Sex flourished in the popular culture like never before. To this day we continue to link the era with carnal images of flappers, dance halls, and the back seats of Fords. The emerging con-sumer society and a new emphasis on leisure cued marketers to promote a more sexu-alized image of the "new woman"—active, flirtatious, daring—and a more sensual portrayal of modern love, including the suggestion of premarital intimacy. In one manifestation of this shift toward more sexual openness, in 1920 the Kimberly-Clark Company introduced Kotex, the first disposable sanitary napkin, "a product," James Reed has written, "that removed one motive for wearing petticoats and reinforced the trend toward less cumbersome clothing." Americans had reached a greater comfort level with sexual hygiene and with their own bodies, which went hand-in-hand with the acceptance of birth control.

Middle- and upper-class women especially, emboldened by new work opportunities and voting rights, sought access to contraception and skirted government prohibitions by supporting a multimillion dollar contraceptive manufacturing industry—dominated by rubber makers and hygiene firms—that was too large and well-rooted for the government to contain. The journalist Ruth Millard recalled that in the early 1920s, "Methods of birth control were discussed over tea cups and featured in correspondence as a problem of legitimate friendly interest." The Comstock laws, she wrote, "were violated hourly, but no charges were pressed." Douches remained the most popular female contraceptive, less so jellies, creams, and suppositories. These methods, which were relatively inexpensive and could be obtained without going to a physician (in drugstores or mail-order catalogs), dwarfed doctor-prescribed diaphragms in popularity during the interwar period. Large numbers of women still relied on withdrawal and some form of periodic abstinence or rhythm. And more men had finally taken to the condom as a birth control method rather than disease preventive; it accounted for roughly 40 percent of all contraceptive use during this era.[3]

In *Middletown*, the classic sociological case study of Muncie, Indiana, interviews and surveys taken from 1924 to 1925 found that all of the women of the "business class" who responded to questions about birth control "used or believed in the use" of a contraceptive method and "took it for granted." Rates of use were considerably lower among the working-class, with slightly less than half employing some means of conception control. However, only 15 out of 77 working-class women disapproved of birth control—less than 20 percent—in this conservative region of the country. In the Midwest as a whole, the average size of the family had shrunk from 5.4 to 3.3 in a single generation. In New York, more than 90 percent of the women who came to the CRB in its first few years had used contraceptives at some time. A 1922 study of 1,000 married women from all parts of the country, a majority of them with college educations, reported a 73 percent contraceptive usage rate. Only 78 of these 1,000 women expressed disapproval of birth control. Most (378) had acquired contraception from a physician. Another survey of just over a 1,000 elderly, white ever-married women, in all economic classes and from all regions of the country, born between 1900 and 1910 (who entered their prime childbearing age between 1920 and 1930), found that 71 percent had used some form of birth control, a figure only slightly lower than that of their daughters' generation. For white collar women in this study the figure was 82 percent, blue collar—70 percent, and farmers—65 percent. Among Catholic women in the study, 60 percent had experience with birth control. More than half of them had ignored church teaching and used a contraceptive device rather than church-sanctioned abstinence. These figures resonate with clinic statistics and the finding that over 30 percent of all birth control clinic patients in the mid-1920s were Catholic.

Of course, it is impossible to know how use rates in the early 1920s compared to contraceptive use in the late 19th century (the Mosher survey, discussed in Chapter 1, measured a very small pool of educated women). We do not know if contraceptive use had significantly increased, and if so, whether it could be explained by the birth control movement's advocacy. It is also difficult to judge if contraceptive use had made any impact on the number of abortions being performed. For obvious reasons, women were reticent about disclosing illegal abortions, even years later. Researchers admitted they were "remarkably unsuccessful" in measuring the number of abortions during this time. Medical experts estimated a ratio of one abortion per every four or five live births, though some thought the rate was much higher.

Overall, birth rate declines leave no doubt that more couples were consciously controlling family size. Between 1895 and 1925 the U.S. birth rate fell roughly 30 percent. Although the first few years of the 1920s saw an inevitable postwar increase, the rates dropped over 20 percent between 1920 and1930. Many factors affect birth rates, but demographic experts have largely rejected other causes as having had a measurable effect in this instance. Historically, an increase in the average marriage age has corresponded with a lower birth rate. However, in the first three decades of the 20th century, the marriage age decreased, yet the birth rate dropped significantly. "Earlier marriage," noted the population experts, Warren Thompson and P. K. Whelpton in 1933, assessing the two decades from 1910 to 1930, "has been taking place concomitantly with the rapid spread of contraceptive information." Birth rate declines were highest among native-born whites and in urban areas, and lower among blacks, recent immigrants, and rural populations, but rates declined across the board.[4]

WOMEN'S SEXUALITY

Alfred Kinsey's pioneering studies on sexuality, covering women who reached sexual maturity in the first decades of the 20th century, not only found a high rate of contraceptive use but also a steady increase over time in the number of women reaching orgasm during intercourse—a correlation that is hard to ignore. However, few early contraception studies provide reliable information on sexual fulfillment. Although birth control had helped broach the topic of women's sexual autonomy, contemporary discussions about contraception rarely touched on sexual satisfaction. Women reported using contraception for economic and health reasons but did not, with few exceptions, disclose an association between birth control and increased sexual enjoyment or frequency. There remained, as well, considerable ignorance on the part of women about their own sexuality. As Sanger wrote euphemistically in 1920,

"Women have not had the opportunity to know themselves, nor have they been permitted to give play to their inner natures, that they might create a morality practical, idealistic and high for their own needs." Women's sexual expression was still repressed by cultural factors, even in this era of comparative sexual liberation. Any acknowledgment of female sexual pleasure had to be muted because of associations with licentiousness and promiscuity—the "wrong kind of woman"—and persistent feelings of guilt. Moreover, the movement's efforts to moderate its feminist rationale to smooth the way for alliances with medicine and eugenics had the effect of desexualizing birth control. Women were in a better position than ever before to experiment with different partners and satisfy sexual desire—before, within, and outside of marriage—but no one in the movement dared to acknowledge this increased freedom. Nor did birth controllers give any serious consideration to openly providing unmarried women with contraception.[5]

THE END OF A SOCIAL MOVEMENT?

Despite its questionable legal status, birth control had become a respectable fixture of American middle-class society, and few outside of the Catholic Church were voicing strong opposition. Sanger's militant call in the pages of *The Woman Rebel* in 1914 to defy the law had quietly come to fruition—anyone involved in sending or receiving contraceptives broke the law on a regular basis. The specter of Comstock that Sanger, Dennett, and others had been projecting to motivate supporters was fading fast. The government rarely enforced the Comstock laws when it came to birth control or, for that matter, abortion. Following the enormous success of the First American Birth Control Conference, the creation of the ABCL, the opening of the first legal clinic, and Sanger's new international standing, she hinted that the movement was nearing its logical culmination. She wrote Havelock Ellis about "finishing up" and enjoying her new marriage and sudden wealth once she helped start a few more clinics. Her plan was for a medical group to take over the New York clinic and any others that formed within the next few years, passing off control from activists to medical professionals and beginning the process of institutionalization she had envisioned since visiting the Dutch clinics in 1915.

Sanger was premature in planning her early retirement but not in signaling the beginning of the end of the social reform movement. Even without reliable polling, it is abundantly clear that the movement had gained broad public acceptance for the use of contraception for family planning and reproductive health. This is borne out by contemporary accounts of the movement, the common use of the term *birth control* in American culture and the media, the anecdotal and cultural evidence indicating a growing social tolerance for erotic enjoyment and nonprocreative sex, and statistical confirmation of the widespread use of contraception and the declining birth rate. The movement's biggest challenge had been achieved: it had made birth control, the term and the concept, familiar and unthreatening to Americans and created an environment where, as Ellis said half jokingly in response to Sanger's retirement tease, the movement "will move by itself."

In many respects it did just that. The ever-increasing demand for contraceptive information largely dictated the movement's approach and growth over the next two decades. The next phase of the social reform was decidedly different and more in line with other well-established reform efforts—featuring professional lobbyists and fund-raisers, media and public relations consultants, expert advisory boards, and high-powered legal counsel. By making birth control a respectable and conventional practice, the movement had entered the final stage in its development—bureaucratization—that heralded its integration into mainstream society, at which point it could no longer be called a social movement.

Enormous challenges remained: the movement had still not obtained an official medical endorsement or made much progress in amending the Comstock laws; it had not adequately reached those sectors of society most in need of access to reproductive control; there was as yet no regulation in the contraceptive industry; and the diaphragm remained the only truly reliable contraceptive method. But the movement had demonstrated that birth control was an irrepressible force for social change, and in an increasingly secular society, there was no going back. The battle now was over the relevance and standing of the law and ease of access.

As the movement entered its mature years, it had to adjust to another change: no longer could leaders rely on sensational events to drive publicity. As one reporter wrote about the early 1920s, "The boisterous early days of the birth control cause seemed over." Sanger, the former woman rebel, had become much like the society women she so depended on. She now looked to push the movement further to the center and stabilize it by using her husband's money and grants from philanthropists like John D. Rockefeller Jr. (the same pillar of capitalism she had wished dead just a decade earlier when she wrote about a failed attack on the Rockefeller family home, bungled by her anarchist comrades). Gravitating to the mainstream, the movement began to respond more forcefully to the public's desire to know rather than directing its focus on the opposition's attempts to impede. Nonetheless, it continued to exploit opposition efforts to restrict speech while at the same time expanding its own channels of communication.[6]

RADIO BIRTH CONTROL

In 1924 birth control went out over the radio, in an address by Margaret Sanger that was deemed safe enough for unknown ears—just two years into the nation's first broadcasting boom. The radio speech in Syracuse, New York, at the conclusion of the New York State Birth Control Conference in February 1924, came after heated Catholic opposition had compelled the city council to pass an ordinance banning the public discussion of birth control. Local Catholic leaders went so far as to have Catholic Boy Scouts distribute a popular anti-birth control tract to Catholic officials, professionals, and businessmen in Syracuse. The Syracuse mayor vetoed the ban, allowing the conference to take place. The publicity generated by the episode ensured a large audience for Sanger's first radio broadcast. She kept it simple and upbeat in an attempt to appeal to an unseen audience that spanned the political spectrum. Sanger presented a vision of America that fell somewhere between 19th century Utopian communities and Lake Wobegon, where citizens "are fighting for better, healthier children, for a race of strong men and beautiful women. . . . We place quality above quantity. We want each child to have proper food, warmth, sunlight and fresh air, devotion and love."

Radio quickly became an important tool for the movement, helping it keep a step ahead of the church. With the film industry moving to adopt decency standards in the early 1920s, the birth control movement avoided the big screen. (Sanger's 1917 film fiasco remained a sore memory.) Radio represented the next media frontier, and Sanger's dignified manner and affected New England Brahmin accent (she sounded a little like Eleanor Roosevelt) proved to be a winning combination in presenting a sensitive subject to the masses. Mail poured in after radio broadcasts and indicated that Sanger was reaching a new audience.

CATHOLIC OPPOSITION

Syracuse was just one of several birth control battlegrounds in the early 1920s. The widespread acceptance of birth control, even among many Catholics, and the postwar revival of regional birth control groups, many of which were affiliated with the ABCL, raised concerns among Catholic organizations. In a relatively short time, anti-birth control Catholic groups became better organized and waged an opposition campaign on multiple fronts. Their efforts were loosely centralized in Washington, D.C., under the direction of the National Catholic Welfare Conference, which marshaled Catholic orders and fraternal groups to lobby against pro-birth control legislation and counter birth control advocates. The Knights of Columbus was particularly aggressive in taking on Sanger and the ABCL at conferences and speaking events. In Cincinnati in November 1922, the Knights threatened to boycott the Hotel Gibson and hold their annual banquet elsewhere if the hotel honored its contract to rent out its ballroom for a birth control conference. The hotel management stood firm, the Knights of Columbus took their business elsewhere, and the ABCL established a Cincinnati branch. Similar circumstances unfolded in Albany, New York, in January 1923, where the mayor succumbed to the pressure tactics of a Catholic police commissioner and his cohorts and stopped Sanger from giving a speech. In Boston in 1924, 1925, and 1926, Mayor Curley made it a chief priority to block Sanger from speaking in a public hall. The ABCL and ACLU worked the press in all of these instances, turning unremarkable public meetings into newsworthy events. Sanger compared the Catholic officials who organized protests to "schoolboys playing with chemicals . . . they have been surprised and shocked by the force and repercussive effect of unexpected detonations . . . they have worked miracles of publicity that would have been impossible to a regiment of press-agents."[7]

Though the Catholic Church was losing ground against the birth control movement in the arena of free speech, it implemented a successful defensive strategy in the state houses and in Congress. Catholic lobbyists and politicians blocked birth control legislation in New York—where Sanger and the ABCL expended considerable resources from 1923 to 1926—New Jersey, and Connecticut, and held back Dennett's bill in Congress. Even non-Catholic lawmakers outside of Catholic districts who understood the need for safe and effective contraception and who had obviously planned their own families (Dennett calculated that Congressmen averaged 2.7 children), sought to avoid a vote on birth control. The perception that birth control was fairly easy to come by and the fact that the prohibition on its circulation was seldom enforced, diminished the urgency of amending the law. Catholic opponents effectively argued that contraceptive use was an unnatural, harmful, indecent, and selfish act that debased marriage and ran counter to the tenets of Christianity. The more that birth control advocates, including many of the eugenicists and social scientists newly enlisted in the movement, emphasized health, population, and economic issues, the more Catholic lobbyists warned of promiscuity, sexual depravity, and moral demise. Beneath the neoclassical domes of capitol buildings, the movement had trouble keeping birth control from sliding off Sanger's "higher plane" and into the gutter. "Blasphermers," one Catholic assemblyman in New York State called the birth controllers, saying that they should be "swept from the face of the earth." The issue was still too politically hazardous for legislators, and the bills that found sponsors were tabled in committee, with the exception of Dennett's federal bill in 1925.

DENNETT'S BILL

Catholic interference stymied Mary Dennett, who ran into one wall after another in directing the Voluntary Parenthood League (VPL) lobbying campaign in Washington in the first few years of the decade. In contrast to Sanger, Dennett had continued to frame birth control as chiefly a free speech and civil liberties issue and was less convincing when she addressed the health and human betterment aspects that had greater political appeal. With the ABCL up and running, the VPL was thoroughly overshadowed as a national organization. Unable to generate much publicity on its own, it struggled to compete with the ABCL in fund-raising and in securing support. Dennett nearly resigned in 1922 when she wearied of paying VPL bills with her own money. In January 1923, she finally had a breakthrough, when Senator Albert Baird Cummins, a progressive Republican from Iowa, agreed to sponsor her open bill, which would excise reference to contraception from the Comstock Act. The same day she found a New York Republican sponsor in the House. The bill was shelved until the next session of Congress when a new sponsor, Colorado Representative William Vaile, joined Cummins. Dennett was on the verge of a breakthrough when the Cummins-Vaile Bill moved to both the Senate and House Judiciary Subcommittees. Growing impatient, she pestered legislators to take immediate action. More delays and a well-orchestrated Catholic assault ensued. In January 1925, the Cummins-Vaile Bill was reported out of the Senate subcommittee without recommendation and failed to get to a floor vote before Congress adjourned that March. The defeat effectively ended Dennett's birth control career, and she faded from public view until her indictment in 1929 under the Comstock law for publication of *Sex Side of Life*. The VPL languished for a number of years before disbanding.[8]

BIRTH CONTROL CONFERENCES

Sanger agreed to pursue legislative change, and in 1925 the League set up a federal lobbying campaign to compete with the VPL. But until the 1930s, Sanger expressed little confidence in a legislative victory. Dennett's setbacks in the early 1920s only hardened Sanger against the political process. For the ABCL in the mid-1920s, lobbying activities were just one part of a sophisticated operation centered on public outreach and education. In 1923 alone, the League's first full year, it boosted membership to over 20,000, sent out more than 200,000 letters, addressed 124 groups and over 60,000 people across the country, and distributed over 600,000 pieces of literature. But it was through conferences that the League created the greatest amount of publicity and strengthened its ties to medicine, eugenics, social welfare, and public health.

The Middle Western States Birth Control Conference in Chicago in September 1923 brought together about 2,500 delegates to discuss how birth control would reduce "the high cost of charities and corrections . . . an ever increasing burden on all American communities." The conference boosted the ABCL's standing among the more conservative leaders of the recently reconstituted Illinois Birth Control League, who had been closely associated with the VPL. More significantly, the conference focused attention on the Illinois league's attempt to open a clinic under the guidance of Rachelle Yarros, a Russian-born physician and leading Chicago-area birth control advocate. The Chicago group had been blocked from obtaining a city permit by the health commissioner, who cited the Comstock Act, city ordinance, and "divine law" in rejecting the clinic application. But Circuit Court Judge Harry Fisher reversed the decision in November 1923, paving the way for the nation's second legal birth control clinic, run out of Yarros's offices. Smaller ABCL conferences in Philadelphia and Cincinnati in 1922 and Albany and Baltimore in 1923 led to organizational activity in those areas. Conferences directly or indirectly resulted in ABCL branches in Pennsylvania, Michigan, Ohio, and Indiana by 1924, joining branches in Massachusetts, Connecticut, and Colorado.

Following the success of the Chicago conference, Sanger convinced reluctant ABCL board members to host the Sixth International Neo-Malthusian and Birth Control Conference in New York in the spring of 1925. A huge undertaking, it confirmed America's emergence as a leader in the international population field. The event linked the American movement with neo-Malthusian birth control activism in Europe, going back to the first such conference in Paris in 1900, the same one that Emma Goldman, then a birth control neophyte, had attended.

Sanger used the international forum to identify the cause with some of the best known figures on both sides of the Atlantic—to have a "brilliant and distinguished array" of men and women "stand in public for what they believed in private." The "vice-presidents" of the conference included Sanger's mentors, Havelock Ellis, and H. G. Wells, as well as the influential British economist, John Maynard Keynes, British novelist Arnold Bennett, and Baron Keikichi and Baroness Shidzue Ishimoto, who had pioneered the birth control movement in Japan. For American sponsors, the ABCL brought well-known eugenists like Herbert Spencer Jennings and Henry Goddard together with suffragists M. Cary Thomas and Harriet Stanton Blatch (Elizabeth Cady Stanton's daughter) and many familiar names in academia. Messages were read and released to the press from the French novelist Henri Barbusse; the American social critic and editor H. L. Mencken; the African American social reformer, historian, and author W.E.B. Du Bois; English philosopher Bertrand Russell; playwright George Bernard Shaw; and 50 other recognized writers, reformers, and leaders in their professions. Delegates from 18 countries took part in sessions ranging from "Fecundity and Civilization," to "Economics—Poverty and Child Labor." A discussion on "Religious and Moral Factors," featured several of the most prominent Jewish and Protestant birth control advocates to counter the condemnation from the Catholic press. A closed medical meeting that attracted over 1,000 physicians included Dr. Aletta Jacobs of the Netherlands, who had started the first contraceptive clinic in the world and who had refused to meet with Sanger in 1915 because Sanger lacked medical credentials.[9]

THE LECTURE CIRCUIT

Sanger claimed that it took her a year to recover from the "strain, physical, nervous, and financial" of the international conference, but she kept up a demanding lecture schedule as did several ABCL officers and board members. ABCL staff addressed women's clubs and political organizations in every state, finding strong pools of support among the professional classes and well-to-do. As in 1916, birth control groups sometimes formed as a result of these gatherings. In 1924 ABCL Executive Secretary Anne Kennedy helped organize five birth control committees in western states on a 10-week lecture tour. Sanger made an effort to reach beyond the clubwoman circuit and speak to college and university groups and many churches and religious organizations. She addressed fewer labor and leftist groups than in the previous decade but sought opportunities to meet with working-class women. She prided herself on a willingness to talk to any audience if they desired knowledge about birth control. "All the world over," she wrote, "I have found women's psychology in the matter of childbearing essentially the same, no matter what the class, religion, or economic status. Always to me any aroused group was a good group. . . ."

Keeping to her word, Sanger agreed to speak to a rally of Ku Klux Klan women in or near Belmar, New Jersey, in May 1926, later calling it "one of the weirdest experiences I had in lecturing." Arriving at a train station, she was taken to an undisclosed location off of a dirt road and left in a car outside a large warehouse. "Occasionally men dropped wives who walked hurriedly and silently within. This went on mystically until night closed down and I was alone in the dark." After a long wait, she was led before a large gathering and introduced. "Never before had I looked into a sea of faces like these," she recounted. "I was sure that if I uttered one word, such as abortion, outside the usual vocabulary of these women they would go off into hysteria. . . . In the end, through simple illustrations I believed I had accomplished my purpose." She never mentioned a possible ulterior motive: to win the support of anti-Catholic groups, including the Klan, in hopes of fending off Catholic opposition to birth control legislation then being debated in New Jersey.[10]

In 1925 Sanger used her husband's money to hire English gynecologist Dr. James F. Cooper, a former missionary in China currently practicing in Boston, as the ABCL's medical director. Taken by his distinguished appearance and British manner, and impressed with the ease with which he could discuss contraception with people as well as fellow physicians, Sanger sent Cooper on a lecture tour of county medical societies, hospital staffs, medical schools, and other medical organizations across the country. In two years he spoke to over 200 medical groups and compiled the names of thousands of doctors willing to prescribe contraception. The names were added to a referral list used by the ABCL when responding to mothers' letters and similar requests, which numbered over 28,000 in 1925. Cooper's discussions with other physicians regarding contraceptives underscored a problem that was becoming more apparent at the CRB. As Sanger put it, "the acceptance of the theory was ahead of the means of practicing it." Reliable contraceptives, particularly diaphragms, were in short supply, and many doctors were not willing to prescribe untested and potentially

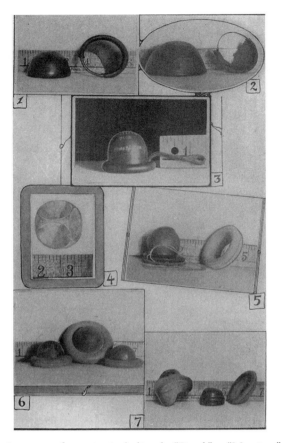

Photograph of various types of pessaries, including the "Dutch" or "Mensinga" style diaphragm (#2), which many birth controllers preferred. From Dorothy Bocker, *Birth Control Methods* (1924). (Courtesy of the Sophia Smith Collection, Smith College.)

harmful devices or douching solutions. Sanger and Bocker had thus far been able to supply the CRB, but as patient loads increased, it was becoming more difficult to get around the importation and mailing bans under the Comstock Act. U.S. Customs was known to check packages addressed to physicians and seize both contraceptives and related publications.[11]

BOOTLEG BIRTH CONTROL

Since the CRB's inception, Sanger had been smuggling diaphragms into the United States from other countries. For instance, when touring British Columbia on a pleasure trip in the summer of 1923, she obtained a dozen pessaries, hid them in "soiled linen," and sent them by post to the clinic. She asked her high society friends traveling in Europe, including Katharine McCormick who had a chateau in Geneva, to return home with rubber souvenirs. J. Noah Slee's Three-in-One Oil Company provided the most productive smuggling system. Slee arranged for supplies from Germany and the Netherlands—500 or more Ramses pessaries at a time—to be sent to his company's branch in Montreal, Canada, where they were stuffed into cartons of the popular household lubricant and shipped to a New York warehouse.

Expense, increased demand from physicians, and the potential for legal problems made it necessary to find an alternative to bootleg birth control. However, Sanger did not want the movement to be associated with commercial concerns and give the impression that she profited from the cause—something her opponents regularly charged. This ruled out a working association with Julius Schmid, one of the condom barons whose company had just started production of a Mensinga-style diaphragm. (The CRB also found his products brittle and inferior to European models.) In the spring of 1925, Sanger brought together Cooper; ABCL publicist Guy Moyston; Herbert Simonds, an old friend with both an engineering and advertising background; Dr. Hannah Stone, who had recently replaced Bocker as CRB medical director; and Slee. Together they conceived of the Holland-Rantos Company, incorporated in October 1925, with Simonds and Moyston as partners and no trace of Sanger's involvement. The new company began experimenting with different designs for a spring-form diaphragm and selling a lactic acid contraceptive jelly originally developed by Cooper and used at the CRB. It took a number of months before the company manufactured enough product to begin to replace imports. By then other firms had started up, especially jelly manufacturers, to take advantage of the clinical success of the diaphragm and jelly method promoted by Cooper on his road tour and Bocker in *Birth Control Methods*, her 1924 published report on the CRB.[12]

GROWTH OF CLINICS

By the end of 1927, a number of independent clinics were in operation across the country, significantly increasing the demand for supplies. The CRB had opened a short-lived clinic in the Columbus Hill section of Manhattan in 1925 and another in Brooklyn in 1926. The Illinois Birth Control League had three clinics in operation by 1927 and assisted with three settlement house clinics, including one in Jane Addams's Hull House. The Los Angeles Mother's Clinic started up in 1925, and the Detroit Mother's Clinic and Baltimore Bureau of Contraceptive Advice opened in 1927. The CRB provided a blueprint for how to start a clinic, right down to the preferred female contraceptive method—the Mensinga-style diaphragm paired with a contraceptive jelly—staff make-up, and oversight board of distinguished medical and community leaders. (Starting in 1924, the CRB included Sanger's four favored eugenicists and several physicians on its advisory board.) Sanger's clinic had also served as a barometer of governmental tolerance. No attempts had been made to interfere with its operation, an assuring sign and a green light for other clinic organizers.

ROBERT DICKINSON AND THE COMMITTEE ON MATERNAL HEALTH

Sixteen hospital-based contraceptive clinics opened in the same time span, 10 of them in New York City. These small, inconspicuous programs were added to maternity care and out-patient departments. They were not, however, connected to the lay birth control movement. In fact, the physician-controlled Committee on Maternal Health (CMH) in New York established all but one of the New York hospital clinics to undertake a scientific investigation of birth control that the CMH argued was not being adequately carried out by movement activists. Longtime physician advocate for contraception, Robert Latou Dickinson (1861–1950), created the CMH just weeks after the CRB began. With funds contributed by early movement supporter Gertrude Pinchot, now estranged from Sanger because of ideological differences, Dickinson brought together a group of prominent physicians to serve on the CMH's executive committee. He persuaded the New York Obstetrical Society to endorse the Committee's research mission to conduct a thorough clinical study of all aspects of human fertility, including birth control.[13]

Dickinson, who had recently served as president of the American Gynecological Society and was an influential voice in the American Medical Association (AMA), had retired from active practice by 1924 to investigate birth control methods and work to legitimize medically-controlled contraception. Although he had prescribed contraceptives to his patients for a number of years, he lamented the lack of sound research on safety and efficacy and sought to develop data sources. He faulted the movement's propaganda tactics and radical leadership for perpetuating physicians' widespread resistance to birth control. Finding Sanger's name to be poisonous among many of his colleagues, Dickinson barred anyone with strong ties to the movement from joining the CMH. He rejected the CRB's research methodology and questioned its seemingly haphazard dispensing of unproven and potentially harmful methods, and treatment of women who did not clearly exhibit a medical condition, required to exempt them from the law. He and his colleagues saw the CRB as an illegal operation and a potential menace to public health.

However, Dickinson soon developed a grudging respect for Sanger and the success of her clinic—relative to the CMH's inability to treat enough women to provide a statistically significant research sample. The CMH was discriminating in patient admittance, only dispensing contraception to those who indicated an obvious illness or disability. Host hospitals feared legal repercussions, and countless women referred by other doctors were turned away. Consequently, after three years, the CMH sample was less than 10 percent of the CRB's, which produced well over 1,000 case records a year. Sanger's clinic accepted most doctor-referred patients and, by the mid-1920s, rejected less than a third of the applicants for contraceptive service—usually only those who were clearly unmarried, pregnant, or had health complications that required further examination. It is unclear how many women the CRB actually turned away for lack of medical indications. Most patients were admitted for gynecological problems, a bona fide disease like tuberculosis, or more nebulous health conditions such as "general debility." Dickinson also experienced a critical shortage of diaphragms after the U.S. Customs confiscated shipments he had ordered from Germany. In 1926 he had no choice but to purchase contraband Ramses pessaries from Sanger.

By this point Dickinson and Sanger, though critical of each other to their respective constituents, had joined together to seek formal medical supervision of the CRB. Dickinson believed that if Sanger could completely separate the ABCL's research and propaganda functions, then the medical community would more readily accept clinical contraception. A medical takeover and tightening of standards would help validate the significant and growing body of CRB case records, which held the key to improving contraceptive safety and effectiveness. For her part, Sanger wanted to proceed with her plan to shift control to a medical body and secure a state dispensary license, a step she believed would offer legal protection and pave the way for medical endorsements. In the spring of 1925, James Cooper and Dickinson were successful in getting the New York Academy of Medicine to support putting the CRB under medical management, as long as the clinic was completely disassociated from the ABCL and properly licensed. To increase the likelihood of securing a license from the State Board of Charities, which had rejected the CRB once, the CMH and the ABCL incorporated a new organization in June 1925, the Maternity Research Council, to oversee the clinic. However, the council, made up of representatives of both organizations and headed by physicians, failed to impress the Charities Board, which again denied the license. Purportedly it had come under considerable pressure from Catholic groups. Over the next few years, Sanger and Dickinson tried several other approaches to a medical merger, but mutual distrust of motives began to fester, and negotiations finally ended in 1929.[14]

The failed medical takeover underscored the obstacles to both medical approval of family planning and medical management of clinics, even as more doctors were prescribing contraception in private practice. Despite Sanger's careful cultivation of scientists and academics of all stripes, conservative medicine still viewed her as a radical and expressed unease with the sexual subtext of birth control—and even hostility toward the idea of women's sexual autonomy. Furthermore, most physicians continued to reject the movement's economic rationale for contraception and preferred to limit access to those who suffered from serious health problems. State and federal laws reinforced this position. Physician groups also struggled with the clinic model offered by the birth control movement in the same way as they resisted the encroachment of social welfare programs that crossed over into the medical realm, such as nutritional, maternal, and infant care initiatives. These efforts often endowed laypeople with a certain degree of medical authority and sometimes competed with for-profit medical services. The medical establishment seemed especially offended by health campaigns with laywomen in leadership positions and excessively critical of women doctors in the birth control movement. Even Dickinson, who frequently defended the movement in medical circles, demeaned the all-women staff at the CRB as unqualified.

Yet Sanger recognized the importance of keeping Dickinson close to the movement—she got him to agree to serve on her clinic's advisory board in 1930—and applauded him for treating birth control as a "clean science, with dignity, decency, and directness." She knew that no one else had the connections and wherewithal to lobby the AMA to recognize birth control. In 1925 Dickinson succeeded in convincing the AMA's gynecology section to accept a resolution to change and clarify relevant laws so that physicians could legally give contraceptive information to any and all patients. Although the Association's governing body, the House of Delegates, refused to take up the resolution, Dickinson had lit a small fire in the conservative organization.

In regard to the Clinical Research Bureau, Dickinson's intrusiveness in the mid-1920s made the clinic into a more professional operation. Changes followed as a result of his surprise inspection in 1924 and his harsh criticisms of Bocker's record-keeping. The clinic physically separated from the ABCL in 1925, moving into its own building, paid for by Slee, on West Fifteenth Street. Newly hired Dr. Hannah Stone, working with Dr. James Cooper, set up a comprehensive contraceptive testing system, standardized patient history records, and carried out assiduous follow-up work. In a short time they established the clinic as the premier contraceptive research center in the world. The valuable case files that Dickinson coveted became the basis of several important studies, including statistician Marie Kopp's 1934 *Birth Control in Practice*, prepared under Dickinson's watchful eye and with Rockefeller foundation money, which analyzed 10,000 CRB case histories.* The findings conclusively refuted baseless opposition claims that contraception caused sterility. They also emphasized the value of the clinic as a health service in detecting early signs of disease. The analyses found

---

* Other important studies that incorporated the CRB data are Hannah M. Stone, *Contraceptive Methods—A Clinical Survey* (New York: Clinical Research Department of the ABCL, 1925); James F. Cooper, *Technique of Contraception* (New York: Day-Nichols, 1928); and Regine K. Stix and Frank W. Notestein, *Controlled Fertility: An Evaluation of Clinic Service* (Baltimore, MD: Williams & Wilkins, 1940).

a high effectiveness rate for the diaphragm and jelly method—well over 90 percent—though there was a fall-off for those with less education and lower incomes.[15]

THE CLINIC RAID

But rather than Dickinson's considerable influence, it was yet another act of government interference that finally compelled the medical establishment into a protective embrace of the birth control movement. On April 15, 1929, agent provocateur Anna K. McNamara, who had posed as a clinic patient the previous month, returned to the CRB with the director of the Women's Bureau of the Police Department and several other officers and detectives, with search and arrest warrants in hand. They interrupted patient consultations, ransacked offices, and confiscated supplies and a selection of case records. The officers then arrested Hannah Stone, another doctor, and three nurses for allegedly giving out contraceptive information without the intention of preventing disease. Sanger accompanied the five women to the police station and oversaw their release on bail.

The raid generated wide coverage in the press and nearly universal criticism of the police action. Most of the editorials and op-ed pieces first acknowledged the legality of the clinic under New York State law and then turned to the question of medical privacy. "Surely a doctor has a right to demand the privilege of keeping his patient from serious illness," wrote Heywood Broun, one of the nation's most widely read syndicated columnists. "Medicine is nothing if this freedom is denied a doctor." The *New York Herald Tribune* added, "Even those doctors who have not agreed with the general position of the birth control clinic are likely to protest against such arbitrary police invasion of medical privacy." Indeed, within two days, more than 40 physicians contacted Sanger or clinic attorneys to offer support. Both the New York County Medical Society and the New York Academy of Medicine adopted resolutions protesting the police seizure of medical records. An Academy committee issued a statement that concluded, "there exists here a definite threat against the public good, and a serious menace to the rights and privileges of the medical profession as granted by law."[16]

On Dickinson's recommendation, Sanger hired attorney Morris Ernst to represent the clinic. An ACLU board member who was just beginning to carve out a legacy as one of the great civil liberties and censorship attorneys of his time, Ernst was a big-picture legal mind, forward-looking, and reformist. On one level he saw the case in the simplest of terms. "All we have to prove," he told the press, is that the doctor was "acting in good faith with the thought that the birth control information will prevent disease. . . . It is the burden of the prosecution to prove the bad faith of the doctor." But he recognized the opportunity to achieve more than a court victory for his clients; he sought to broaden the 1918 Crane decision, which permitted contraceptive information to be dispensed for disease prevention. In fashioning a long-term approach to securing reproductive rights, Ernst fostered the process of judicial nullification. He believed the courts would whittle away the state and federal Comstock laws until they became irrelevant to birth control. "In the United States," he wrote, "we seldom, if ever, repeal moral legislation. It is my belief that long before all the birth-control laws now on the statute books have been repealed they will have been openly nullified."

The two-day trial concluded on April 24, with Ernst calling to the witness stand some of the most prominent physicians in New York, including Dickinson; Louis Harris, the former city health commissioner; and Foster Kennedy, the chief neurologist at Bellevue Hospital. All testified that the clinic staff acted legally and appropriately in treating the undercover officer. As the mother of three children, the youngest being just one-year-old, she had been given contraceptive information and advised to wait before having another child. Although she was also diagnosed with a minor pelvic disorder, the physician witnesses for the defense argued that child-spacing was a legitimate disease preventive and should exempt her from the law. "The possibility of recuperation for the mother," gynecologist Frederick Holden told the court, "depends upon proper spacing." Dr. Louis Harris discussed the benefit of spacing to a child's health, and Ernst augmented the testimony with statistical evidence from the Department of Labor's Children's Bureau, showing that children born at short intervals had a higher mortality rate than those spaced further apart.

On the last day of the trial, the police commissioner issued a public apology and instigated an internal investigation, though not much came of it. Officers involved were demoted or reprimanded, but the police never fully disclosed what triggered the raid. According to private detectives hired by the ABCL, Catholic officials may have leaned on the police to try to shut down the CRB, after learning from Catholic social workers that many parishioners were attending the clinic. Under terrific pressure from medical groups and the press, the police returned the patient records and other confiscated data, except for 150 patient record cards that were never accounted for. On May 14, Magistrate Abraham Rosenbluth dismissed the charges against the clinic workers, writing in his decision that "physicians, and nurses who act upon the instructions of physicians, are absolved from the prohibitions of Section 1142 . . . if they act in good faith in instructing a married woman in the use of contraceptives. Good faith, in these circumstances, is the belief by the physician that the prevention of conception is necessary for the patient's health and physical welfare." Not only had he relaxed Crane's disease requirement to include general health, but his ruling, based on the expert testimony of physicians, also permitted contraceptive use for the planned spacing of children. Sanger wrote Havelock Ellis, "It put us ahead ten years especially because of the medical testimony. . . ." Ernst later noted that another "big section was taken out of the law."[17]

SANGER'S RESIGNATION FROM THE ABCL

The clinic raid came in the middle of a tumultuous time in the movement. Just two days before, Sanger had finalized her break from the ABCL, resigning as a board member and as the editor of the *BCR*. She had stepped down as president of the League in June 1928 following a protracted power struggle with Eleanor Dwight Jones, the board chair who assumed increasing authority in 1926 to 1927, when Sanger was off in Europe organizing the first World Population Conference in Geneva. Jones, a veteran of the women's suffrage movement, was an exacting, by-the-rules administrator, and demanded that the League's Board of Directors place limits on Sanger's unchecked presidential powers. Sanger had no intention of altering her highly independent leadership style and blamed Jones and several of Jones's cronies for allowing rival factions to form within the League. "I could have fought it," Sanger wrote to Juliet Rublee, who resigned with Sanger, "& pushed them out but what for?"

Sanger was clearly relieved to be done with the ABCL, but she gave mixed signals as to why she left. In her resignation letter she said she wished to pursue contraceptive research and international work, yet she had no clear plan in mind. She stated elsewhere that she found organizational work onerous and boards and committees inhibiting, yet just a few months later, she would establish a new national organization with a formal organizational structure. Sanger's correspondence suggests that she had entered a kind of mid-life crisis in her leadership of the movement, impatient with the pace of reform on the legislative and medical fronts and unconvinced that the more professional movement organizers of the 1920s were zealous enough. "The old spirit is gone," she wrote to Juliet Rublee about the ABCL on her resignation. Kitty Marion was the only holdover from the radical *BCR* crowd of the late 1910s and her days were numbered, as Jones disapproved of the confrontational activism that was Marion's trademark. Most of the new supporters offered money and name— such as Eleanor Roosevelt, who was elected at the 1928 annual meeting as an "active member"—but not the kind of selfless commitment exhibited by many of the earlier activists. Sanger feared that the movement had grown complacent under the ABCL's "more or less doctrinaire program of social activity," which was "efficient . . . for routine results" but "could be a drag or a weight upon effective, spontaneous, aggressive action."[18]

Sanger consolidated her support around the New York clinic, which she wrestled away from the ABCL and renamed the Birth Control Clinical Research Bureau (BCCRB). As in the immediate post-World War I years, there were again two distinct camps in the movement, and Sanger thrived whenever she was engaged in a rivalry. Within a year, she had siphoned funders (her husband's money most immediately), members, and staff from the ABCL, though many in the movement supported both organizations. The ABCL was destabilized by the loss of its chief fund-raiser and newsmaker, the editor of the *Review*, and its research arm (though it did retain an affiliation with the BCCRB). Eleanor Jones was forced to downsize the League and limit its objectives. A few years later she even considered a merger with the American Eugenics Society in an act of financial desperation. One measurement of the sudden impact of Sanger's absence on the ABCL: in 1929 incoming mail dropped from nearly 33,000 letters to just over 19,000.

THE HARLEM CLINIC

The publicity created by the clinic raid helped further consolidate support for Sanger and the BCCRB and keep her well-positioned as the face of the movement. She moved quickly in 1929 on several initiatives, including contraceptive research projects abroad and an expansion of the BCCRB, this time to Harlem. Although the midtown satellite clinic in the mostly black neighborhood of Columbus Hill—one of many social reform efforts at the time to reduce the alarmingly high infant and maternal mortality rates in the black community—had failed in 1925, Sanger was committed to finding ways to bring contraceptive services to poor and working-class women wherever they lived. She responded to a community-based effort in Harlem, spearheaded by the New York Urban League, to open a branch of the BCCRB. She found two philanthropists who had made their fortunes in retail, Julius Rosenwald of Sears-Roebuck and Caroline Bamberger Fuld of Bamberger Department Stores, to initially fund the clinic, which opened in February 1930. The clinic had its own medical staff and a largely black advisory council that included a number of local black professionals and community leaders. Along with benefitting thousands of black and white women in northern Manhattan, the Harlem Clinic demonstrated that black women had the same desire for reproductive autonomy and the same success rates using a diaphragm as white women. Such evidence contradicted the prevalent racist assumption that, as eugenicist Raymond Pearl put it, black women inherently lacked "intelligent foresight" in matters of sex. Although the Harlem Clinic did steady business, it ran on voluntary fees and contributions. The facility succumbed to financial problems in the mid-1930s, in the midst of the Depression, with Slee's fortune decimated by the market collapse and the BCCRB on shaky ground. The New York City Committee of Mother's Health Centers, an ABCL offshoot, secured outside funding and took over the clinic in 1935, and it functioned until the mid-1940s.[19]

FEDERAL LOBBYING

Just two weeks after the clinic raid, Sanger quietly launched a new organization, the National Committee on Federal Legislation for Birth Control (NCFLBC), charged with reforming the Comstock law to legalize the distribution of contraceptives and contraceptive information through the mails. Plans for the lobbying group had been hatched in the fall of 1928 by Sanger and Helen Graham Carpenter, the head of the Illinois Birth Control League, though they initially envisioned the Committee as a subgroup of the ABCL. Sanger's inability to work with the new ABCL leadership and the League's indifference to federal legislative work set Sanger on an independent path with this new endeavor.

In the past, Sanger had avoided any serious commitment to changing the federal law, concentrating on agitation and education and believing she would have more success through the courts than in Congress. However, by the end of the 1920s, she came to understand that medical conservatism, not the Catholic Church, posed the most significant impediment to the expansion of medically-controlled contraceptive services. Her dealings with the state licensing board and medical groups in New York in the failed efforts to negotiate a merger between the CRB and a medical organization underscored the complexity of the current legal climate and physicians' reluctance to publicly support birth control. "In my conversation with members of the profession," Sanger wrote to Dickinson, "I am told repeatedly that 'the doctor's job is to obey the laws.'" Even in the 28 states that had no laws on the books regarding birth control, the local medical establishments were deterred from endorsing contraception because of its codified federal status as obscene material, and they still had to contend with the federal ban on mailing contraceptive information or devices. In 1928, the respected Johns Hopkins obstetrician, John Whitridge Williams, expressed to his colleagues his regret that dispensing contraceptives

> . . . often must imply a certain feeling of degradation on the part of the person securing them from semibootleg sources. I feel very strongly that our state and national laws should be amended so as to make it possible for physicians to prescribe contraceptive means with the same freedom and decency as any other prophylactic or medical device, and I resent very strongly the attempt of the government to interfere in this respect, as I regard it as an unwarrantable aspersion against the integrity and bona fides of the medical profession.

Because laws differed from state to state, considerable confusion existed among doctors about their legal rights. Although 28 independent clinics had opened by 1929, there could easily have been more, if not for uncertainty and intransigence on the part of doctors. Sanger believed that to "move forward constructively into the larger sphere where birth control is included with public health activities," the Comstock Law had to be amended. At the same time, she and Morris Ernst kept apprised of potential test cases with which to challenge the statute.[20]

The NCFLBC was headquartered in Washington, D.C., and divided into four national regions, each with its own director. Here Sanger surrounded herself with faithful friends and activists who had money, including Frances Ackermann, the former ABCL treasurer; philanthropist Ethel Clyde; Dorothy Hamilton Brush, a wealthy Cleveland socialite who was instrumental in establishing that city's first clinic; and Connecticut suffrage leader Katharine Houghton Hepburn, mother of the actress, who grew up on the right side of the tracks in Sanger's hometown of Corning, New York. The Committee pursued an education campaign that was strikingly similar and in competition with the ABCL's—distributing educational literature, organizing conferences, and sending out field workers to attract members, money, and endorsements. Sanger and several professional lobbyists traced Mary Dennett's steps in the halls of Congress to find bill sponsors and relevant committee support. Sanger had learned from Dennett's legislative defeats that she needed to bring pressure to bear from outside the nation's capital. Therefore the NCFLBC concentrated on winning both endorsements from so-called "outstanding citizens"—325,000 between 1929 and 1936—and from medical, scientific, fraternal, business, and religious organizations—nearly 1,000 in seven years. The NCFLBC wanted to demonstrate to legislators that birth control enjoyed wide support from influential leaders and groups in their respective constituencies. Winning endorsements from large and politically powerful organizations may have been the NCFLBC's greatest contribution to the movement. The Committee received the approval of the General Federation of Women's Clubs, the League of Women Voters, and the Committee on Marriage and the Home of the Federal Council of the Churches of Christ in America—the largest and most influential American Protestant organization to endorse birth control. Within organized religion, only the Catholic Church and several Lutheran groups actively opposed contraception.

Committee attorneys drafted a doctors-only bill that addressed pertinent sections of the Criminal Code under the Comstock Act and a section of the Tariff law regarding the importation of contraceptives. Between May 1930 and February 1936, the NCFLBC secured seven different sponsors to introduce House or Senate versions of the bill a total of 10 times. By 1935 every single congressman, according to Sanger, had been approached and asked for support. And not a few uncomfortable meetings—often in hallways and on the run—took place. "We should let it alone," South Carolina Senator Ellison Smith told a Committee member. "It jars me. It is revolting to interfere in people's personal affairs." "I'm not ready to teach our children to become whores yet," offered Senator William Dieterich, an Illinois Democrat. "We have not the right to deny the joy of life to millions," Kentucky Republican Charles Finley asserted. Quite a few lawmakers were sympathetic but either feared political repercussions or believed that contraception was already readily available to most Americans. "I'm a Jew," said Connecticut Representative William Citron, a Democrat, "and the Catholics would crucify me if I voted for this bill." Representative Henry Ellenbogen, a Pennsylvania Democrat, said, "You haven't a chance this session. The R.C. [Roman Catholics] have been busy getting all their people to write letters, and even friendly Congressmen are afraid." Senator Hugo Black, the feisty Alabama Democrat, tried to dodge lobbyist Hazel Moore, calling out, "I have all the information I need and so do you."

Only one bill survived committee hearings, the 1933 Hastings Bill (S.1842), which was reported favorably out of the Senate Judiciary Subcommittee in April 1934 and put on the Senate docket. On June 13, 1934, in the frenzied atmosphere of a final session day, the bill miraculously passed without objection or amendment. But within minutes, Senator Pat McCarren, a Democrat from Nevada and a Catholic, called under Senate rules for an immediate vote to recall the bill. It passed, and the bill was returned to die in committee. Hazel Moore, who had been largely responsible for shepherding the bill this far and witnessed its momentary passage, wrote immediately afterward, ". . . why couldn't every man in favor have jumped to their feet and shouted "No"—but men are men—and Senators are Cowards." After seven years of intense lobbying, the much-heralded NCFLBC legislative campaign, which dwarfed the VPL efforts of the early 1920s, ended with exactly the same result.[21]

Despite the legislative failures, the NCFLBC's work resulted in six Congressional hearings between 1931 and 1934, during some of the darkest days of the Depression and with a backdrop of unprecedented government expansion under President Roosevelt's New Deal program. Hearings before committees in both the House and Senate provided dramatic public forums on the morality of birth control, the urgency for changing the law, and the idea of birth control as a relief measure—a theme that the NCFLBC aggressively promoted in mailings and public events. As an editorial in the *Dallas Morning News* stated, "In these days of depression with their burden of charity the need of exact information becomes a social necessity. . . . Quality, not quantity is the modern demand." The Committee assembled several dozen expert witnesses—from well-known eugenicists like Henry Pratt Fairchild, physicians such as Hannah Stone, and abortion expert Frederick Taussig, to attorney Morris Ernst, religious leaders including Rabbi Sidney Goldstein and the Reverend Charles Francis Potter, and the feminist reformer and writer Charlotte Perkins Gilman—to present the broad rationales for birth control, but especially to emphasize the economic burdens posed by large families surviving on government relief. Sanger argued for—and others echoed the need—to incorporate birth control programs into President Roosevelt's ambitious reform agenda. The opposition, tightly organized and wholly dominated by the Catholic Church, countered with doctors and social scientists of their own, prepared with the well-honed arguments that contraception was harmful, led to promiscuity, and defied not only church teaching but also natural law.

The debate over the birth control bills received extensive press coverage that peaked during the January 1934 hearings when Father Charles Coughlin, the demagogic and bigoted Detroit radio priest, came before the House Judiciary Committee, his glare focused on Sanger, who was sitting just a few feet away. Coughlin reminded the packed hearing room of "God's fundamental command, 'Increase and multiply,' not 'Control and destroy.'" And he characterized nonprocreative marital sex as "legalized prostitution." Reporters recorded "scornful laughter," groans, and a woman who called out, "You're ridiculous." Sanger later called Coughlin's testimony a "half-hour of grossness." The press, which showed little patience for Coughlin's line of attack or Catholic opposition arguments in general, expressed a matter-of-fact advocacy during the hearings of what sounded a lot like reproductive rights, although no one yet used that phrase. For example, an editorial in the *News and Observer* of Raleigh, North Carolina, criticized Coughlin for deflecting attention from the crux of the issue, which was "whether or not the Congress of the United States shall continue to say that it is a crime to disseminate a phase of man's knowledge to people who as free agents, men and women, are entitled to shape their families and their lives in terms of their own judgment and not in terms of a dictatorial government or church."

Even when sparring with Catholic lawmakers, both Sanger and Katharine Houghton Hepburn, who took turns anchoring the proponents' side of the testimony, remained remarkably restrained and conciliatory toward the Church. They avoided easy rejoinders and steered the questioning toward common ground, such as safeguarding women from unscrupulous dealers and unregulated drugstore contraception. Toward the end of the January 1934 hearings, Sanger confounded opposition Congressmen by declaring the two sides to be essentially in agreement. This came in response to Catholic claims that a "natural" birth control method—rhythm—was highly effective and made the bill in question unnecessary. Though women had followed various safe period schedules before, an improved rhythm calendar based on new research and explained in a 1932 how-to guide by Chicago physician Leo Latz, had recently received ecclesiastical approval.* The door had been opened by Pope Pius XI in his 1930 *Encyclical on Christian Marriage*, in which he allowed for marital relations during infertile periods. Sanger, taking stock of these revisions in Catholic teaching on birth control and an acceptance in some Catholic circles of child-spacing for health and economic reasons, told the House Committee, "We are both together on the principles, and we separate on the question of methods." Disbelieving Congressmen refused to equate so-called natural birth control with artificial contraception. But Sanger had made her point that even the Church now acknowledged the benefits of family planning and had been forced to respond to the laity's widespread use of birth control.[22]

---

* Leo J. Latz, *The Rhythm of Sterility and Fertility in Women* (Chicago: Latz Foundation, 1932). Most doctors and birth control advocates rejected the method as unreliable.

THE ABCL WITHOUT SANGER

Though the ABCL endorsed the doctors-only bill in the early 1930s, Jones and the League viewed the federal laws as an inconvenience but not a significant obstacle for physicians, and did not believe the movement should expend resources on lobbying Congress. Under Jones's direction, the League sought to shift the emphasis from "propaganda to action," to make an immediate difference in the lives of those most adversely affected by the Depression by fostering more leagues and clinics, and working with public health agencies in an attempt to add contraceptive services to public clinics and hospitals. Starting in 1935, the League instigated a clinic affiliation program to advise clinics, ensure they met professional standards, and collect much needed dues. As Carole McCann has written, the League established itself as "a responsible public health agency" and played a role in helping to cultivate, by 1936, an estimated 30 contraceptive outlets operating in tax-supported institutions in 17 states—the first stage of public health birth control. But the League ultimately fell short of its goals, particularly in failing to partner with state public health departments. It was held back in large part by funding problems, exacerbated by having to compete with the more media savvy NCFLBC and the BCCRB, which, despite its own budget crisis, also started a clinic affiliation program in 1935 and, like the ABCL, sent workers out into the field.

EUGENICS AND STERILIZATION

The ABCL, especially under Jones's direction from 1929 to 1935, demonstrated a strong eugenic motivation in trying to deliver birth control to the poorest and least-educated Americans. At the same time, the League encouraged the middle- and upper-classes to have larger families. "More well born . . . fewer ill born," Jones wrote in 1931. The League won support from eugenic groups that had come to recognize the potential of birth control but remained aloof from the NCFLBC and BCCRB because of Sanger's refusal to encourage any woman to have more children. Reports in the mid-1930s that the birth rate was 60 percent higher among families receiving government assistance spurred the League to follow Sanger's example in promoting birth control as a savings to the taxpayer. Unlike Sanger, the ABCL at times blurred separation between the poor and the unfit, lumping the groups together under the umbrella of relief families.

On the question of negative eugenics, movement leaders in the 1930s pushed for a strong public policy on limiting, through birth control, the fertility of the mentally and physically disabled, and those with hereditary defects. However, neither the NCFLBC nor ABCL leaders endorsed compulsory sterilization programs, which were legal in 30 states. The Supreme Court upheld such laws in *Buck v. Bell* (1927), an 8–1 decision made emphatic by Justice Oliver Wendell Holmes Jr.'s, blunt majority opinion: "The principle that sustains compulsory vaccination is broad enough to cover the fallopian tubes."* By 1940, at least 35,000 Americans—nearly half of them in California—had been sterilized without their consent. The ABCL believed that birth control and voluntary sterilization campaigns would be sufficient to address the problem of "the dysgenic multiplication of the unfit" if given public support. Sanger suggested that the government pay a yearly pension to "paupers, morons, feeble-minded, mentally and morally deficient persons, who will submit to sterilization."

The movement's eugenic stance became problematic in light of press coverage in 1934 to 1935 about Nazi Germany's eugenic courts and sterilization policies and successful efforts by several leading scientists in the United States and Britain in the late 1930s to expose eugenics as a sham science motivated by class bias and racism. Nevertheless, the movement continued to press eugenic themes, still well received in many quarters during the difficult economic years leading up to World War II.[23]

THE BUSINESS OF BIRTH CONTROL

The ABCL was not alone in criticizing Sanger for forging ahead with the lobbying campaign, even after several failed attempts to get a bill out of committee. Others in the press and Congress in particular questioned the logic of creating such a ruckus over restrictions on mailing contraceptive information when the birth control business was booming. The contraceptive industry had received a big boost in December 1930, when yet another court decision chiseled a chunk out of the Comstock laws. In a trademark suit between two condom manufacturers, *Youngs Rubber Corporation v. C. I. Lee and Co., Inc.*, the U.S. Court of Appeals for the Second Circuit ruled that condom manufacturing was a legal enterprise and therefore entitled to trademark protection. More importantly, the court questioned why contraceptives should be barred from the mails "merely because they are capable of illegal uses." The decision signaled the need for further judicial clarification. In the short term, it gave manufacturers some leeway in mailing information to physicians and pharmacists and advertising more widely in newspapers and other serial publications, though the industry held fast to its euphemistic synonyms for birth control, "feminine hygiene" and "marriage hygiene." Even the tony *New York Times* ran ads for birth control, including one for the clumsily named contraceptive jelly "birconjel"—"the practice of feminine hygiene can have an aesthetic as well as practical side."

The *Youngs Rubber* decision not only contributed to the rapid expansion of the contraceptive industry in the early 1930s, it also opened up new channels of

---

* Most states eventually either repealed or overturned compulsory sterilization laws, but the Supreme Court decision has never been reversed.

distribution. A 1932 survey taken in western Florida found "prophylactics" for sale in 376 retail outlets other than drugstores, including "gas stations, garages, restaurants, soda fountains, barber shops, pool rooms, cigar stands, news stands, shoe-shine shops, grocery stores." In certain parts of the country, saleswomen peddled contraceptive jellies and even diaphragms and IUDs door-to-door. Condom-dispensing machines were installed in some men's rooms and in businesses where men gathered. By 1938, birth control industry sales were estimated to be over $250 million per year, just a bit less than the jewelry business. Four-fifths of the money went to manufacturers of an astounding 600 brands of female contraceptives, mostly jellies and douching solutions. Men spent less than women, but still paid out twice as much money on condoms than on shaving needs. Although the number of nonprofit birth control clinics had soared to over 300 by the late 1930s, there were by then over 400 contraceptive makers, including fly-by-night operations and physician-run businesses. As an article in the *New Republic* concluded, "What has happened is that the contraceptive business has outgrown the birth-control movement."[24]

JUDICIAL NULLIFICATION AND THE *ONE PACKAGE* CASE

The absurdity of the legal situation surrounding contraception and the failure of legislators to take action put pressure on the courts to determine the Comstock law's relevance to a society steeped in birth control. Several cases in the early 1930s reinforced judgments rendered in the *Young's Rubber* case and in Dennett's defense of her *Sex Side of Life* indictment (*U.S. v. Dennett*) in 1930: there must be illegal intent for the federal obscenity laws to have bearing on the exchange of contraceptive information (*Young's*) and context, above all else, determines whether or not a work is indecent (*Dennett*). In *U.S. v. One Book Entitled "Contraception* (1931)," the U.S. District Court for the Southern District of New York exempted the importation of printed contraceptive information from prohibition under the Tariff Act. In *Davis v. United States* (1933), the Sixth Circuit Court of Appeals ruled that the interstate transportation of a contraceptive device was legal unless evidence could be furnished to show a misuse of the product.

Morris Ernst, who had served as Dennett's lead attorney in 1930, apprised Sanger of the relevant cases making their way through the courts, and the two schemed about ways to instigate a more clear-cut test case that involved the medical profession. Hannah Stone and Sanger went so far as to draft a dummy contraceptive pamphlet designed to lure the authorities. They backed off that plan when, in January 1933, U.S. Customs confiscated a package of about 120 "Koyama Suction" pessaries sent from a Japanese doctor to Hannah Stone at the BCCRB. Sanger had requested the shipment, having a legitimate interest in testing this unusual, cone-shaped diaphragm. Ernst believed that the package should have been lawfully admitted into the country and, with Sanger's authorization, contested the seizure.[25]

After nearly three years of procedural activity, the case came to trial on December 10, 1935, before Judge Grover M. Moscowitz of the U.S. District Court for the Eastern District of New York. Ernst, representing the claimant, reprised part of his 1929 defense in the clinic raid trial, calling many of the same doctors to explain the medical indications for contraception and to vouch for Hannah Stone's legitimate intentions in prescribing the devices in question. The district attorney's office seated only one expert, Dr. Frederic Bancroft, a New York City surgeon who frequently prescribed contraceptives for specific health problems and endorsed child-spacing. Why the government enlisted his expertise is a bit of a mystery, since he supported the claimant's case. Stranger yet, the evidence—samples of the Japanese pessaries—disappeared after Bancroft's testimony, leading some trial observers to believe he pocketed them out of professional interest. Following the testimony, Ernst laid out the higher court opinions that provided a foundation for his argument: because contraceptives "can be used legally and illegally it is not to be presumed that Congress intended to condemn their use for decent public health purposes." The assistant district attorney held that the statutes must be interpreted literally and that Congress' recent inaction on the proposed birth control bills should inform the court's decision. Moving quickly, Judge Moscowitz dismissed the jury since the facts of the case were not in question, only the interpretation of the law.

On January 6, 1936, Judge Moscowitz decided in favor of Hannah Stone. He quoted extensively from both *Young's Rubber* and *Davis*, and referenced *Bours v. United States* (1915), which exempted doctors from the law when they performed an abortion to save a woman's life. Moscowitz ruled that Section 305(a) of the Smoot-Hawley Tariff Act of 1930, a descendant of the Comstock Act and the specific law under which the pessaries were confiscated, must be "given a reasonable construction" that allows for the importation of articles intended for the prevention of disease, "a lawful purpose." The government filed for appeal, and nearly another year passed before the Second Circuit Court of Appeals upheld the decision on December 7, 1936. In his historic opinion, Judge Augustus Hand treated all of the federal prohibitions on birth control that originated from the 1873 Comstock Act as "part of a continuous scheme to suppress immoral articles and obscene literature and should so far as possible be construed together and consistently." The court believed that the design of the Comstock law, written before Congress could have "understood all the conditions" under which contraception would be used, "was not to prevent the importation, sale, or carriage by mail of things which might intelligently be employed by conscientious and competent physicians for the purpose of saving life or promoting the well being of their patients."[26]

Ernst wasted no time in declaring that the decision "means the end of birth control laws." He emphatically pointed to what the court left out of its opinion: it did not specify under what circumstances a physician could prescribe birth control. "The inference was clear," Ernst later wrote, "that the medical profession was to be sole judge of the propriety of a prescription in a given case, and that as long as a physician exercised his discretion in good faith the legality of his action was not to be questioned." Initially, Sanger reacted more guardedly in public, telling reporters, "This decision definitely clarifies the situation. . . ." By the end of January 1937, after the Attorney General announced that it would not appeal the case to the Supreme Court, she was more triumphant. "There is no further question as to the rights of the medical profession in regard to contraception," she wrote to NCFLBC supporters. "The birth control movement is *free*."

AMERICAN MEDICAL ASSOCIATION ENDORSEMENT

The AMA was tepid in its initial response to the *One Package* decision, failing to see how it changed anything but importation law. Just a few months earlier, an AMA Committee to Study Contraceptive Practices, created in 1935 after years of prodding from Dickinson and the CMH (now known as the National Committee on Maternal Health), submitted its first report. The language sounded contemptuous of the birth control movement. The report could not justify birth control for economic or eugenic reasons and blamed birth control activists for reducing the birth rate of the best and brightest. The AMA committee concluded that neither state nor federal laws interfered with a doctor's prerogative to prescribe contraceptives. But when the committee reported back to the AMA annual conference in June 1937, its tone had softened, due in part to an intense lobbying effort by Dickinson, who had met individually with committee members.

For the medical establishment, the *One Package* decision had removed a haze of confusion and lifted the stigma associated with birth control's uncertain legality. Physicians seemed relieved to have clarity. Many doctors had also expressed growing concern over the commercial exploitation of contraceptives, convincing a greater number of their colleagues that the AMA must become actively involved in developing contraceptive standards. The Committee to Study Contraceptive Practices issued a series of recommendations—including that the AMA promote contraceptive instruction in medical schools and advise doctors on their legal rights—that together constituted a cautious endorsement of birth control. Most significantly, it stated, "The intelligent voluntary spacing of pregnancies may be desirable for the health and general well being of mothers and children." The committee also proposed that the AMA undertake a thorough analysis of contraceptive methods. That investigation ended up under Robert Dickinson's direction and took several years to complete. On June 8, 1937, the AMA's House of Delegates unanimously adopted the committee's report, having taken 90 years to formally recognize birth control as a proper medical practice.[27]

"We believe in the long run," ran an editorial in the *New York World-Telegram*, that the AMA action "will be counted as a milestone of progress toward a healthier and better country." Allison Pierce Moore, chairman of the ABCL wrote, "We welcome the progressive leadership of the American Medical Association." Moore added, "Lay support and education behind the physician and the public health agency is the cornerstone of national health." When she first heard the news, Sanger told reporters, "This is an overwhelming victory." She called the country's largest medical body "the last stronghold" of birth control resistance, dismissing the opposition of the Catholic Church, which she said, "no longer has a leg to stand on." In a radio speech a few days later Sanger stated that the AMA endorsement "marks the end of a long and arduous fight against fear and taboo, inertia, and bigotry. . . . Birth control, 20 years ago outlawed, reviled, has won its place in the sun."

MASSACHUSETTS AND CONNECTICUT

Despite the movement's dual victories, in the courts and in the medical establishment, that liberating sun still only shone in the doctor's office or medical clinic. And several states had misgivings about the nullification of the federal laws, accusing the courts of overreach—what today would be called judicial activism. While 21 states had no provisions against contraception, 18 states exempted physicians, 6 restricted advertising, and 3—Massachusetts, Connecticut and Mississippi—banned contraception with no exemptions. Not long after the *One Package* decision, Massachusetts and Connecticut reaffirmed their sweeping prohibitions on birth control, preserved like fossils in the bedrock of Catholic political power. On June 3, 1937, police raided the North Shore Mothers' Health Office in Salem, Massachusetts, the first of a series of raids in the Commonwealth that summer that led to the arrest and convictions of clinic doctors and staff. In August, the Birth Control League of Massachusetts, also raided by police, closed its remaining clinics and focused its resources on mounting a legal defense. In May 1938, the Massachusetts Supreme Judicial Court upheld the Salem convictions, finding no medical exemption in the law. Other appeals were withdrawn or denied, and the birth control clinics never reopened. Connecticut followed suit in June 1939 when police raided the Waterbury Maternal Health Clinic and later arrested the clinic staff. The Connecticut Supreme Court, like its northern neighbor, refused to grant a medical exception. Activists in both states tried repeatedly to pass amendments in the state legislatures in the late 1930s, to no avail.[28]

THE BIRTH CONTROL FEDRATION OF AMERICA

The *One Package* decision and AMA endorsement did little in the short term to expand or improve access to contraception. The most immediate effect was on the organizational makeup of the movement. Sanger declared mission accomplished and disbanded the NCFLBC in April 1937—even though it had failed to achieve its stated goal in Congress. Strategy sessions for the *One Package* case had drawn the two remaining national organizations, the ABCL and BCCRB, which shared legal counsel, closer together. This cooperation led to the formation in May 1937 of the Birth Control Council of America, a kind of joint advisory board charged with eliminating redundancies and coordinating publications, field work, and clinic affiliations. The meetings were testy and combative, and the Council dissolved a few months later. However, the ABCL knew it could not long survive the difficult economic times without a recognized national leader to compete with Sanger's fund-raising prowess. For her part, Sanger seemed ready to let others run the day-to-day activities of the movement. With various health problems and an elderly husband to care for, she wished to spend more time in Tucson, Arizona, where she had recently settled.

An outside consulting firm coordinated a joint committee formed between the two groups in 1938, and negotiations led to a merger. The Birth Control Federation of America (BCFA) was established in January 1939.* Public relations executives and physicians were placed in the BCFA leadership positions, and Sanger assumed an advisory role, serving on the executive committee and as an honorary chair. A number of her closest supporters, including Juliet Rublee, took positions on the board, and several of her key staff, such as her indispensable secretary, Florence Rose, tried with mixed success to fit in to the corporate-style structure of the Federation. Surprisingly few of the ABCL leaders survived the transition. Sanger may have had some influence in pushing out several ABCL officers whom she had grown to distrust, including the former president Allison Pierce Moore and executive director Marguerite Benson, who ran the League after Eleanor Jones left in 1935.[29]

When the merger took place there were over 400 birth control clinics in the country. A majority of them later affiliated with the BCFA to form an impressive national health organization with representation in every state and strong medical support both nationally and regionally. The new Federation also had what its precursor organizations lacked when they first formed, credible poll numbers to attest to the widespread approval of birth control. There had been some earlier polling of specific groups, such as medical societies, and nonscientific surveys (for instance, in 1935 a New Jersey radio station asked listeners to call in for or against birth control—over 87 percent approved). But the first truly national poll with a significant sample,

---

* While the BCCRB, which had absorbed many NCFLBC staff, became part of the new Federation, the clinic itself remained independent and under Sanger's direction and Hannah Stone's medical oversight.

conducted by the American Institute of Public Opinion, was not completed until 1936. Based on 100,000 respondents, the poll found that 70 percent of the American public thought birth control should be legal, with a pro–birth control majority in every state. Of the largest cities, only Boston voters said no, 55 percent to 45 percent. Not surprisingly, the approval among women, young people, and college students rated higher than the national average. In 1938, 79 percent of women said they were in favor of contraception in a *Ladies' Home Journal* poll.[30]

BIRTH CONTROL AND PUBLIC HEALTH

While these surveys represented independent confirmation that the movement's public outreach and education efforts had succeeded in winning acceptance for birth control, they did not measure contraceptive knowledge, which was still sorely lacking in underprivileged America. Despite the legal advances, the spread of clinics, and the sharp growth of the contraceptive industry in the interwar years, effective and afford- able birth control remained beyond the economic—and sometimes geographic— reach of many poor women, especially in rural areas and in immigrant and African American communities. Most clinics were established to serve the working class and those who could not afford a private doctor, and they eliminated or reduced fees for the poor. Yet, for a number of reasons they did not tend to reach the poorest popula- tions, which continued to rely on withdrawal and abortion for limiting family size.

The movement's near fixation with the diaphragm was a main stumbling block. The lower the education and income level, the less likely a woman would use the diaphragm, though this was the method most preferred by clinics and prescribed by doctors. At about $5 a unit, the supplies were too expensive for many women to obtain from a doctor. Even when offered for free or at a reduced rate, the diaphragm not well suited to poor women. As Linda Gordon has pointed out, it "was difficult to use without privacy, running water, and a full explanation and fitting, luxuries not available to most Americans." Doctors were also reluctant to spend the considerable time it took to fit the diaphragm if they were not getting properly reimbursed. They had little faith, based partly on experience and influenced by prejudice, in unedu- cated women learning the proper insertion and care procedure and then sticking with the method over time. In fact, studies in the 1930s found that about half of all women gave up on the diaphragm because of discomfort and the hassle factor. Physicians were often unwilling to offer other contraceptives because of a lack of reli- able data on safety and effectiveness. The Consumers Union *Analysis of Contraceptive Materials*, the first guide to specific brands, was not published until 1937. It disclosed up front that "such knowledge as exists is so qualified as to render it only partially useful." The AMA did not issue standards and recommendations for contraception until 1943. Erratic pricing and distribution further dissuaded the medical profession from expanding contraceptive choices. Although the availability of condoms and suppositories had increased in most areas, at about $1 per dozen, they cost too much for many Americans to buy on a regular basis.[31]

Following the *One Package* decision, Sanger pushed for the movement to turn its full attention to linking with state public health services and interesting federal agencies in reaching poor communities not served by independent clinics, even though in the past leaders had failed miserably in trying to secure state and federal funds for birth control work. Most notably, Sanger and Dennett had been rebuffed in the 1920s by the Children's Bureau, a division of the U.S. Department of Labor. The two advocates had lobbied to have contraceptive services added to state health programs on birth hygiene, funded under the breakthrough Sheppard-Towner Maternity and Infant Protection Act (1921). Before its passage, the controversial act, designed to reduce infant and maternal mortality rates, was fought on the grounds that it was a birth control bill in disguise. This left the bureaucrats at the Children's Bureau no real choice but to reject entreaties by birth control activists, even though the Bureau received thousands of requests each year for contraceptive information. Although Sheppard-Towner was underfunded and excluded contraception, it established the first federally-funded social welfare program in the United States and marked the first time that the government responded specifically to women's health issues. Discontinued in 1929, it nevertheless had created a template for preventive and women's health programs in many states, a number of which found alternative funding to continue maternal and infant care programs. With legal barriers removed, birth controllers believed the time was ripe to embark on birth control as public health, tapping into existing social welfare and public health services created under Sheppard-Towner and New Deal programs.[32]

Physician and medical researcher Clarence Gamble (1894–1966) devised plans to increase access to contraception for the poor using the immunization model of mobile and local clinic-based distribution. Gamble, who worked most directly with the CMH but also through the BCCRB and ABCL in the mid-1930s, was an heir to the Proctor and Gamble fortune and dedicated his career and his philanthropy to finding better birth control for the masses. His motivations were strongly eugenic, and his gung-ho approach and impatience with medical bureaucracy bedevilled organizations and institutions that partnered with him. Gamble was convinced that "doctorless" birth control—simple methods such as a contraceptive jelly used alone—though inferior to the diaphragm, could markedly lower birth rates in impoverished regions. He instigated field trials in the mid-1930s in Appalachia to make his case. A three-year project in Logan County, West Virginia, demonstrated that some birth control was better than no birth control, but it was not an unqualified success. Women generally disliked the contraceptive jelly alone, and a majority ceased using it. However, the West Virginia study and other field work at the time did prove that very poor women, white and black, wanted increased access to contraception and were willing to try different methods.

Sanger, Gamble, and Dickinson had been investigating new contraceptives, both in the United States and abroad, with an eye out for less expensive methods. Sanger held out hope that a biological contraceptive involving hormonal manipulation or the production of sperm antibodies—something she had discussed with researchers at the Seventh International Birth Control Conference in Zurich in 1930—might lead to an inexpensive contraceptive pill or injection. Others found such ideas farfetched. Dickinson questioned the wisdom of letting imagination interfere with the rational scientific approach and warned Sanger about exposing the movement to ridicule. But both Sanger and Gamble were determined to discover innovative ways of preventing pregnancy, not only to expand the contraceptive revolution in the United States, but also to enable population control in the developing world. They were willing to follow any leads, from herbal remedies, to common table salt as a spermicide added to a paste or jelly.[33]

By the late 1930s, a simple foaming powder paired with a natural sponge emerged as the most promising method for mass distribution. Developed in the early 1930s by Dr. Lydia Allen DeVilbiss, who had settled into a clinical practice in Miami after running out on Sanger's proposed clinic in 1921, the foam powder method was cheap and easy and did not require a medical examination. Users simply moistened a sponge, sprinkled powder on it, and kneaded it a few times to produce lather before inserting it into the vagina. The method was both occlusive and spermicidal—blocking and killing the sperm—and fared well in clinic testing. Sanger quickly set up foam powder field trials in several Asian countries and in a number of states, where, costing only a few cents per use, the sponge and foam powder became the preferred method for U.S. public health providers.

Birth controllers zeroed in on southern state public health programs in the mid- and later 1930s because of the alarmingly high birth rates in many poor, rural communities in the region, weak Catholic opposition, and willing public health officials. Starting in 1937, Clarence Gamble helped pay for and organize birth control work in North Carolina, one of the few states to have full-time public health officers in every county. Following successful pilot projects in a few county health centers, George M. Cooper, the assistant director of the North Carolina State Board of Health, expanded the contraceptive program to three-fourths of the state's counties. Health officers, working with birth control field workers, prescribed foam powder for most women but also dispensed condoms and fitted diaphragms. The program had the potential to reach two-thirds or more of the rural poor in the state. However, relatively few took advantage of the service owing to cultural pressures (agricultural communities valued large families), ineffective outreach, lack of transportation to the clinics, and other factors. Nevertheless, North Carolina's nationally publicized public birth control program (articles appeared in *Life Magazine, Reader's Digest,* and many news-papers), the first in the nation, served as a model for other states in the South. By the early 1940s, six southern states had established contraceptive services as part of their public health programs.[34]

THE NEGRO PROJECT

After 1939, the BCFA helped coordinate public health efforts, including what became known as the Negro Project, a series of demonstration clinics in South Carolina and Tennessee designed to provide a model for how contraceptive clinics could serve African American communities. Conceived by Sanger; Mary Reinhardt, a BCFA executive committee member; and Florence Rose, Sanger's close assistant, the Negro Project was, at its most basic, Sanger's attempt to deliver contraception to abject black poverty pockets in the South. Several Southern tours beginning in 1919 and field reports on the birth control public health work in Virginia, Kentucky, and other southern states in the 1930s had made Sanger acutely aware that black women's reproductive health had been neglected by the white medical establishment in segregated areas.

On another level, the project aimed to do its part in addressing the so-called *Negro problem,* the post-Reconstruction term that referred to the enduring, economic, and social challenges created by poverty and racism. An influential government report in 1938 by the National Resources Committee underscored the correlation between high birth rates and poverty—both white and black—in the South and its increas-ing financial toll on the rest of the country. Sanger, Reinhardt, and Rose drafted a detailed proposal that identified Southern blacks "as the group among which the greatest misery exists" and recommended a birth control program to "increase the cultural, as well as the health and economic advancement of the negro race." They outlined an education campaign whereby black ministers and medical professionals would first speak to the community about the benefits of birth control before contra-ceptive services were established. In part, they hoped community involvement would stem any backlash from black residents who had a legitimate fear of white health administrators. There had been a long history of contempt toward blacks on the part of the medical establishment and incidents—some just coming to light—of medical malfeasance. More importantly, Sanger knew from her experience in New York that a black clinic would succeed only if the community had a stake in it.[35]

After the proposal received funding from philanthropist Albert Lasker, the BCFA leadership decided to forgo Sanger's planned educational approach and add contra-ceptive services to existing public health facilities with no concrete plans to prime the community first or directly involve community leaders. Sanger was irate, but in her diminished role at the BCFA she lacked the power to change policy. In late 1940,

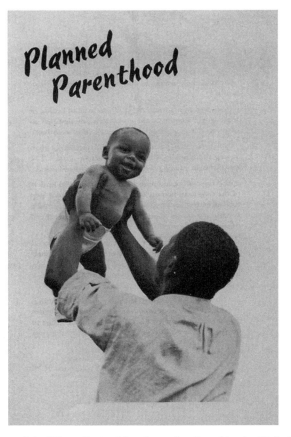

An example of one of the "Negro Project" brochures distributed by the Birth Control Federation of America (1940). (Courtesy of the Sophia Smith Collection, Smith College.)

she did raise additional funds to have Florence Rose launch a national education program under the BCFA's Division of Negro Service, the department that oversaw the demonstration clinics for African Americans. Rose sent to black professionals and organizations educational publications that underscored the relevance of reproductive health and family planning to racial progress. She also created an impressive national advisory council of black leaders, including Du Bois; Mary McLeod Bethune, the prominent black educator; and the Rev. Adam Clayton Powell Jr., the civil rights leader and politician. Rose secured the endorsements of major black civic, educational, and medical organizations. Meanwhile, the demonstration clinics, which dispensed foam powder or the diaphragm, functioned for about two years before the grant money ran out. Although they did employ a troop of black visiting nurses in South Carolina and black physicians and nurses in the two clinics in Nashville, the clinics had trouble attracting and keeping patients. Only about 2,000 women received contraception in the two states combined.[36]

The BCFA and state health administrators hailed the Negro Project and other state-supported, public health-based birth control programs in the South as success stories and a significant advancement for the movement. But the work brought to light some troubling questions. Methods continued to disappoint, leading to high dropout rates in most of the public health programs. The diaphragm presented its usual problems, and foam powder proved irritating to some and too messy to many. Clinic workers were slow to substitute other methods, like the condom. Although the condom's effectiveness and quality had improved significantly by this time, it remained in disfavor among the medical profession and many birth control activists.

More problematic was the lack of any long-term commitments to the Southern white and black communities served or any permanent footprint. Most of these campaigns and trial clinics shut down when funding ceased; the rest vanished with World War II. There was little effort on the part of those in charge to combine contraceptive services with infant and maternal health care to create a holistic approach to family planning that could have created lasting community benefits. Eugenic motivations narrowed the vision of the organizers, who tended to focus on reducing the birth rate among indigent populations—a good percentage of whom were considered "unfit"—instead of quality of life issues. An article about the North Carolina program in the *Atlantic Monthly* casually slipped in the prevailing outsider bias, commenting that in the state's poor mountain regions, "human life has never been given a particularly high valuation." As historian Johanna Schoen has written, these birth control programs "emphasized controlling the reproduction of the poor rather than extending reproductive control to poor women." This was especially true for the Negro Project. Although there is little evidence of overt racism among organizers and clinic workers, a demeaning paternalism informed nearly every planning decision and consigned black women to a special category of contraceptive user. Despite the hard work of many nurses and social workers to connect with patients, public health projects in general—and African American programs especially—were not structured to respond to individual needs.[37]

FEDERAL FUNDING

Birth controllers hoped that state programs would pave the way for federal funding of contraceptive services, but President Roosevelt's administration continued to resist taking a public stand for fear of a Catholic backlash at the polls. That did not stop Farm Security Administration agents, starting in 1937, from working with the

BCCRB, the ABCL, and then the BCFA to give contraceptive advice to migrant workers, mainly in the Southwest and California. By the end of 1940, over 3,000 migrant families received birth control information and supplies—foam powder in most cases. But government involvement was kept quiet. Despite Eleanor Roosevelt's public disclosure in 1940 that she had in earlier years contributed to "the maintenance of clinics in New York City" and favored "the planning of children," the Roosevelt administration would not allow federal public health agencies to incorporate contraceptive services.[38]

PLANNED PARENTHOOD

Noticeably absent from the documentary record of the public health programs and the Negro Project is any mention of a woman's right to birth control. In fact, that observation could be applied to the movement as a whole as it entered the 1940s. Apart from Sanger, the major voices for birth control, including Dickinson, Gamble, and the doctors leading the BCFA, seldom, if ever, referred to women's autonomy or reproductive freedom. In its 1940 annual report, the BCFA listed nine steps toward furthering the cause, and not one of them included women or motherhood.

After a decade of economic depression, at the onset of another world war, and with the medical takeover of birth control complete, the BCFA promoted family planning for economic well-being, national security—stronger families make a stronger nation—and for health reasons. However, the Federation did not advocate reproductive rights. Its gender-neutral marketing and messaging centered on family planning and child-spacing. The BCFA used the term *birth control* selectively, almost nostalgically at times, as if it referred to another era. The phrase had lost its relevance in an organization that now encouraged middle-class childbearing. In 1941, the BCFA committed itself to "planned parenthood in its widest sense," declaring that it was "the duty and responsibility of parents to have as many children as their health or economic circumstances justify." It was only a matter of time before the Federation abandoned any reference to "control" as it related to the organization's aims and principles. In discussing possible name changes with affiliates in 1941, the Federation argued that the phrase *planned parenthood* better suited its objectives and appealed more to men and the male-dominated public health departments, hospitals, legislatures, and government agencies that were integral to the future success of the movement. *Birth control* sounded disparaging of the family and still carried the residue of extremism. In February 1942, the BCFA became the Planned Parenthood Federation of America (PPFA).[39]

Sanger contested every Federation decision that distanced the movement from its women-centered, activist roots, including the pronatalist appeals for increased middle-class childbearing and attempts by Federation physicians to limit and tighten the accepted medical indications for contraception. She called the name change a "very weakening influence on the future of the movement." But the decision had been made despite her protests and with few Sanger loyalists left to assert her position. Besides, Sanger's own policies had brought about the accommodations and alliances that, by design, gradually obscured her feminist vision of voluntary motherhood. Since the early 1920s, the movement, under Sanger's leadership, sought acceptance for the concept of family planning as a social responsibility rather than a woman's right. Sanger continued to emphasize that the movement's fundamental task was to ensure that every woman had access to birth control and remind supporters that, above all else, "Women must be relieved of the fear of the unwanted child." However, the Federation steadfastly avoided the issue of reproductive freedom, finding it too bound up in the radical feminist origins of the movement. It would take a new generation of activists in the 1960s and a series of historic court rulings to reassert and legally establish birth control as a basic human right.[40]

Institutionalization brought with it the realization of broad and solid approval of birth control, but it also marked the passing of a dynamic, woman-led movement for women's sexual liberation.

CONCLUSION

The new era of planned parenthood, underscored by the Federation's name change in 1942, was profoundly shaped by World War II. The war forced the Planned Parenthood Federation of America (PPFA) to further retool its message to emphasize family, security, health, and productivity even over its branded words *choice* and *spacing*. The PPFA also expanded its program to meet wartime needs. It reached out to women working in the war industries who needed to delay childbirth. And it became one of the largest organizations to get into the marriage counseling business, turning out publications geared toward war brides and returning soldiers and training clergymen to give marriage advice.

In the baby boom years of the late 1940s and the 1950s the Federation sought to "build happy families" by offering marriage and parenthood education programs and special fertility clinics along with traditional "child-spacing assistance." PPFA became one of the most recognized and established health organizations in the country with over 100 affiliates by 1957 and support from across the political spectrum. On the whole, the Federation and regional groups had largely abandoned the women-centered approach of the earlier birth control movement, promoting instead a combination of family services and public education. The family planning movement steered clear of the association between birth control and sexual liberalism that was growing among the public. But there were rumblings within the PPFA in late 1950s about changing the policy that forbid clinics from serving unmarried women. By the early

1960s, with the advent of the contraceptive pill—approved by the Food and Drug Administration in 1960—and signs of changing sexual mores, the movement was forced to adjust not only to increased demand for services, but a renewed call for securing reproductive freedom.[1]

THREE YEARS

Several events during the years 1965 to 1967 laid down the framework for the modern-day movement for reproductive rights. Earlier efforts of the birth control movement, especially Sanger's decision to encourage medical authority over reproductive control, brought about or influenced the rapid series of events that unfolded during these three years. Developments in this short span of time related to the legality, federal support, and technological improvement of birth control and abortion have affected every issue regarding women's reproductive health and decision making since then.

In November 1965, the White House held the first-ever government-sponsored public discussion on family planning, at which Dr. Alan Guttmacher, the PPFA president stated "if we are going to give birth control to the underprivileged group, it's going to have to be done by the government." That meeting and a report issued in May 1965 by the National Academy of Sciences that called for "a far-reaching birth control program to extend the basic human right of family planning to all" helped expedite government action. President Johnson had begun providing limited family planning funds to public clinics in 1964 as part of his War on Poverty program. In a message to Congress in March 1966, he included family planning among four urgent American health problems and promised to increase government involvement in contraceptive services.

On September 6, 1966, the Department of Health, Education, and Welfare announced that it would hold a series of regional conferences to help communities develop family planning programs and "remove a barrier of silence" that still hampered access to contraceptives in many impoverished regions. That same day Margaret Sanger died in a Tucson nursing home, just shy of her eighty-seventh birthday. Though she had been too ill to be aware of the changes taking place that resulted from her activism, she had lived to a day that she thought might never come, when the government that had persecuted her took up her cause.[2]

While obituaries and editorials honored Sanger's contribution to improving women's lives and noted the vindication of her once controversial ideas, many also emphasized her work to curb population growth in a crowded world, a central concern of the time. Sanger's efforts to organize and lead a postwar international birth control movement (she remained president of the International Planned Parenthood Federation until she was 80) were integral to the establishment of a population control movement that began to coalesce in the late 1950s. American fears of a population explosion in the developing world compelled PPFA to extend its program to support population planning abroad. The Federation even changed its name for several years, starting in 1961, to Planned Parenthood-World Population after merging with a fund-raising organization seeking solutions to the population "crisis." The expansion of the American family planning movement to take on global population concerns was widely endorsed by birth control advocates even though the population control movement, with its emphasis on demographic change and fertility rates, was often at variance with the promotion of family planning and its assertion of individual choice. The population control movement strengthened in the years following Sanger's death and with the publication of Paul Ehrlich's seminal book, *The Population Bomb* in 1968.[3]

Sanger also survived long enough to witness the revolutionary impact of the contraceptive pill on American society. By 1965, just five years on the market and despite persistent reports of health concerns and side effects, the birth control pill had become the most widely used contraceptive method in the country, even showing up in the mid-1960s in Catholic medical institutions. Here was the nearly foolproof birth control that the movement had long sought. The pill put women in complete control and did not delay or interfere with sex, a huge drawback with most other methods. Coming on the market in the early 1960s, the pill helped create and sustain an environment conducive to the sexual revolution and the women's movement, as it forced society to confront woman's sexual freedom and the changing dynamic of the American family.

Sanger had played a key role in the development of the pill, linking long-time supporter and medical philanthropist Katharine Dexter McCormick with biologist Gregory Pincus and the Worcester Foundation for Experimental Biology. Pincus, receiving funding from PPFA starting in 1948, had been studying the hormone progesterone as an ovulation suppressant for several years. But the Federation proceeded cautiously on contraceptive research and expressed skepticism toward Pincus's work. Pincus and his colleagues needed significantly more money to take a promising idea and make it a practical reality. In 1953, Sanger arranged for McCormick to meet with Pincus in Massachusetts, at which time McCormick pledged substantial support. In all she gave about $2 million to finance the research and testing of the pill. Though both activists were well into their seventies, Sanger and McCormick kept in close contact with Pincus and the physician John Rock, who was instrumental in moving the concept from the laboratory to tests on human subjects. They had a hand in bringing in other experts and working with U.S. and international family planning organizations to coordinate controversial field trials. Together they fostered one of the most significant medical discoveries in history. McCormick and Pincus both died in 1967, a year after Sanger.[4]

With the pill grabbing headlines, the Supreme Court completed the judicial nullification of the provisions regarding contraception in the Comstock laws in its June 1965 ruling in *Griswold v. Connecticut*, a landmark legal decision. The case dealt with the arrest and conviction of Dr. C. Lee Buxton, a Yale professor and the medical director of the Planned Parenthood League of Connecticut, and Estelle Griswold, the director of the League, for giving contraceptive advice to three married couples in 1962. Buxton and Griswold were attempting to create a test case. The use of contraception remained illegal under Connecticut's draconian antiobscenity law passed in 1879 and inspired by the federal Comstock Act. In a 7–2 decision, the Supreme Court struck down the Connecticut law, declaring that it "unconstitutionally intrudes upon the right of marital privacy" and invades "the zone of privacy created by several fundamental constitutional guarantees." Writing for the majority, Justice William O. Douglas asked rhetorically, "Would we allow the police to search the sacred precincts of marital bedrooms for telltale signs of the use of contraceptives? The very idea is repulsive to the notions of privacy surrounding the marriage relationship."

In this historic decision the court cobbled together a right of privacy—first articulated in 1890 by a young attorney and later a Supreme Court Justice, Louis Brandeis, and his law partner, Samuel Warren—from language and clauses in the Bill of Rights and the due process clause of the Fourteenth Amendment. This adaptable right, with judicial roots in a number of birth control cases, including the 1936 *One Package* decision, has profoundly shaped American jurisprudence since *Griswold*, underpinning assertions of gay rights and the right to die, as well as the reproductive rights of women. Most immediately, however, the Griswold decision once and for all legalized birth control, though prohibitions in Massachusetts remained on the books and states ranging from Maryland to Mississippi still had statutes in effect that limited access to contraception.*

In May 1966, the Massachusetts legislature, well aware of the commonwealth's black sheep status as the only remaining anti–birth control state, amended the state's Comstock's laws to allow for contraceptives to be given to married persons. A little less than a year later, on April 6, 1967, the issue again came to the forefront when William Baird, a self-promoting birth control activist out of the mold of Sanger and Goldman, was arrested for handing a foam contraceptive to a young woman following a lecture he gave at Boston University. Though the Massachusetts law had been modified, it still prohibited laymen from distributing birth control and unmarried persons from using it. The case, *Eisenstadt* (the Suffolk County sheriff) *v. Baird*, was decided by the U.S. Supreme Court on March 22, 1972. In a 6–1 ruling, the court

---

* In 1970, Congress finally stripped out all reference to contraception in the 1873 Comstock Act.

overturned Baird's conviction and extended the right to privacy in reproductive decisions to unmarried persons, though it left intact a state's legal prerogative to determine who dispenses birth control. "If the right to privacy means anything," wrote Justice William J. Brennan, the only Catholic on the court at the time, "it is the right of the individual, married or single, to be free from unwarranted governmental intrusion into matters so fundamentally affecting a person as the decision whether to bear or beget a child." At the time the court announced the *Eisenstadt* decision, Justice Harry Blackmun was already drafting the majority opinion legalizing abortion in *Roe v. Wade*.[5]

The highest court's assertion of privacy rights dovetailed with increased public and medical support for legal therapeutic abortion, permitted in many states but only to protect the life of the mother. In the mid-1960s, serious outbreaks of rubella (German measles), a major cause of birth defects, following on the heels of thalidomide babies—infants born in the late 1950s and early 1960s with serious defects after their mothers took the sedative thalidomide during pregnancy—stepped up demands for safe and legal abortions. In 1966, a group of doctors in California publicly admitted to performing abortions in cases where women suffered from rubella in the first trimester of pregnancy, prompting other doctors to come forward. The American Medical Association passed a resolution in 1967 calling for a softening of the abortion laws in cases where a baby would likely be born with a severe or life-threatening disability. Medical groups joined legal associations, health workers, and many other organizations in seeking reform, before women activists took hold of the cause.

In 1966, a group of moderate feminists established the National Organization for Women, and by 1967 radical feminists began to split off from New Left organizations to devote themselves to a liberation campaign centered on issues related to gender, sexuality, and reproduction. By the end of the decade, this second wave of the women's movement had redefined the abortion reform campaign as a repeal movement, declaring an unconditional right to abortion and reasserting Sanger's now decades-old feminist decree that every woman must own and control her own body. The activism culminated in 1973 with the Supreme's Court's decision in *Roe v. Wade*, which ended most restrictions on abortions and opened the way for safe abortion practices.[6]

A major scientific breakthrough that dramatically changed the way in which many couples approached childbearing was pushed to the back pages of newspapers when it was first announced in October 1966. Geneticists had discovered a process by which amniotic fluid cells could be "cultured," enabling an analysis of chromosomes and certain enzymes. This led physicians to offer women a chromosomal prenatal diagnosis that allowed for early detection of certain fetal abnormalities and genetic disorders, and in some states (all by 1973), the choice to terminate the pregnancy. The technology led one scientist to boast later that year "that man may someday be able to direct his own evolution," while others feared a return to the monstrous eugenic policies of the Nazis. The term *eugenics*, like the name "Adolf," had understandably gone out of fashion with World War II. However, the birth control movement's fundamental eugenic objective—to give women more control in ensuring the health of their children—had gradually been achieved through effective birth control and medical abortion, prenatal testing, greater acceptance of voluntary sterilization, improvements in artificial insemination, and a better understanding of hereditary disorders and disease.[7]

The present-day reproductive rights movement, like its predecessor, is dedicated to increasing access to safe and effective birth control and to keeping abortion legal and available, at a time when recent court decisions have severely undermined a woman's right to choose. PPFA remains at the forefront of a battle against a resurgent conservative Christian morality and an antichoice movement focused on repealing *Roe v. Wade*. The political and legal strategies and publicity tactics are not all that different now from when the Catholic Church confronted the birth control movement in the 1920s.

This time the determining factor in the debate may not be public acceptance and demand or a media-savvy social movement, but a much less predictable force: medical technology. After a lull of more than a century between the discovery of vulcanized rubber and the birth control pill, medical-technological breakthroughs in reproductive control have occurred with increased frequency. Just as the pill and the patch and other hormonal contraceptives made birth control nearly invisible, so have recent drugs, like Mifepristone (Ru486) and Misoprostol, provided women with a nonsurgical, discreet method of early abortion. In August 2010, the Food and Drug Administration approved ulipristal acetate (ella®), a prescription-only, nonhormonal emergency contraceptive that blocks conception if taken up to five days after sex. It joins Plan-B, the so-called "morning after pill," that is available over the counter. Other drugs that blur the line between contraception and abortion will undoubtedly make reproductive control not only more morally ambiguous but also more private. A male contraceptive drug is probably not far in the future. Medical technology in this age of biology has dramatically expanded birth control choices and improved reproductive and women's health. By sheer effectiveness, efficiency, and pervasiveness, technology just might ensure an inviolable reproductive freedom.[8]

NOTES

INTRODUCTION

1. Margaret Sanger, *Woman and the New Race* (New York: Brentano's, 1920), 1.

2. Margaret Sanger, "The Aim," *The Woman Rebel* (March 1914): 1 (quotation 1); Margaret Sanger, *My Fight for Birth Control* (New York: Farrar & Rinehart, 1931), 83 (quotations 2, 3); Otto Bobsien to Sanger, October 24, 1953, in *The Margaret Sanger Papers Microfilm Edition: Smith College Collections*, eds. Esther Katz, Peter C. Engelman, Cathy Moran Hajo and Anke Voss Hubbard (Bethesda, MD: University Publications of America, 1996), Reel 41: 956 (hereafter *MSPME-SCC*); Esther Katz, Cathy Moran Hajo, and Peter C. Engelman, eds. *The Selected Papers of Margaret Sanger,* vol. 1, *The Woman Rebel, 1900–1928* (Urbana: University of Illinois Press, 2003), 52, 68, 104; Max Eastman, *Love and Revolution: My Journey through an Epoch* (New York: Random House, 1964), 262–64.

3. Janet Farell Brodie, *Contraception and Abortion in 19th Century America* (Ithaca, NY: Cornell University Press, 1994), 5; Sanger, *My Fight*, 83 (quotations); Katz, Hajo, and Engelman *Selected Papers I*, 70.

4. Fred Pearce, *The Coming Population Crash and Our Planet's Surprising Future* (Boston: Beacon Press, 2010), v–vii, 96.

5. See, for instance, Angela Frank's *Margaret Sanger's Eugenic Legacy: The Control of Female Fertility* (2005) and Dinesh D'Souza's *End of Racism* (1995). An Internet search of Sanger will turn up dozens of sites linking the birth control movement with extermination campaigns and mass abortion policies; for an example see www.blackgenocide.org. For the perspective of reproductive rights supporters, see Gloria Feldt, *The War on Choice: The Right-Wing Attack on*

Women's Rights and How to Fight Back (2003), and the history section on Planned Parenthood's Web site: www.plannedparenthood.org.

6. While a number of sources on social movements influenced my thinking, I relied most closely on Donatella Della Porta's and Mario Diani's *Social Movements: An Introduction* (Malden, MA: Blackwell Publishing, 2006).

7. Lenore Guttmacher, *Planned Parenthood Beginnings: Affiliate Histories* (New York: PPFA, 1979), 59–60.

CHAPTER ONE

1. Dr. N. Allen, "The New England Family," *New Englander and Yale Review* 41 (March 1882): 151.

2. Norman Himes, *Medical History of Contraception* (New York: Schocken Books, 1970; reprint of 1936 edition), xii–xviii, 3–5; Angus McLaren, *A History of Contraception from Antiquity to the Present Day* (Oxford: Blackwell, 1990), 2–5; the story of Onan is from Genesis 38:8–10.

3. Himes, *Medical History*, 59–66; Linda Gordon, *The Moral Property of Women* (Urbana: University of Illinois Press, 2002), 14, 18–21; Andrea Tone, *Devices and Desires: A History of Contraceptives in America* (New York: Hill & Wang, 2001), 13–14; Abraham Stone and Norman E. Himes, *Planned Parenthood: A Practical Guide to Birth-Control Methods* (New York: Macmillan, 1951), 13–17; Peter Fryer, *The Birth Controllers* (London: Secker & Warburg, 1965), 32–34.

4. Gordon, *Moral Property of Women,* 16; Margaret Sanger to Clarence Gamble, August 15, 1939, in Esther Katz, Peter C. Engelman, and Cathy Moran Hajo, eds., *The Selected Papers of Margaret Sanger,* vol. 2, *Birth Control Comes of Age, 1928–1939* (Urbana: University of Illinois Press, 2006), 495–96; Gary N. Clarke, "Etiology of Sperm Immunity in Women," *Fertility and Sterility* 91 (Feb. 2009): 639–43; Paul S. Henshaw, "Physiologic Control of Fertility," *Science* 117 (May 29, 1953): 572–82; Bernard Asbell, The *Pill: A Biography of the Drug That Changed the World* (New York: Random House, 1995), 70–73, 82–83, 109–110, 368.

5. McLaren, *History of Contraception*, 157–58; Janet Farell Brodie, *Contraception and Abortion in 19th Century America* (Ithaca, NY: Cornell University Press, 1994), 205–210; Stone and Himes, *Planned Parenthood*, 22–23.

6. Brodie, *Contraception and Abortion* 38–44; The Bradford quotation from *Of Plymouth Plantation* was referenced in Himes, *Medical History*, 224–225; Cornelia Hughes Dayton, "'Taking the Trade': Abortion and Gender Relations in an Eighteenth-Century New England Village," *William and Mary Quarterly* 48 (1991): 19–25.

7. John D'Emilio and Estelle B. Freedman, *Intimate Matters: A History of Sexuality in America* (Chicago: University of Chicago Press, 1988), 41–42, 57–59; Brodie, *Contraception and Abortion*, 41, 56; McLaren, *History of Contraception*, 178–79.

8. James Reed, *The Birth Control Movement and American Society: From Private Vice to Public Virtue* (Princeton, NJ: Princeton University Press, 1978), 3–5. See Carl N. Degler, *At Odds: Women and the Family in America from the Revolution to the Present* (New York: Oxford University Press, 1980), 178–209, for an insightful discussion of the demographic transition and fertility control in 19th century America.

9. Brodie, *Contraception and Abortion*, ix (quotation), 87–88; Degler, *At Odds*, 211–12; Gordon, *Moral Property of Women*, 24.

10. Robert Dale Owen, *Moral Physiology; or, A Brief and Plain Treatise on the Population Question* (Boston: J. P. Mendum, 1875 [10th ed.]), 13, 19, 58–69; Himes, *Medical History*, 224; Fryer, *Birth Controllers,* 89–98.

11. Himes, *Medical History*, 212–18; Charles Knowlton, *Fruits of Philosophy, or, The Private Companion of Adult People* (Mt. Vernon, NY: Peter Pauper Press, 1937; reprint of 1839 edition), 6 (quotation 2), 5–25, 60 (quotation 1)–68; Fryer, *Birth Controllers,* 99–106; C. Thomas Dienes, *Law, Politics and Birth Control* (Urbana: University of Illinois Press, 1972), 22–26.

12. Fryer, *Birth Controllers,* 103 (quotation), 104–106; Brodie, *Contraception and Abortion*, 89–105.

13. Rosanna Ledbetter, *A History of the Malthusian League, 1877–1927* (Columbus: Ohio University Press, 1976), 6–7, 29–41.

14. Brodie, *Contraception and Abortion*, 106–135; Reed, *Birth Control Movement*, 11–13.

15. Brodie, *Contraception and Abortion*, 64, 71–72, 231, 163; Himes, *Medical History*, 262–63; Gordon, *Moral Property of Women*, 36–37.

16. Reed, *Birth Control Movement*, 13–16; Tone, *Devices and Desires*, 14–15; Esther Katz, Cathy Moran Hajo, and Peter C. Engelman, eds. *The Selected Papers of Margaret Sanger,* vol. 1, *The Woman Rebel, 1900–1928* (Urbana: University of Illinois Press, 2003), 325.

17. William Alcott, *The Physiology of Marriage* (Boston: J. P. Jewett & Co., 1856), 180–81, 183 (quotation)–85; James C. Mohr, *Abortion in America: The Origins and Evolution of National Policy* (New York: Oxford University Press, 1978), 46–60, 239; *The Pittsfield Sun*, September 28, 1854; *New York Times*, February 26, 1864; *Lowell Daily Citizen and News*, February 4, 1864; *The Barre Gazette*, September 20, 1861; Fryer, *Birth Controllers,* 113–16; F. Barham Zincke, *Last Winter in the United States* (London: John Murray, 1868), 293–94; Brodie, *Contraception and Abortion*, 180–81, 201.

18. Degler, *At Odds*, 222–23, 262–65; Brodie, *Contraception and Abortion*, 57–58, 182–88.

19. Brodie, *Contraception and Abortion*, 143–44, 153; Leslie Woodcock Tentler, *Catholics and Contraception: An American History* (Ithaca, NY: Cornell University Press, 2004), 15–16; John Todd, *Serpents in the Dove's Nest* (Boston: Lee & Shepard, 1868), 18–22 (quotation); D'Emilio and Freedman, *Intimate Matters*, 72–73, 145–46; Reed, *Birth Control Movement*, 16–17, 33; Carroll Smith-Rosenberg, *Disorderly Conduct: Visions of Gender in Victorian America* (New York: Alfred A. Knopf, 1985), 218–20; Mohr, *Abortion in America*, 147–56, 200–204; Gordon, *Moral Property of Women*, 105–107.

20. Brodie, *Contraception and Abortion*, 253, 262; Reed, *Birth Control Movement*, 34–37, 35 (quotation); D'Emilio and Freedman, *Intimate Matters*, 150–56; Dienes, *Law, Politics and Birth Control*, 30–32.

21. D'Emilio and Freedman, *Intimate Matters*, 139–67; Gordon, *Moral Property of Women*, 55–71, includes a provocative chapter on feminist advocacy of voluntary motherhood in the late 19th century.

22. "The Comstock Act of 1873," reprinted in Andrea Tone, ed., *Controlling Reproduction: An American History* (Wilmington, DE: Scholarly Resources Inc., 1997), 140–41; Bottom

of Form Ralph K. Andrist, "Paladin of Purity," *American Heritage* 24 (October, 1973): 5–7, 84–89; Dienes, *Law, Politics and Birth Control,* 32–39; Tone, *Devices and Desires,* 3–13; Anthony Comstock, *Traps for the Young* (New York: Funk & Wagnalls, 1883), 6 (quotation).

23. Mary A. Hopkins, "Birth Control and Public Morals," *Harpers Weekly* 60 (May 22, 1915): 490 (quotation 1); Fryer, *Birth Controllers,* 117–18; Dienes, *Law, Politics and Birth Control,* 58–59; Brodie, *Contraception and Abortion,* 281; *New York Times,* Apr. 2, 1878 (quotations 2–3); Andrist, "Paladin of Purity," 87 (quotation 4).

24. *New York Times,* Sept. 25, 1905; Dienes, *Law, Politics and Birth Control,* 58–63; Mohr, *Abortion in America,* 226; Himes, *Medical History of Contraception,* 282–83; Brodie, *Contraception and Abortion,* 286–88, 352; Gordon, *Moral Property of Women,* 111–13.

25. Tone, *Devices and Desires,* 25–32, 38 (quotations); Brodie, *Contraception and Abortion,* 281–86.

26. Joanne E. Passet, *Sex Radicals and the Quest for Women's Equality* (Urbana: University of Illinois Press, 2003), 2–6, 14–16, 147–50; D'Emilio and Freedman, *Intimate Matters,* 161–66; Himes, *Medical history of Contraception,* 269–71; Fryer, *Birth Controllers,* 195–96; Comstock, *Traps for the Young,* 164 (quotation); Carol Flora Brooks, "The Early History of the Anti-Contraceptive Laws in Connecticut and Massachusetts," *American Quarterly* 18 (Spring 1966): 15–20; Angela T. Heywood, "Editorial: The Obscenity Raid," *The Word* 8 (January 1880): 1 (quotation).

27. D'Emilio and Freedman, *Intimate Matters,* 175–78; Margaret Sanger, National Committee on Federal Legislation for Birth Control, *A New Day Dawns for Birth Control* (New York, July 1937), 9, in *MSPME-SCC,* Reel 64: 742.

CHAPTER TWO

1. Margaret Sanger, *Family Limitation* (New York, privately printed, 1914), 3 (complete first edition in *MSPME-SCC,* Reel 76: 842).

2. Margaret Sanger, "Suppression," *The Woman Rebel* (June 1914): 25.

3. David M. Rabban, *Free Speech in Its Forgotten Years* (New York: Cambridge University Press, 1997), 23–26, 41–48, 66–67; *New York Tribune,* October 18, 1902; Craddock quotation in John D'Emilio, and Estelle B. Freedman, *Intimate Matters: A History of Sexuality in America* (Chicago: University of Chicago Press, 1988), 161; Ralph K. Andrist, "Paladin of Purity," *American Heritage* 24 (October 1973): 87; Moses Harman, "Ruminations," *Lucifer the Light-Bearer* (June 5, 1902): 161, quotation in Rabban, *Free Speech,* 46.

4. Rabban, *Free Speech,* 47; Emma Goldman, *Living My Life,* vol. 1 (New York: Alfred A. Knopf, 1931), 137, 170–74, 185–86 (quotations 1–3), 187, 272–73 (quotation 4), 274–78; James Reed, *Birth Control Movement and American Society: From Private Vice to Public Virtue* (Princeton, NJ: Princeton University Press, 1978), 47–48; Candace Falk et al., eds., *Emma Goldman: A Documentary History of the American Years,* vol. 1, *Made for America, 1890–1901* (Urbana: University of Illinois Press, 2003), 509, 526; Emma Goldman, *Living My Life,* vol. 2 (New York: Alfred A. Knopf, 1931), 552–53 (quotation 5).

5. Rabban, *Free Speech,* 66–67, 76; Christine Stansell, *American Moderns: Bohemian New York and the Creation of a New Century* (New York: Henry Holt, 2000), 76 (quotation).

6. Margaret Sanger, *An Autobiography* (New York: W. W. Norton, 1938), 11–92 (quotations on 21, 69, 88); Margaret Sanger, *My Fight for Birth Control* (New York: Farrar & Rinehart, 1931), 3–57 (quotations on 47, 49, 56); *Corning Leader*, January 30, 1917 (quotation); Harold B. Hersey, "Margaret Sanger: The Biography of the Birth Control Pioneer" (1938 unpublished manuscript, New York Public Library), 13–21, 25–26; Esther Katz, Cathy Moran Hajo, and Peter C. Engelman, eds. *The Selected Papers of Margaret Sanger,* vol. 1, *The Woman Rebel, 1900–1928* (Urbana: University of Illinois Press, 2003), 3–5, 15–19.

7. Sanger, *Autobiography,* 68–74, 92 (quotation), 70 (quotation); Paul Avrich, *The Modern School Movement: Anarchism and Education in the United States* (Princeton, NJ: Princeton University Press, 1980), 69–70, 79–80; Katz, Hajo, and Engelman, *Selected Papers* 1, 17–18; Mabel Dodge Luhan, *Movers and Shakers* (Albuquerque: University of New Mexico Press, 1985; reprint of 1936 edition), 82–91, 83.

8. Avrich, *Modern School Movement*, 80; Margaret Sanger to Nancy Pearmain, November 4, 1912, and Emma Goldman to Margaret Sanger, April 9, 1914 in Katz, Hajo, and Engelman, *Selected Papers* 1, 39–40, 75–76 (quotation), 96 (quotations); Alice Wexler, *Emma Goldman: An Intimate Life* (New York: Pantheon Books, 1984), 167–69; *Los Angeles Times*, May 4, 1912 (quotations); *Washington Post*, April 10, 1909; *San Francisco Bulletin*, June 7, 1916.

9. Candace Falk et al., eds., *Emma Goldman: A Documentary History of the American Years,* vol. 2, *Making Free Speech, 1902–1909* (Urbana: University of Illinois Press, 2005), 503; D'Emilio and Freedman, *Intimate Matters*, 223–26; Edward Carpenter, *Love's Coming of Age* (New York: Vanguard Press, 1926; first published in 1896), 144; Linda Gordon, *Moral Property of Women: A History of Birth Control Politics in America* (Urbana: University of Illinois Press, 2002), 126 (quotation); Havelock Ellis, *Studies in the Psychology of Sex,* vol. I: *The Evolution of Modesty* (Philadelphia: F. A. Davis, 1910), vi, and vol. VI: *Sex in Relation to Society* (Philadelphia: F. A. Davis, 1913), 601 (quotations).

10. Ellen Kay Trimberger, *Intimate Warriors: Selected Works of Neith Boyce and Hutchins Hapgood* (New York: The Feminist Press, 1991), 10–13; Luhan, *Movers and Shakers*, 70 (quotation); Katz, Hajo, and Engelman, *Selected Papers* 1, 18, 24, 30, 41, 46, 54; Sanger, *Autobiography*, 76–77, 80–85; Joyce L. Kornbluh, "Industrial Workers of the World," in Mari Jo Buhle et al., eds., *Encyclopedia of the American Left* (Urbana: University of Illinois Press, 1992), 354–58; Ellen Chesler, *Woman of Valor: Margaret Sanger and the Birth Control Movement in America* (New York: Simon & Schuster, 1992; revised 2007), 66; *The Call*, December 29, 1912 and March 2, 1913.

11. Paul S. Boyer, *Purity in Print: The Vice-Society Movement and Book Censorship in America* (New York: Charles Scribner's Sons, 1968), 23–28; D'Emilio and Freedman, *Intimate Matters*, 207–08; Francis M. Vreeland, "The Process of Reform with Especial Reference to Reform Groups in the Field of Population" (PhD dissertation, University of Michigan, 1929), 54–55; Allan M. Brandt, *No Magic Bullet: A Social History of Venereal Disease in the United States Since 1880* (New York: Oxford University Press, 1987), 45–47.

12. Hersey, "Margaret Sanger," 101, 110 (quotations); Sanger, *Autobiography*, 93–96, 87 (quotation).

13. Sanger, *My Fight*, 57–61; Theodore Schroeder, *List of References on Birth Control* (New York: H. W. Wilson, 1918); Alkaloidal Clinic Editorial Staff, *Sexual Hygiene* (Chicago: The

Clinic Publishing Co., 1902), 184 (quotation)–89; C. F. Taylor, ed., *Medical World* 15 (1897) (yearly index indicates several articles on prevention of conception and a number are reviewed in *Sexual Hygiene*, above); *Love without Danger: Secrets of the Alcove* (Paris: privately issued, 1904; copy in the Countway Library of Medicine), 89.

14. Vreeland, "Process of Reform, 50–53; Norman Himes, *Medical History of Contraception* (New York: Schocken Books, 1970 (reprint of 1936 edition), 310–12; William J. Robinson, "Few or Many Children," *Critic & Guide* 4 (Oct. 1904): 81–84 (quotation); Charles R. Parmele to Editor, *BCR* 15 (Dec. 1931): 363; Gordon, *Moral Property of Women*, 115–118, 142; William J. Robinson, *Practical Eugenics: Four Means of Improving the Human Race* (New York: Critic & Guide Co., 1912), 17–35, 17–18 (quotations).

15. William Robinson to May Cobb, December 7, 1910, quotation in Brandt, *No Magic Bullet*, 49; *New York Times*, October 1, 1913; Vreeland, "Process of Reform," 44; *Journal of the American Medical Association* 58 (June 8, 1912): 1736 (quotation).

16. Himes, *Medical History of Contraception*, 312–13; Robinson, *Practical Eugenics*, 17–18, 34 (quotations).

17. A. L. Goldwater to Editor, *BCR* 15 (Nov. 1931): 331–32; Margaret Sanger to Roma Brashear, Dec. 12, 1931, Margaret Sanger Papers Microfilm, Library of Congress, Reel 67: 41 (hereafter MSP-LC); Reed, *Birth Control Movement*, 81 (quotation).

18. Andrea Tone, *Devices and Desires: A History of Contraceptives in America* (New York: Hill & Wang, 2001), 81–82; Katz, Hajo, and Engelman, *Selected Papers* 1, 18–19, 52; Sanger, *My Fight*, 65–75, quotation on 68; Robert Jütte, *Contraception: A History* (Malden, MA: Polity Press, 2008), 166–67.

19. Avrich, *Modern School Movement*, 121–124; Sanger, *Autobiography*, 106–07; William Sanger to Margaret Sanger, January 11 and February 3, 1914, in *MSPME-SCC,* Reel 1: 71, 132; and February and March 12, 1914 in Katz, Hajo, and Engelman, *Selected Papers* 1, 62–68; Paul Avrich, *Anarchist Voices: An Oral History of Anarchism in America* (Princeton, NJ: Princeton University Press, 1995), 114.

20. Margaret Sanger, "Why the Rebel Woman," "The Aim," "A Woman's Duty," "The New Feminists," "On Picket Duty," and "The Prevention of Conception," *The Woman Rebel* (March 1914): 1, 3, 8; "Woman Rebel Wanted," *The Woman Rebel* (April 1914): 16, all in Esther Katz, Peter C. Engelman, Cathy Moran Hajo, eds., *Margaret Sanger Papers Microfilm Edition: Collected Documents Series* (Bethesda, MD: University Publications of America, 1997), Reel 16: 515–23 (hereafter *MSPME-CDS*); Sanger, *Autobiography*, 108–112 (quotation on 110).

21. Edward M. Morgan to Margaret Sanger, April 2, 1914 and Emma Goldman to Margaret Sanger, April 9, 1914 in Katz, Hajo, and Engelman, *Selected Papers* 1, 74–75 and 75–76 (quotation), also 81–82; *Washington Post*, April 5, 1914; *New York Times*, April 4, 1914; *New York Tribune*, April 4, 1914; *Pawtucket Evening Times*, April 16, 1914; *Pittsburgh Sun* editorial quotation in Lawrence Lader, *The Margaret Sanger Story and the Fight for Birth Control* (New York: Doubleday, 1955), 54; Bertram Wolfe, *A Life in Two Centuries* (New York: Stein & Day, 1981), 27; Margaret Sanger, "Humble Pie," *The Woman Rebel* (April 1914): 9; Margaret Sanger, "Abortion in the United States," *The Woman Rebel* (June 1914): 25; Sanger, *Autobiography*, 111; Emma Goldman to Margaret Sanger, June 22, 1914, in MSP-LC, Reel 8:894; Margaret Sanger to Reginald Kaufman, April 19, 1914, in *MSPME-SCC,* Reel 1:31 (quotations).

22. *Boston Journal*, August 26, 1914; *Philadelphia Inquirer*, August 23, 1914; J.M.R. to "Woman Rebel, n.d., in "Some Letters," *The Woman Rebel* (Sept.–Oct): 55; Sanger, "Why the Rebel Woman," 8; Margaret Sanger to Theodore Schroeder, August 19; Margaret Sanger to Upton Sinclair, September 23; James F. Morton, Jr. to Margaret Sanger, September 8, 1914; Margaret Sanger to Comrades and Friends, October 28, 1914 in Katz, Hajo, and Engelman, *Selected Papers* 1, 81–91; Rabban, *Free Speech*, 50; Avrich, *Modern School Movement*, 120; Sanger, *Autobiography*, 119.

23. Katz, Hajo, and Engelman, *Selected Papers* 1, 87–90; Joan M. Jensen, "The Evolution of Margaret Sanger's *Family Limitation* Pamphlet, 1914–1921," *Signs* 6 (Spring 1981): 548–55; Sanger, *Family Limitation*, 2–16.

24. Harold Content to Margaret Sanger, October 13, 1915 in Katz, Hajo, and Engelman, *Selected Papers* 1, 166–67; also 93–97, 103,150–51; Sanger, *Autobiography*, 120, 144–48, 153–72; Himes, *Medical History of Contraception*, 321.

25. Sanger, *Autobiography*, 133–41; Margaret Sanger, *English Methods of Birth Control*, (quotation) excerpt in Katz, Hajo, and Engelman, *Selected Papers* 1, 118–120, see also 94–5, 103; Havelock Ellis, *My Life: Autobiography of Havelock Ellis* (Boston: Houghton Mifflin, 1939), 520; Ellis, *Sex in Relation to Society*, 586–87 (quotations); Phyllis Grosskurth, *Havelock Ellis: A Biography* (New York: Alfred A. Knopf, 1980), 242–45, 409–12; Havelock Ellis/Margaret Sanger correspondence in MSP-LC, Reel 4.

26. Margaret Sanger to Anna Higgins, March 25 or 26, 1915 (quotation); Margaret Sanger to Comrades, Feb. 4, 1915 (quotation); and Margaret Sanger to the Editor of *Mother Earth* 10 (February 1915), in Katz, Hajo, and Engelman, *Selected Papers* 1, 123–30; Leonard Abbott to Mabel Dodge, Feb. 3, 1915 (quotation), Mabel Dodge Luhan Papers, Yale Collection of American Literature, Beinecke Rare Book and Manuscript Library, Yale University; "The Control of Births," *The New Republic* 2 (March 6, 1915): 115 (quotation); Mary Alden Hopkins, "Spacing Out Babies," *Harper's Weekly* 60 (April 24, 1915): 401(quotation); *New York Tribune*, May 21, 1915 (quotation); *Daily Herald* (Biloxi, MS.), April 15, 1915 (quotation); *Kansas City Star*, May 22, 1915 (quotation).

27. Leonard Abbott, "The Conviction of William Sanger," *Mother Earth* 10 (October 1915): 268–71; Steward Kerr, "The Woman Rebel," *Modern School* 1 (November 1914), 6–7; FSL, "The Latest Comstock Case—The Arrest of William Sanger," January, 1915, and Leonard Abbott to Theodore Schroeder, April 19, 1915 (quotations), in *MSPME-CDS*, Reel 15: 55, 67.

28. Robyn L. Rosen, "Mary Coffin Ware Dennett," *American National Biography Online* (February 2000); Vreeland, "Process of Reform," 68–71; Constance M. Chen, *The Sex Side of Life: Mary Ware Dennett's Pioneering Battle for Birth Control and Sex Education* (New York: New Press, 1996), 159–66, 180–82; Mary Ware Dennett, "Speech at the Meeting Which Organized the National Birth Control League," March 1915, Papers of Mary Ware Dennett and the Voluntary Parenthood League, Schlesinger Library, Radcliffe College, Harvard University (Women's Studies Manuscript Collection Microfilm, Series 3, Part B; Reel 13: 679–81) (quotations); "Films and Births and Censorship," *The Survey* 34 (April 3, 1915): 4–5.

29. Caroline Nelson to Margaret Sanger, June 12, 1915, in Katz, Hajo, and Engelman, *Selected Papers* 1 136–42; *New York Times*, May 27, 1915; *New York Tribune*, May 21 and 27, 1915 (quotations).

30. *New York Tribune*, May 22, 1915 (quotations); D'Emilio and Freeman, *Intimate Matters*, 230–31 (quotation); *The Ledger* (Columbus Georgia), Nov. 22, 1915 (quotation); Mary Alden Hopkins, "What Doctors Say of Birth Control," *Harper's Weekly* 61 (October 16, 1915): 380 (Kelly quotation); Mary Alden Hopkins, "The Catholic Church and Birth Control," *Harper's Weekly* 60 (June 26, 1915): 609–10 (Ryan quotation).

31. *Atlanta Constitution*, March 8, 1914 (Roosevelt quotations); *Washington Post*, March 14, 1915 (Carver quotations); Henry F. Pringle, *Theodore Roosevelt: A Biography* (New York: Harcourt & Brace, 1931), 332; David M. Kennedy, *Birth Control in America: The Career of Margaret Sanger* (New Haven, CT: Yale University Press, 1970), 42–50.

32. *Chicago Daily Tribune*, March 19, 1915 (quotation); Vreeland, "The Process of Reform," 67–71; Roger A. Bruns, *The Damndest Radical: The Life and World of Ben Reitman, Chicago's Celebrated Social Reformer, Hobo King, and Whorehouse Physician* (Urbana: University of Illinois Press, 1987), 168–71 (quotation); Gordon, *Moral Property of Women*, 148; Ben Reitman, "The Tour," *Mother Earth* 10 (September, 1915): 269–70 (long quotation); *Morning Oregonian*, August 7 (quotation), 8, 1915; *New York Times*, August 8, 1915.

33. William Sanger to Margaret Sanger, September 12, 1915 in Katz, Hajo, and Engelman, *Selected Papers* 1, 158–60; and September 14, 1915 (quotations) in *MSPME-SCC*, Reel 1: 462; *New York Times*, September 11, 1915 (quotations); *New York Tribune*, September 11, 1915 (long quotation).

34. *New York Times*, September 22, 1915; *The Masses* 6 (September 1915): 9.

35. William Sanger to Margaret Sanger, September 12, 1915 (quotation); Margaret Sanger to "Comrades and Friends," August 1, 1915; and Elizabeth Gurley Flynn to Margaret Sanger, August 1915 (quotation) in Katz, Hajo, and Engelman, *Selected Papers* 1, 158–60, 152–53; *The Call*, September 11, 1915 (Robinson quotation); *New York Tribune*, September 11, 1915; "Report of Mr. Sanger's Trial," *The Malthusian* (October 1915): 82; "Birth Control and the New York Courts," *The Survey* 34 (September 25, 1915): 567.

36. Sanger, *Autobiography*, 180 (quotations)–82; Harold Content to Margaret Sanger, October 13, 1915, in Katz, Hajo, and Engelman, *Selected Papers* 1, 168–69.

37. *Chicago Daily Tribune*, Nov. 18 and 20 (Gibbons quotation), 1915; *Salt Lake Telegram*, November 28, 1915 (quotation); *New York Times*, November 18, 1915 (Haiselden, Addams, Fallows quotations); Helen Keller, "Helen Keller, Blind, Deaf and Dumb Genius, Writes for Daily Ledger on Defective Baby Case," *The Ledger* (Columbus, Georgia), November 26, 1915 (quotations); Martin S. Pernick, *The Black Stork: Eugenics and the Death of 'Defective' Babies in American Medicine and Motion Pictures Since 1915* (New York: Oxford University Press, 1996), 3–7.

38. Pernick, *The Black Stork*, 3–7, 33–35, 68–70; *The Ledger* (Columbus Georgia), November 22, 1915 (quotation); Victor Robinson, *Pioneers of Birth Control in England and America* (New York: Voluntary Parenthood League, 1919), 76–78 (quotations).

39. Leonard Abbot to Theodore Schroeder, November 26, 1915 (quotation), in Katz, Hajo, and Engelman, *Selected Papers* 1, 171, note 2; Margaret Sanger to Leonard Abbott, November 26 and Emma Goldman to Margaret Sanger, December 7, 1915 (quotations); Margaret Sanger to Friends and Comrades, January 5, 1916 (quotation), all in, *Selected Papers I*, 170–176; *New York Tribune*, Feb. 15, 1916 (quotation); *New York Times*, January 15, 18 and

February 15, 1916; Sanger, *Autobiography*, 182–89; for samples of support letter and resolutions see *MSPME-CDS*, Reel 15.

40. H. Snowden Marshall to U.S. Attorney General Thomas W. Gregory, July 13, 1916 (quotations), *MSPME-CDS*, Reel 15: 156; *New York Tribune*, February 19 and 21 (quotation) 1916; Kathleen L. Endres and Therese L. Lueck, eds., *Women's Periodicals in the United States: Consumer Magazines* (Westport, CT: Greenwood Press, 1995), 274–77; "What Shall We Do about Birth-Control," *Pictorial Review* (October 1915), (February 1916), and (March 1916): 24–26, 76 (quotation on 25); Samuel Untermyer to Margaret Sanger, December 6, 1915 (quotation), in Katz, Hajo, and Engelman, *Selected Papers* 1, 172.

41. "Observations and Comments," *Mother Earth* 11 (March 1916): 422 and Margaret Sanger to Editor, *Mother Earth* 11 (April 1916): 402–03; Wexler, *Emma Goldman*, 212–215; *New York Tribune*, February 21, March 2 (quotation), April 21 and 28, May 9 and 21, 1916; *Chicago Daily Tribune*, May 6, 1916; *New York Times*, June 6, 1916.

42. *Chicago Daily Tribune*, May 21, 1916; Goldman, *Living My Life, Vol. 2*, 576–79; Chen, *Sex Side of Life*, 181–194.

43. Sanger, "Birth Control," April 1916, in MSP-LC, Reel 129: 12; *Aberdeen Daily News*, April 1, 1916; *Denver Post*, May 27, 1916; *Detroit Journal*, May 3, 1916; Kevin E. McClearey, "The Noonday Devil: Margaret H. Sanger's 1916 American Lecture Tour," (1999 manuscript in author's possession), "Descriptions," 1–14.

44. McClearey, "Noonday Devil," 3:1–3 and 4:17–22; Sanger, *My Fight*, 146–47 (quotations); *St. Louis Globe–Democrat*, May 2 and 25, 1916; Robert C. Cottrell, *Roger Nash Baldwin and the American Civil Liberties Union* (New York: Columbia University Press, 2000), 43.

45. Vreeland, "Process of Reform," 410–15; McClearey, "Noonday Devil," 4:29–39; Margaret Sanger to Marie Equi, July, 1916 and to Charles and Bessie Drysdale, August 9, 1916, in Katz, Hajo, and Engelman, *Selected Papers* 1, 184–93; *Portland Morning Oregonian*, June 20, 22, 24, 30, July 1, 2, 8 (Sanger quotation); *Portland Evening Telegram*, July 2, 6; *Portland News*, July 1, 8.

46. Sanger, *Autobiography*, 196 (quotation)–97; McClearey, "Noonday Devil," 4: 3–5, 7–9, 29; *Chicago Daily Tribune*, April 11, 26 (quotation), 27 and May 10 (quotation), 1916; Margaret Sanger to Charles and Bessie Drysdale, August 9, 1916, in Katz, Hajo, and Engelman, *Selected Papers* 1, 184–93 (quotation); Rev. J. F. Duggan, "A Dangerous Doctrine," *The Monitor* (June 10, 1916): 4, quotation in McClearey, 4:4; Margaret Sanger, "Birth Control," April 1916, in MSP-LC, Reel 129: 12 (quotations).

47. Vreeland, "Process of Reform," 401–03; Sanger, *Autobiography*, 198–99 (quotation); Margaret Sanger to Charles and Bessie Drysdale, August 9, 1916, in Katz, Hajo, and Engelman, *Selected Papers* 1, 186–93; Birth Control League of Ohio, *Birth Control News* 1 (July 1916): 1–8 (quotations); Jimmy Elaine Wilkinson Meyer, *Any Friend of the Movement: Networking for Birth Control, 1920–1940* (Columbus: Ohio State University Press, 2004), 23–25.

48. *Boston Journal*, July 12, 13, 14, 15, 20, 21 (quotations), 24, 25, 31 (quotations), August 14 (quotations), September 6, 13, 1916; *Philadelphia Inquirer*, July 24, 1916; *New York Tribune*, November 22, 1916; Vreeland, "The Process of Reform," 388–92; Jack Beatty, *The Rascal King: The Life and Times of James Michael Curley, 1874–1958* (Reading, MA: Addison-Wesley, 1992), 172–75; Gordon, *Moral Property of Women*, 142, 184–85; Cerise Carman Jack, "Massachusetts," *BCR* 2 (April 1918): 7–8 (quotation).

49. Margaret Sanger to Edith How-Martyn, July 18, 1916, in *MSPME-CDS,* Reel 1: 139; Cathy Moran Hajo, *Birth Control on Main Street: Organizing Clinics in the United States, 1916–1939* (Urbana: University of Illinois Press, 2010), 25; Caroline Nelson to Margaret Sanger, June 12, 1915, in Katz, Hajo, and Engelman, *Selected Papers* 1, 136–42; Sanger, *My Fight,* 149–50.

CHAPTER THREE

1. Alexander Berkman, "The Birth Control Fight," *The Blast* 1 (July 1, 1916): 5.

2. Margaret Sanger to Comrades and Friends, August 1, 1915, in Esther Katz, Cathy Moran Hajo, and Peter C. Engelman, eds. *The Selected Papers of Margaret Sanger,* vol. 1, *The Woman Rebel, 1900–1928* (Urbana: University of Illinois Press, 2003), 152–53; Margaret Sanger, *An Autobiography* (New York: W. W. Norton, 1938), 178–80.

3. Dorothy Bocker, *Birth Control Methods* (New York: CRB, 1924), 4–8; Andrea Tone, *Devices and Desire: A History of Contraceptives in America* (New York: Hill & Wang, 2001), 55–77; Abraham Stone and Norman E. Himes. *Planned Parenthood: A Practical Guide to Birth-Control Methods* (New York: Macmillan, 1951), 123–40; Robert Dickinson, *Techniques of Conception Control* (Baltimore, MD: Williams & Wilkins, 1942), 9–38; Margaret Sanger, *The Case for Birth Control: A Supplementary Brief and Statement of Facts* (New York: privately printed, 1917), 185–93; Marie Stopes, *Married Love: A New Contribution to the Solution of Sex Difficulties* (New York: G. P. Putnam's Sons, 1931), 89–94.

4. *Boston Journal,* November 14, 1916; *New York Tribune* and *Kansas City Star,* July 22, 1916; Sanger, *Autobiography,* 213–14.

5. C. Thomas Dienes, *Law, Politics and Birth Control* (Urbana: University of Illinois Press, 1972), 43–44, 82 (quotation), 320–21; Proceedings of the First American Birth Control Conference, November 11, 1921, Second Session, 40–41, in *MSPME-SCC* Reel 67: 837 (quotation); William Robinson to Margaret Sanger, September 13, 1916, in, Katz, Hajo, and Engelman, *Selected Papers* 1, 198 (quotations); Sanger, *Autobiography,* 211 (quotation)–12.

6. Linda Gordon, *The Moral Property of Women: A History of Birth Control Politics in America* (Urbana: University of Illinois Press, 2002), 167–8 (quotation); Margaret Sanger, *My Fight for Birth Control* (New York: Farrar & Rinehart, 1931), 153–56; Ellen Chesler, *Woman of Valor: Margaret Sanger and the Birth Control Movement in America* (New York: Simon & Schuster,1992; revised 2007), 151; *New York Tribune,* September 6, 1916.

7. Sanger, *Autobiography,* 210–18; Brownsville Clinic Flyer, October 1916, in *MSPME-SCC,* Reel 62: 835; Kevin Starr, *Inventing the Dream: California through the Progressive Era* (New York: Oxford University Press, 1985), 212; Elizabeth Stuyvesant, "The Brownsville Birth Control Clinic," *BCR* 1 (March 1917): 6–8 (quotation); New York v. Sanger, 222 NY 192, 118 N. E. 637 (Court of Appeals 1917), National Archives, Records of the U.S. Supreme Court, RG 267, in *MSPME*-CDS, Reel15: 298–362 (hereafter N.Y. v. Sanger, 1917); *Salt Lake Telegram,* November 12, 1916 (quotations); *Brooklyn Daily Eagle,* October 24, 1916 (long quotation); *New York Tribune,* October 20, 24 (quotation), 1916; *Washington Post,* October 22, 1916.

8. *Washington Post,* Oct. 22, 1916 (quotation; this article also appeared in many newspapers across the country); Stuyvesant, "Brownsville," 8 (quotation); *New York Tribune,* October

20 and 27 (quotation), 1916; Katz, Hajo, and Engelman, *Selected Papers* 1, 199–202; Peter C. Engelman, "Margaret Sanger Opens the First Birth Control Clinic in the U.S.," in *Great Events from History: Human Rights*, ed. Frank Northen Magil (Pasadena, CA: Salem Press, 1992), 184–89.

9. *New York Times*, October 13 (quotations), 28 and 31, 1916; *New York Tribune*, October 13 (quotations), 21 and 24, 1916; *Aberdeen Daily News*, October 14, 1916; *Columbus* (GA) *Daily Enquirer*, October 20, 1916 (the same photo and article found in several different papers); Committee of One Hundred, *The Birth Control Movement* (New York: privately printed, 1917), 8–9, in *MSPME-CDS*, Reel 12: 1085.

10. *Boston Journal*, November 14, 1916 (quotation); *The Call*, November 13, 15 and 17, 1916; *New York Tribune*, November 18, 1916; Cathy Moran Hajo, *Birth Control on Main Street: Organizing Clinics in the United States, 1916–1939* (Urbana: University of Illinois Press, 2010), 24–25; Gordon, *Moral Property of Women*, 156; Sanger, *Autobiography*, 212, 227.

11. *New York Tribune*, November 27, 1916 (quotation); David J. Garrow, *Liberty and Sexuality: The Right to Privacy and the Making of Roe v. Wade* (New York: MacMillan, 1994), 12–13 (December hearing quotations); Katz, Hajo, and Engelman, *Selected Papers* 1, 208; Jonah J. Goldstein, "The Birth Control Clinic Cases, *BCR* 1 (February, 1917): 8; Sanger, *Autobiography*, 225–29; Chesler, *Woman of Valor*, 152–53; *New York Times*, January 5, 9, 23, 24, 25, 26 (health bulletin), 27, 28, 29 1917; *Corning* (N.Y.) *Leader*, January 27, 1917.

12. *New York Tribune*, January 5 and 9, 1917 (quotations); *The Call*, November 29, 1916; Committee of One Hundred, Minutes, January 21, 1917, in *MSPME-CDS*, Reel 12: 1072; Sanger, *Autobiography*, 229–30 (quotations); Susan Ware, "Florence Jaffray Hurst Harriman," in *Notable American Women, The Modern Period*, Barbara Sicherman, and Carol Hurd Green, eds., (Cambridge: Harvard University Press, 1980), 314–15; Committee of One Hundred, *Birth Control Movement*, 42–3.

13. Katz, Hajo, and Engelman, *Selected Papers* 1, 219; *Philadelphia Inquirer*, January 25, 1916; Paul Marashio, Interview with Horace Rublee, Apr. 19, 1980, Juliet Rublee Papers, Dartmouth College; Peter Engelman, "Katharine Dexter McCormick," in *Encyclopedia of Birth Control*, Vern L. Bullough, ed. (Santa Barbara, CA: ABC-CLIO, 2001), 169–71.

14. N.Y. v. Sanger, 1917; *New York Times*, January 29, 30 (quotation), 31, and February 1, 2, 1917; *New York Tribune*, January 30, 31, February 1, 2, 3, 6 (quotations) 1917; *Corning* (NY) *Leader*, January 30 and February 2, 1917; Francis M. Vreeland, "The Process of Reform with Especial Reference to Reform Groups in the Field of Population" (PhD diss., University of Michigan, 1929), 89–90; Edward F. Mylius, "Hunger-Striking Against an Unjust Law," and na, "The Sanger Clinic Cases," *BCR* 1 (March, 1917): 10 (quotation), 13; *San Jose Mercury News*, January 30, 1917 (quotations); *New York Evening Post*, January 27, 1917; Sanger, *Autobiography*, 230–37. Access to hundreds of articles on Byrne's hunger strike and the clinic trial is available through the online database, America's Historical Newspapers.

15. "Birth Control Centers in the United States," *BCR* 1 (February 1917): 2 and (December 1917): 2; *Lexington* (KY) *Herald*, April 22, 1917 and May 6, 1917 (quotations); Frederick Blossom, "Growth of the Movement," *BCR* 1 (March 1917): 4; David. M. Kennedy, *Birth Control in America: The Career of Margaret Sanger* (New Haven, CT: Yale University Press, 1970), 174–75; *New York Times*, Dec. 27, 1916; A. L. Goldwater, "Symposium on Birth

Control," *Medical Review of Reviews* 25 (March 1919): 143–43 (quotation); *Chicago Tribune*, February 17, 1916; Robert Dickinson, "Simple Sterilization of Women by Cautery Stricture of Intra-uterine Tubal Openings," *Surgery, Gynecology and Obstetrics* 23 (1916): 185–90, quoted in James Reed, *The Birth Control Movement and American Society: From Private Vice to Public Virtue* (Princeton, NJ: Princeton University Press, 1978), 167.

16. Sanger, *Autobiography*, 251–52; *Chicago Tribune*, April 22, 1917, (quotations); "What the Birth Control Leagues Are Doing," *BCR* 1 (February 1917): 10–11 and (April–May, 1917):14–15; Blossom, "Growth of the Movement," *BCR* 1 (March 1917): 4; Virginia Heidelberg to Mary Ware Dennett, March 1, 1917 (Mary Ware Dennett Papers, Schlesinger Library, Radcliffe Institute, Harvard University, Series 4, Folder 169 (hereafter "Dennett Papers").

17. *Dallas Morning News*, October 26, 1915 (quotation); Pernick, *The Black Stork*, 143–44; *Chicago Daily Tribune*, October 17 and 22, 1916; *Philadelphia Inquirer*, November 7, 1916 (quotation); Kevin Brownlow, *Behind the Mask of Innocence* (New York: Alfred A. Knopf, 1990), 47–55; *Variety*, April 13 and May 11, 1917; Martin F. Norden, "Birth Control," in *Censorship: A World Encyclopedia, Vol. 4, S–Z*, Derek Jones, ed. (Chicago: Fitzroy Dearborn Publishers, 2001), 2137–38; *New York Tribune*, May 7, 1917 (quotation); *New York Times*, March 28, May 7, 10, June 7 (quotation) and 14 (quotation), 1917.

18. "More Spies," *BCR* 1 (March 1917): 16; Roger A. Bruns, *The Damndest Radical: The Life and World of Ben Reitman, Chicago's Celebrated Social Reformer, Hobo King, and Whorehouse Physician* (Urbana: University of Illinois Press, 1987, 180–88; *Philadelphia Inquirer*, June 13, 1917; "What the Birth Control Leagues Are Doing," *BCR* 1 (April–May 1917): 14; *New York Times*, March 8, 1917; "In Our Morning Mail," *BCR* 1 (February 1917): 14 (quotation); *Boston Journal*, February 28, 1917 (Pope quotation); "Editorial Comment," *BCR* 2 (June 1918): 16 (quotation); Leslie Woodcock Tentler, *Catholics and Contraception: An American History* (Ithaca, NY: Cornell University Press, 2004), 16–19, 26–31, 37–40.

19. *New York Tribune*, June 2, 1917 (quotation); "Take It from Billy," *BCR* 1 (June, 1917): 6; Paul Popenoe, "Birth Control and Eugenics," *BCR* 1 (April–May, 1917): 6 (quotation); Warren S. Thompson, "Race Suicide in the United States," *Scientific Monthly* 5 (July, 1917): 22–35; Carole R. McCann, *Birth Control Politics in the United States, 1916–1945* (Ithaca, NY: Cornell University Press, 1994), 16–21.

20. Frederick Blossom to Virginia Heidelberg, December 8, 1916 and Heidelberg to Mary Ware Dennett, March 1, 1917 (Dennett Papers, Series 4, Folder 169); Margaret Sanger to Gertrude Pinchot, April 16 and May 6, 1917; to Juliet Rublee, July 13, December 4 and 29, 1917, and August 10, 1918; to Frederick Blossom, October 22, 1917, in Katz, Hajo, and Engelman, *Selected Papers* 1, 213–16, 218–20, 224–28, 232–36; Gertrude Pinchot to Margaret Sanger, April 17, 1917 and Frederick Blossom to Margaret Sanger, October 18, 1917, in MSP-LC, Reel 9: 1140 and Reel 7: 1012; Vreeland, "Process of Reform," 90–92; Emma Goldman, *Living My Life*, Vol. 2 (New York: Alfred A. Knopf, 1931), 590 (quotation); *New York Tribune*, July 8, 1918; *Evening Leader* (Corning, NY), July 9, 1918 (quotation).

21. Margaret Sanger to Juliet Rublee, December 4 and 29, 1917 and January 22, 1918, in Katz, Hajo, and Engelman, *Selected Papers* 1, 224–31; NYWPC, Certificate of Incorporation, February 26, 1918, in *MSPME*-SCC, Reel 62:640; Jared L. Manley, "Crusader," *The New Yorker* (July 4, 1936): 22; Kitty Marion, ""Ye That Pass By," *BCR* 7 (February 1923): 45

(quotation); "Judges with Small Families Jail Kitty Marion," *BCR* 2 (November 1918): 5; Sanger, *Autobiography*, 257 (quotation); Janice R. MacKinnon and Stephen R. MacKinnon, *Agnes Smedley: The Life and Times of an American Radical* (Berkeley: University of California Press, 1988), 46–49 (quotations on 48–49).

22. Margaret Sanger, "Editorial Comment," *BCR* 2 (January 1918):16 (quotation); N.Y. v. Sanger, 1917; Sanger, *Case for Birth Control*, 3; People of New York v. Margaret Sanger, Court of Appeals of New York, 222 N.Y. 192; 118 N.E. 637, 1918 (decision) (quotations); McCann, *Birth Control Politics*, 63–65; *New York Tribune*, January 9, 1918; Dienes, *Law, Politics and Birth Control*, 85–88; Margaret Sanger, "Why Not Birth Control Clinics in America?" *BCR* 3 (May 1919): 10; Margaret Sanger to Juliet Rublee, January 22, 1918, in Katz, Hajo, and Engelman, *Selected Papers* 1, 228–31 (quotation on 230).

23. Sanger, *Autobiography*, 296–97; Hajo, *Birth Control on Main Street*, 30 (quotation); Mary Halton, "The Investigation of the Hospitals," *BCR* 3 (December 1919): 5 (quotations).

24. Margaret Sanger to Juliet Rublee, December 4, 1917 and August 10, 1918, in Katz, Hajo, and Engelman, *Selected Papers* 1, 224–26, 232–36; Sanger, *Family Limitation*, 5th ed., 1916 and 6th ed., 1917, in *MSPME-SCC*, Reel 76: 901, 911; Jensen, "Evolution of Sanger's *Family Limitation*," 551.

25. "The Fight from Coast to Coast," *BCR* 2 (April 1918): 5; "The National Birth Control League," *BCR* 2 (July 1918): 15 (quotations); Constance M. Chen, *The Sex Side of Life: Mary Ware Dennett's Pioneering Battle for Birth Control and Sex Education* (New York: The New Press: 1996), 171–77, 205–17 (quotation on 215), 241–43, 332–33; Rosen, "Mary Coffin Ware Dennett"; Minutes of the Eastern Conference on Birth Control, May10–11, 1918, in *MSPME-CDS*, Reel 14: 918; Mary Ware Dennett, *Birth Control Laws: Shall We Keep Them, Abolish Them or Change Them?* (New York: Frederick H. Hitchcock, 1926), 170–75 (quotations on 171, 173); Mary Ware Dennett, *The Sex Side of Life: An Explanation for Young People* (New York: privately printed, 1919) (quotation on 15); Sanger, *Autobiography*, 262, 181 (quotations); Margaret Sanger to Juliet Rublee, December, 1917 in Katz, Hajo, and Engelman, *Selected Papers* 1, 224–26 (quotation p. 225).

26. Bianca Van Beuren, "*Married Love*—A Review," *BCR* 2 (August 1918): 6; Melvyn Dubofsky, *We Shall Be All: A History of the Industrial Workers of the World* (Urbana: University of Illinois Press, 2000), 215–60; Christine Stansell, *American Moderns: Bohemian New York and the Creation of a New Century* (New York: Henry Holt, 2000), 312–18; Goldman, *Living My Life, Vol. 2*, 602–12; *New York Times*, June 16, 1917, April 15, 1918; *New York Herald Tribune*, April 8 (quotation) and May 27, 1918; Chesler, *Woman of Valor*, 160–62.

27. Olive Schreiner, "Breeding Men for Battle," *BCR* 1 (April–May 1917): 5; Margaret Sanger, "Woman and War," (quotation) *BCR* 1 (June 1917): 5; Margaret Sanger "Let's Have the Truth," *BCR* 2 (August 1918): 8; Sanger. "A Victory, A New Year and A New Day," *BCR* 3 (February 1919): 3; Sanger, *Autobiography*, 255 (quotation)–56; Chesler, *Woman of Valor*, 161–62, 531; Joint legislative Committee to Investigate Seditious Activities, Investigation Subject Files, 1919–1920, New York State Archives.

28. Allan M. Brandt, *No Magic Bullet: A Social History of Venereal Disease in the United States Since 1880* (New York: Oxford University Press, 1987), 52–95, 164 (quotation on 59); Tone, *Devices and Desires*, 51, 98–106 (quotation on 106); John Parascandola, *Sex, Sin, and*

Science: A History of Syphilis in America (Westport, CT: Praeger, 2008), 48–65; *New York Times*, October 28, 1917 (Zinsser quotation); Louis Schwartz, "Comment and Criticism," *The Military Surgeon* 42 (May 1918): 569 (quotation); Margaret Sanger to Katharina Lipinski Stützin, March 22, 1932, in Esther Katz, Peter C. Engelman, and Cathy Moran Hajo, eds., *The Selected Papers of Margaret Sanger,* vol. 2, *Birth Control Comes of Age, 1928–1939* (Urbana: University of Illinois Press, 2006), 169 (quotation); Regine K. Stix and Frank W. Notestein, *Controlled Fertility: An Evaluation of Clinic Service* (Baltimore, MD: Williams & Wilkins, 1940), 51.

29. Tone, *Devices and Desires,* 51, 102–03, 106 (quotation)–09; Antoinette Konikow (Pseudo. "Woman Physician"), *Voluntary Motherhood; A Study of the Physiology and Hygiene of Prevention of Conception* (Boston: privately printed, 1928), 11; Hannah M. Stone, *Contraceptive Methods—A Clinical Survey* (New York: CRB, 1925), 5; Bocker, *Birth Control Methods,* 5.

30. Margaret Sanger, "Birth Control and Women's Health," *BCR* 1 (December 1917): 7–8; Margaret Sanger, "When Should a Woman Avoid Having Children?" *BCR* 2 (November 1918): 6–7; Margaret Sanger, "Birth Control or Abortion?" *BCR* 2 (December 1918): 3–4; Margaret Sanger, "Birth Control and Racial Betterment," *BCR* 3 (February 1919): 11–12; Margaret Sanger, "The Tragedy of the Accidental Child," *BCR* 3 (April 1919): 5–6.

31. "Birth Control Organizations," *BCR* 3 (July 1919): 20; Sanger, *Autobiography,* 266–67; Margaret Sanger to Edward Mylius, September 14 and to Juliet Rublee, November, and to William Sanger, December 1, 1919, in Katz, Hajo, and Engelman, *Selected Papers* 1, 260–61, 266–70; Margaret Sanger to Walter Roberts, September 24, 1919, in *MSPME-SCC,* Reel 1: 869.

32. "The Voluntary Parenthood League," *BCR* 3 (May 1919): 18; Mary Ware Dennett, *Birth Control Laws: Shall We Keep Them, Abolish Them or Change Them?* (New York: Frederick H. Hitchcock, 1926), 68, 94–96; McCann, *Birth Control Politics,* 68–73.

33. Margaret Sanger, "How Shall We Change the Law," *BCR* 3 (July 1919): 8 (first two quotations and long quotation); Margaret Sanger, "Meeting the Need Today," *BCR* 3 (October 1917): 14–15 (quotation); Dennett, *Birth Control Laws,* 59, (quotation), 68, 94–96, 201 (quotation), 203 (long quotation), 271.

34. James F. Morton, Jr., "Shall We Have a Limited Birth Control?" *BCR* 3 (October 1919): 12 (quotation)-14; Chen, *Sex Side of Life,* 213–15, 219; Margaret Sanger, "Editorial: The Sweep of the Movement," *BCR* 4 (February 1920): 3 (quotations); Sanger, *Woman and the New Race,* 224 (quotation).

35. Margaret Sanger, "Editorial: A Birth Strike to Avert World Famine," *BCR* 4 (January 1920): 3; Mary Ware Dennett to the NYWPC, January 20, 1920 and Dennett, Report to the Council of the VPL, February 6, 1920, in MSP-LC, Reel 10: 1002, 1004; Mary Ware Dennett to Margaret Sanger, March 19, 1920, in *MSPME-CDS,* Reel 1: 441; Margaret Sanger to Mary Ware Dennett, March 19, 1921, in Katz, Hajo, and Engelman, *Selected Papers* 1, 294–96.

36. Sanger, *Woman and the New Race,* (quotations on 208, 234, 117, 214, 7, 94); Sanger, *Autobiography,* 362; Carrie Chapman Catt to Margaret Sanger, November 24, 1920, in Katz, Hajo, and Engelman, *Selected Papers* 1, 290; Chesler, *Woman of Valor,* 192 (quotation)–94; *New York Tribune,* October 3, 1920.

37. Vreeland, "Process of Reform," 100, 273; Brentano's to Anne Kennedy, April 20, 1921, reprinted in *BCR* 5 (August 1921): 4; Margaret Sanger, *Motherhood in Bondage* (New York: Brentano's, 1928), xi–xii; Mrs. (name withheld) to Margaret Sanger, June 23, 1924, in

MSPME-SCC, Reel 2: 606; for last quotation see countless examples in *Motherhood in Bondage*, and many variations, such as "I'd rather be dead than have a wee-one," Client to Margaret Sanger, May 31, 1921, in Katz, Hajo, and Engelman, *Selected Papers* 1, 296.

38. Margaret Sanger, ed., *Appeals from American Mothers* (New York: New York Women's Publishing Company, 1921), 11–12 (first letter), 4–5 (second letter); Mrs. (name withheld) to Margaret Sanger, April 23, 1924 in *MSPME-SCC*, Reel 2: 572; Mary Sumner Boyd, "Analysis of Typical Letters," included in Sanger, *Motherhood in Bondage*, 439–46.

39. Frederick J. Taussig, *Abortion: Spontaneous and Induced* (St. Louis: C.V. Mosby, 1936), 25–6; Leslie J. Reagan, *When Abortion Was a Crime: Women, Medicine, and Law in the United States, 1867–1973* (Berkeley: University of California Press, 1997), 109–111; Sanger, *Motherhood in Bondage* (quotations on 399, 405, 404, 403); Sanger, *Woman and the New Race*, 129 (quotation).

40. Dennett, *Birth Control Laws*, 110–14; Sanger, *Appeals from American Mothers*; Vreeland, "Process of Reform," 276 (Boyd quotation).

41. Vreeland, "Process of Reform," 101; Sanger, *Autobiography*, 296–97, 300 (quotation); NYWPC, Board of Directors, minutes, November 25, 1919 and Margaret Sanger to Friend, September 1921, in *MSPME-SCC*, Reel 62:708 and S67:741; Margaret Sanger to Mrs. William C. Peirce, December 7, 1920, in MSP-LC, Reel 9: 1079; Margaret Sanger to Friend, April 20, 1921, in *MSPME-CDS*, Reel 1: 659; "Outline of Margaret Sanger's Work Since Her Return from England," *BCR* 5 (May 1921): 2; Nancy Cott, *The Grounding of Modern Feminism* (New Haven, CT: Yale University Press, 1987), 68–69; Margaret Sanger to Juliet Rublee, July 20, 1921, in Katz, Hajo, and Engelman, *Selected Papers* 1, 301–02.

42. *New York Times*, November 9 and 14, 1921; Harold Hersey, "First American Birth-Control Conference," *BCR* 5 (August 1921): 3 (quotation); Margaret Sanger to Friend, October 1921, in *MSPME-SCC*, Reel 67: 743 (quotation); Advertisement in *BCR* 5 (October 1921): 3 (quotation).

43. Margaret Sanger to Friend, September 1921 in *MSPME-SCC*, Reel 67: 741 (quotation); "Outline of Legislative Work in Albany," *BCR* 5 (May 1921): 11; Margaret Sanger, "Editorial," *BCR* 5 (March 1921): 3; Margaret Sanger to Mary Ware Dennett, March 19 and October 31, 1921, and Margaret Sanger to Marie Stopes, July 29 (quotation) and October 29, 1921 (quotation), in Katz, Hajo, and Engelman, *Selected Papers* 1, 294–96, 318–19, 304–05, 316–18; Mary Ware Dennett to *BCR* Board of Directors, July 25, 1921, in MSP-LC, Reel 10: 1017 (quotation); Mary Ware Dennett to Margaret Sanger, July 29, 1921, in *MSPME-CDS* Reel 1:752 (quotations).

44. *New York Times*, November 12, 1921; Program, First American Birth Control Conference, November 11–13, 1921, and Medical Session, November 11, 1921, in *MSPME-SCC*, Reel 67: 745–783, 791–93; MS, *Autobiography*, 290, 301; "Methods of Birth Control Used by 1,250 Families," 1921, in MSP-LC, Reel 34: 69.

45. *New York Times*, November 13, 1921 (quotations); *Kansas City Star*, November 13, 1921; MS, *Autobiography*, 297–98; Pearl Safford, "An Interview," *Medical Women's Journal* (October 1944): 31–32.

46. *New York Times*, November 10 (advertisement quotation), 14 (quotations), 1921; *New York Tribune*, November 14 (long quotation), 1921; Transcription of Hearing Held at Office

of Commissioner of Accounts, February 17, 1922, in LC-MSP, Reel 28: 301–21; Mary Ware Dennett, Note, November 13, 1921, Dennett Papers, Series IV, Folder 277; Mary Ware Dennett to Juliet Rublee, November 13, 1921, in *MSPME-CDS*, Reel 1: 885; Margaret Sanger to Henry John Gibbons, December 7, 1921, in Katz, Hajo, and Engelman, *Selected Papers* 1, 331–32.

47. *New York Times*, November 15, (quotations), 22, 1921 (New York Academy quotation); *New York Tribune*, November 14 (long quotation), 15 (editorial quotations), and 19, 1921 and January 13, 1922; *Tulsa Daily World*, November 21, 1921 (quotation); Margaret Sanger, *Autobiography*, 302–05; Kennedy, *Birth Control in America*, 181–82; Margaret Sanger to Archbishop Patrick Joseph Hayes, November 15, 1921, in Katz, Hajo, and Engelman, *Selected Papers* 1, 327; Margaret Sanger, "Closing Remarks," First American Birth Control Conference, November 18, 1921, in *MSPME-SCC*, Reel 67: 916 (long quotation).

48. *New York Tribune*, November 16, 19, 21 (Hayes quotations); *New York Times*, November 19, 21, 22 (Sanger quotations), December 18 (Hayes Pastoral Letter quotations), 20 (Sanger quotations in response to Pastoral Letter), 1921; *Dallas Morning News*, November 21, 1921.

49. *New York Times*, November 23, 25, December 3, 4, 8, 10, 18, 1921 and February 18, 21 and May 20, 1922; *New York World*, December 3, 1921 (quotation); "Mrs. Rublee's Arrest: A Record and a Protest," *BCR* 6 (January 1922): 5–6; Sanger, *Autobiography*, 315 (quotation); *New York Tribune*, November 17, 1921 (Field quotation); "Church Control?" *BCR* 5 (December 1921): 3 (long quotation); Sanger, *My Fight*, 237 (quotation); Tentler, *Catholics and Contraception*, 53 (quotation).

50. *New York Tribune*, January 13, 1922; "One Million Members!" *BCR* 5 (December 1921): 20; "ABCL," *BCR* 6 (September 1922): 187 (ABCL quotations and long quotation); "First American Birth Control Conference," *BCR* 5 (August 1921): 3 (quotation).

51. Daniel J. Kevles, *In the Name of Eugenics: Genetics and the Uses of Human Heredity* (New York: Knopf, 1985), 3–5, 42–44, 82–90; Carl N. Degler, *In search of Human Nature: The Decline and Revival of Darwinism in American Social Thought* (New York: Oxford University Press, 1991), 11, 38–44; Peter S. Harper, *A Short History of Medical Genetics* (New York: Oxford University Press), 407–12.

52. Kevles, *In the Name of Eugenics*, 55–63; Harper, *Short History of Medical Genetics*, 267–71; *Miami Herald*, July 9, 1920.

53. Diane B. Paul, *Controlling Human Heredity, 1865 to the Present* (Amherst, NY: Humanity Books, 1995), 5; Robinson, *Practical Eugenics*, 92; S. Adophus Knopf, "Birth Control: Its Medical, Social, Economic and Moral Aspects," *The Survey* 37 (November 18, 1916): 161 (quotation); Emma Goldman, "The Social Aspects of Birth Control," *Mother Earth* 11 (April 1916): 469 (quotation); Mary Ware Dennett and Frederic H. Robinson, "Foreword" to "A Symposium on Birth Control," *Medical Review of Reviews* 25 (March 1919): 132 (quotation); Robyn L. Rosen, "Federal Expansion, Fertility Control, and Physicians in the United States: The Politics of Maternal Welfare in the Interwar Years," *Journal of Women's History* 10 (Autumn 1998): 73.

54. Margaret Sanger, "Birth Control and Racial Betterment," *BCR* 3 (February 1919): 11–12 (quotation); Margaret Sanger, *The Pivot of Civilization* (Amherst, NY: Humanity Books;

reprint of 1922 edition), quotations on 64, 65, 123; Margaret Sanger to Sydney L. Lasell, Jr., February 13, 1934, in Katz, Engelman, and Hajo, *Selected Papers* 2, 278 (quotation).

55. Havelock Ellis, *The Task of Social Hygiene* (New York: Houghton Mifflin, 1913), 46 (quotation); Sanger, "The Eugenic Value of Birth Control Propaganda," *BCR* 5 (Oct 1921): 5 (quotation); Sanger, *Pivot of Civilization*, quotations on pp. 122, 133, 138; Kevles, *In the Name of Eugenics*, 78; *Philadelphia Inquirer*, February 4, 1921 (quotations).

56. Margaret Sanger, "Birth Control and Racial Betterment," *BCR* 3 (February 1919): 11 (quotation); "Intelligent or Unintelligent Birth Control?" *BCR* 3 (May 1919): 12 (quotation).

57. Sanger, *Pivot of Civilization*, 121–23, 173–87 (quotations on pp. 186, 182, 181, 122); Margaret Sanger, "Birth Control and Racial Betterment," *BCR* 3 (February 1919): 11–12 (for her views on sterilization); Kevles, *In the Name of Eugenics*, 75 (quotation), 103; Elof Axel Carlson, *The Unfit: A History of a Bad Idea* (Cold Spring Harbor, NY: Cold Spring Harbor Laboratory Press, 2001), 258–61; Paul, *Controlling Human Heredity*, 17–18, 108–09.

58. Sanger, *Woman and the New Race*, 32 (quotation); Sanger, *Pivot of Civilization*, 252 (quotation).

59. McCann, *Birth Control Politics*, 119–22; Chesler, *Woman of Valor*, 216–17; Margaret Sanger to James A. Field, June 5, 1923, and Havelock Ellis to Margaret Sanger, December 19, 1921, in Katz, Hajo, and Engelman, *Selected Papers* 1, 367–70, 333–34; Sanger, *Autobiography*, 364; *Morning Oregonian*, October 4, 1921; Richard A. Soloway, *Demography and Degeneration: Eugenics and the Declining Birthrate in Twentieth Century Britain* (Chapel Hill: University of North Carolina Press, 1995), 96, 108; *New York Times*, September 27, 1921.

60. Margaret Sanger, "The Eugenic Value of Birth Control Propaganda," *BCR* 5 (Oct 1921): 5 (quotation); Kennedy, *Birth Control in America*, 121 (quotation); Margaret Sanger to Hugh de Selincourt, July 15, 1922, in Katz, Hajo, and Engelman, *Selected Papers* 1, 345.

61. Sanger, *Autobiography*, 358–60; Richard Wallace, State Board of Charities to Anne Kennedy, May 16, 1922 and Margaret Sanger, "Clinical Research Fund," 1923, in MSP-LC, Reel 33: 553 and 34: 179; Margaret Sanger to Dorothy Bocker, October 17, 1922, in Katz, Hajo, and Engelman, *Selected Papers* 1, 351–53.

62. Margaret Sanger to William J. Fielding, February 10, 1923 (quotation) and to Charles H. Johnson, January 17, 1924 (quotation), in Katz, Hajo, and Engelman, *Selected Papers* 1, 360, 382; Sanger, *Autobiography*, 359–60 (quotations); Bocker, *Birth Control Methods*, 1–31; Anne Kennedy, ABCL, "Summary of Events for 1923," December?, 1923, in *MSPME-SCC*, Reel 61: 172; *Los Angeles Times* and *New York Times*, December 6, 1923.

CHAPTER FOUR

1. *Birth Control Hearings before the Committee on the Judiciary, House of Representatives*, 73rd. Congress, 2d sess., on H.R. 5978, Jan. 18–19, 1934 (Washington, D.C., 1934), 233–239, in MSPME-SCC, Reel 69: 506.

2. Annie G. Porritt, "Publicity in the Birth Control Movement," *BCR* 7 (April 1923): 88–89 (quotation); *New York Times*, September 9, 1923 (business quotation); "Calls Rebuilt Dwellings 'Birth Control Houses,'" *The American Architect* 117 (April 28, 1920): 525; Edwina

Davis, "Birth Control of the Seas," *Life Magazine* 82 (August 2, 1923): 5; "Book Reviews," *Coast Artillery Journal* 57 (August, 1922): 188; Francis M. Vreeland, "The Process of Reform with Especial Reference to Reform Groups in the Field of Population" (Ph.D. dissertation, University of Michigan, 1929), 299.

3. John D'Emilio and Estelle B. Freedman, *Intimate Matters: A History of Sexuality in America* (Chicago: University of Chicago Press, 1988), 239–41 (quotation); James Reed, *The Birth Control Movement and American Society: From Private Vice to Public Virtue* (Princeton, NJ: Princeton University Press, 1978), 54–63 (quotation on p. 60); Andrea Tone, *Devices and Desires: A History of Contraceptives in America* (New York: Hill & Wang, 2001), 136–37, 152–53; Dorothy Bocker, *Birth Control Methods* (New York: Birth Control Clinical Research Bureau, 1924), 4–8; *World Telegram*, March 27, 1931 (quotations).

4. Robert and Helen Merrell Lynd, *Middletown: A Study in Contemporary American Culture* (New York: Harcourt, Brace, 1929), 123–24; *New York Times*, March 27, 1925; Katharine Bement Davis, "A Study of the Sex Life of the Normal Married Woman," *Journal of Social Hygiene* 8 (April, 1922): 173–89; Deborah Dawson, et al., "Fertility Control in the United States before the Contraceptive Revolution," *Family Planning Perspectives* 12 (March–April, 1980): 76–86 (abortion quotation on 85); Caroline Robinson, *Seventy Birth Control Clinics* (Baltimore, MD: Williams & Wilkins, 1930), 62–64, 66–67, 224–25; Kristen Luker, *Abortion and the Politics of Motherhood* (Berkeley: University of California Press, 1984), 48–54; Warren S. Thompson and P. K. Whelpton, *Population Trends in the United States* (New York: McGraw-Hill, 1933), 212–13, 226 (quotation), 285–87, 266.

5. Alfred C. Kinsey et al., *Sexual Behavior in the Human Female* (Philadelphia: W. B. Saunders, 1953), 300–301, 327, 356–57; Reed, *Birth Control Movement*, 124; Donald Porter Geddes, ed., *An Analysis of the Kinsey Reports on Sexual Behavior in the Human Male and Female* (New York: E. P. Dutton, 1954), 58, 152; Margaret Sanger, *Woman and the New Race* (New York: Brentano's, 1920), 177 (quotation).

6. Havelock Ellis to Margaret Sanger, December 8, 1923, in Esther Katz, Cathy Moran Hajo, and Peter C. Engelman, eds., *The Selected Papers of Margaret Sanger,* vol. 1: *The Woman Rebel, 1900–1928* (Urbana,: University of Illinois Press, 2003), 379 (Ellis and Sanger quotation); Leslie Woodcock Tentler, *Catholics and Contraception: An American History* (Ithaca, NY: Cornell University Press, 2004), 44–45; Carole R. McCann, *Birth Control Politics in the United States, 1916–1945* (Ithaca: Cornell University Press, 1994), 77–78; Donatella Della Porta and Mario Diani, *Social Movements: An Introduction* (Malden, MA: Blackwell Publishing, 2006) 150–51; *World Telegram*, March 27, 1931 (quotation); Margaret Sanger, "Tragedy," *The Woman Rebel* 1 (July 1914): 33.

7. Margaret Sanger, "The Meaning of Radio Birth Control," February 29, 1924, in Katz, Hajo, and Engelman, *Selected Papers* 1, 384–87; *Syracuse Post-Standard*, February 28, 1924; Tentler, *Catholics and Contraception*, 56; Margaret Sanger, *My Fight for Birth Control* (New York: Farrar & Rinehart, 1931), 200–202; *New York Times*, January 24, 1923; Margaret Sanger, *An Autobiography* (New York: W. W. Norton, 1938),411; *Boston Globe*, February 16, 1925; "News Notes," *BCR* 10 (January 1926): 30; Margaret Sanger, "The War against Birth Control," *The American Mercury* (June 1924): 231–36 (quotation).

8. *New York Times*, April 11, 1923 (quotation); Mary Ware Dennett to Friends, September 29, 1922 and Dennett to John Favill, November 6, 1923, in MSP-LC, Reel 10: 1038 and 1042; Rosen, "Mary Coffin War Dennett"; Constance M. Chen, *Sex Side of Life: Mary Ware Dennett's Pioneering Battle for Birth Control and Sex Education* (New York: The New Press: 1996), 230–38; Mary Ware Dennett, *Birth Control Laws, Shall We Keep Them, Abolish Them or Change Them?* (New York: Frederick H. Hitchcock, 1926), 298.

9. Anne Kennedy, ABCL Report for 1923, in *MSPME-SCC*, Reel 61: 172; *Chicago Daily Tribune*, September 20 (quotation), October 28 and November 24, 1923; Middle Western States Birth Control Conference Program, October 29–31, 1923, in *MSPME-SCC*, Reel 67: 936; Lenore Guttmacher, *Planned Parenthood Beginnings: Affiliate Histories* (New York: PPFA, 1979), 40;Vreeland, "Process of Reform," 379–80; Sanger, *Autobiography*, 370 (quotation)–75; *New York Times*, March 27 and 29, 1925; *Washington Post*, March 30, 1925; Sixth Neo-Malthusian and Birth Control Conference Program, March 25–31, 1925, in *MSPME-SCC*, Reel 67: 70.

10. Sanger, *My Fight*, 294 (quotation); Sanger, *Autobiography*, 366–67 (quotations); ABCL, Summary of Events, 1924 and 1924 Calendar, in *MSPME-SCC*, Reel 61: 176 and 78: 556–87; Margaret Sanger, 1926 Calendar, in MSP-LC, Reel 1: 596; Editorial, *BCR* 10 (April 1926): 113.

11. Sanger, *Autobiography*, 362–63 (quotation); Reed, *Birth Control Movement*, 116; ABCL Motherhood Department Report, January 12, 1926, in *MSPME-SCC*, Reel 61: 190; James F. Cooper, *Technique of Contraception* (New York: Day-Nichols, 1928), xv; Ellen Chesler, *Woman of Valor: Margaret Sanger and the Birth Control Movement in America* (New York: Simon & Schuster,1992; revised 2007), 276.

12. Margaret Sanger to Anne Kennedy, July 22, 1923 and to Agnes Smedley, January 8, 1925, in Katz, Hajo, and Engelman, *Selected Papers* 1, 370, 414–15; Reed, *Birth Control Movement*, 336; Sanger, *Autobiography*, 363–64; J. Noah Slee to Murray Agency, October 16, 1924, to Carl Schmid, May 19, 1926, and untitled statement, November 25, 1925, in MSP-LC, Reel 11: 579, 590, 584; Anne Kennedy, "History of the Development of Contraceptive Materials in the United States," *American Medicine* 41 (March 1935): 159–61; "Accident of Birth," *Fortune Magazine* 17 (February 1938): 112; Tone, *Devices and Desires*, 127–32; Herbert Simonds, "Reminiscences of Herbert Simonds," n.d. (Margaret Sanger Papers, Sophia Smith Collection, Smith College), 82–83.

13. Robinson, *Seventy Birth Control Clinics*, 23–34; Cathy Moran Hajo, *Birth Control on Main Street: Organizing Clinics in the United States, 1916–1939* (Urbana: University of Illinois Press, 2010), 24; Clara Taylor Warne, "Making Birth Control Respectable," *BCR* 14 (April 1930): 110–11; Cooper, *Technique of Contraception*, 217–25; Margaret Sanger to ABCL Members, March 1926, in Katz, Hajo, and Engelman, *Selected Papers* 1, 437–38 (quotation); Reed, *Birth Control Movement*, 143, 168; Linda Gordon, *The Moral Property of Women: A History of Birth Control Politics in America* (Urbana: University of Illinois Press, 2002), 181–82.

14. Robert Dickinson, "Contraception—A Medical Review of the Situation," *American Journal of Obstetrics and Gynecology* 8 (November 1924): 583–605; McCann, *Birth Control Politics*, 79–91; Reed, *Birth Control Movement,* 168–180; Marie E. Kopp, *Birth Control in*

Practice: An Analysis of Ten Thousand Case Histories of the Birth Control Clinical Research Bureau (New York: Robert M. McBride & Company, 1934), 160; Maternity Research Council Minutes, Nov. 12 and 24, 1925, in *MSPME-CDS*, Reel 13: 787 and MSP-LC, Reel 32: 39; Robert Dickinson to ABCL, Dec. 1, 1925; Margaret Sanger to Robert Dickinson, Dec. 9, 1925; "Testimony of Robert L. Dickinson," Jan. 15, 1926; and "Stenographer's Minutes of Public Hearing, State Board of Charities," Jan. 15, 1926, in MSP-LC, Reel 32: 51–53, 72–77.

15. Kopp, *Birth Control in Practice*, 57–66, 210–12; McCann, *Birth Control Politics*, 90; Margaret Sanger, "Contraception: A Medical Review of the Situation," *BCR* 9 (January 1925): 20–21 (quotation); "Section on Obstetrics, Gynecology & Abdominal Surgery," *JAMA* 84 (June 13, 1925): 1833; Margaret Sanger to Hannah Stone, June 11, 1926, in Katz, Hajo, and Engelman, *Selected Papers* 1, 442–45; Joyce M. Ray and F. G. Gosling, "American Physicians and Birth Control, 1936–1947," *Journal of Social History* 18 (Spring 1985): 399–400; Chesler, *Woman of Valor*, 295.

16. *New York Times*, April 17 and 19, 1929; *New York Telegram*, April 17, 1929 (Broun quotation); *New York Herald Tribune*, April 17, 1929 (editorial quotation); "The Raid," *BCR* 13 (June 1929), 155 (Academy of Medicine quotation).

17. *New York Times*, April 25, 1929; Sanger, *Autobiography*, 404–408; *New York Times*, April 20, 1929 (first Ernst quotation) and May 15, 1929; Morris Ernst, "How We Nullify," *The Nation* 134 (Jan. 27, 1932): 113 (second and third Ernst quotations)–14; Hannah M. Stone, "The Birth Control Raid," *Eugenics* 2 (August 1929): 2–3 (Holden quotation); "The Raid," *BCR* 13 (June 1929): 154–55; "Judge Rosenbluth's Opinion," *BCR* 13 (July 1929): 194 (quotation); Margaret Sanger to Havelock Ellis, May 20, 1929, in Esther Katz, Peter C. Engelman, and Cathy Moran Hajo, eds., *Selected Papers,* vol. 2, *Birth Control Comes of Age, 1928–1939* (Urbana: University of Illinois Press, 2006), 33.

18. Margaret Sanger to Juliet Rublee, June 28, 1928, in Katz, Engelman, and Hajo, *Selected Papers* 2, 3–4 (quotation); Margaret Sanger to ABCL Board of Directors, June 8, 1928, in Katz, Hajo, and Engelman, *Selected Papers* 1, 480–81 (quotation); Margaret Sanger to Juliet Rublee, May 20, 1928, in *MSPME-CDS,* Reel 4: 640; ABCL, Annual Meeting Minutes, January 12, 1928, PPFA (I) Records, Sophia Smith Collection, Smith College; Sanger, *My Fight*, 329 (quotations).

19. McCann, *Birth Control Politics*, 177–81, 147–59; Penelope B. P. Huse, "Report of the ABCL Executive Secretary for the Year 1929," in *MSPME-SCC,* Reel 61: 213; Margaret Sanger to Edward Murray East, December 31, 1929, in Katz, Engelman, and Hajo, *Selected Papers* 2, 55–57; Marie Pichel Levinson Warner, "Birth Control and the Negro," in BCCRB Progress Report, June 1935, in *MSPME-SCC,* Reel 61: 790; Raymond Pearl, "Contraception and Fertility in 2,000 Women," *Human Biology* 4 (September 1932): 395 (quotation); Invitation, New York City Committee on Mother's Health, Commemoration of Ten Years of Service in Harlem, 1945, Florence Rose Papers, Sophia Smith Collection, Smith College (hereafter Rose Papers).

20. Margaret Sanger to Robert Dickinson, October 3, 1929, in Katz, Engelman, and Hajo, *Selected Papers* 2, 43 (quotation); ABCL, "Prospect and Retrospect," *BCR* 13 (February 1929): 57–60; Helena Huntington Smith, "Birth Control and the Law," *The Outlook* 149 (August 29, 1928): 686–87, 718; J. Whitridge Williams, "Indication for Therapeutic Sterilization in Obstetrics," *JAMA* 91 (October 27, 1928): 1242; NCFLBC, *A New Day Dawns for Birth*

Control (New York: NCFLBC, July 1937), 10 (Sanger quotation), 16, in *MSPME-SCC* Reel 64:742.

21. Sanger, *Autobiography*, 417–27; Margaret Sanger to Penelope B. P. Huse, January 29, 1931, in Katz, Engelman, and Hajo, *Selected Papers* 2, 89–92; NCFLBC, *New Day Dawns*, 17–21, 33–36; "Birth Control and the Good Old Boys in Congress," *Margaret Sanger Papers Project Newsletter* 26 (Winter 2000/2001): 1–5; NCFLCBC Lobbying Reports, 1930–1935 (quotations), in MSP-LC, Reel LCM 82: 183, 78: 260, 77:457, 82: 50, 77: 99; Hazel Moore, "Year of the Devil and Roman Catholics," June 13, 1934, in MSP-LC, Reel 68: 349 (quotation).

22. For source information on hearing transcripts see Katz, Engelman, and Hajo, *Selected Papers* 2, xxxiv–xxxv; *Dallas Morning News*, December 12, 1933 (quotation); NCFLBC, *New Day Dawns*, 22; *Chicago Daily Tribune*, January 19, 1934 (Coughlin and hearing room quotations); *Washington Post*, January 19, 1934; "Extract from Testimony on H. R. 5978," January 19, 1934, in Katz, Engelman, and Hajo, *Selected Papers* 2, 252–63 (quotation on 257); *The News and Observer* (Raleigh, N.C.), January 20, 1934 (quotation); Sanger, *Autobiography*, 424–26 (quotation on 425); John T. Noonan, Jr., *Contraception: A History of Its Treatment by the Catholic Theologians and Canonists* (Cambridge, MA: Harvard University Press, 1986), 442–47.

23. ABCL, "The Next Step Forward," 1933, Margaret Sanger Papers, Unfilmed Portion, Sophia Smith Collection, Smith College; McCann, *Birth Control Politics*, 181–87 (quotations on 180, 183); Hajo, *Birth Control on Main Street*, 176–83; Allison Pierce Moore, ABCL Report for 1936, PPFA (I) Records, Sophia Smith Collection, Smith College; Eleanor Dwight Jones, "Birth Control on the Air," *BCR* 15 (December 1931), 341–42 (quotation); *New York Times*, January 20, 1933 and January 25, 1935; Elof Axel Carlson, *The Unfit: A History of a Bad Idea* (Cold Spring Harbor, NY: Cold Spring Harbor Laboratory Press, 2001), 12, 15, 215, 255 (Holmes quotation); Margaret Sanger, "For International News Service on Sterilization Symposium," February 7, 1934, in Katz, Engelman, and Hajo, *Selected Papers* 2, 273 (quotation); *Los Angeles Times*, August 11, 1935.

24. NCFLBC, *New Day Dawns*, 8; McCann, *Birth Control Politics*, 178–79; "News Notes," *BCR* 14 (February 1930): 55; David J. Garrow, *Liberty and Sexuality: The Right to Privacy and the Making of Roe v. Wade* (New York: MacMillan, 1994), 26; *Youngs Rubber Corporation v. C. I. Lee and Co., Inc, et al. 45 F. 2d 103; 1930 U.S. App. LEXIS 3582* (quotation); *New York Times*, October 28, 1934 (quotation); "The Accident of Birth," *Fortune* 17 (February 1938): 83–86, 108, 110, 112, 114; Elizabeth H. Garrett, "Birth Control's Business Baby," *The New Republic* 77 (January 17, 1934): 269–72 (quotations on 270, 271).

25. *New York Times*, July 18, 1931; Anthony M. Turano, "Birth Control and the Law," *American Mercury* (April 1935): 466–72; C. Thomas Dienes, *Law, Politics and Birth Control* (Urbana: University of Illinois Press, 1972), 110–11; David. M. Kennedy, *Birth Control in America: The Career of Margaret Sanger* (New Haven, CT: Yale University Press, 1970), 243–45; Margaret Sanger to Morris Ernst, March 28, 1932; Florence Rose, "Summary of Correspondence dealing with Customs Interference," n.d.; Sakae Koyama to Sanger, October 17, 1931, all in MSP-LC, Reel 59: 166, 60: 108, and 18: 1083; Florence Rose to Morris Ernst, February 8, 1933, in *MSPME-CDS,* Reel 5: 501.

26. Florence Rose, Memorandum: U.S. vs. Japanese Pessaries, December 10, 1935, in Katz, Engelman, and Hajo, *Selected Papers* 2, 353–55; "Transcript of Record," *U.S. v. One Package, containing 120, more or less, rubber pessaries to prevent conception*, 86 F. 2d 737 (May 23, 1936), in *MSPME-CDS,* Reel 15: 571–574 (quotation on frame 561); *United States v. One Package*, in *MSPME-SCC,* Reel 69: 372 (quotations).

27. *New York Times*, December 8, 1936 (first Ernst quotation; first Sanger quotation); Morris Ernst and Alexander Lindey, *The Censor Marches On* (New York: Doubleday, 1940), 165 (second Ernst quotation); "Editorial," *National Birth Control News* (February 1937): 3 (second Sanger quotation)–4, in *MSPME-CDS,* Reel 16: 400; Reed, *Birth Control Movement*, 187; "Resolutions on Contraception," *JAMA* 104 (June 22, 1935): 2268–69; "Report of Committee to Study Contraceptive Practices and Related Problems," *JAMA* 106 (May 30, 1936): 1910–11; "Report of Reference Committee on Executive Session," *JAMA* 108 (June 26, 1937): 2217 (quotation)–18.

28. *New York World-Telegram*, June 10, 1927; Allison Pierce Moore, "What of the Future?" *BCR* 4 (June 1937): 2–3 (quotation); *New York Post*, June 9, 1937 (quotations); Margaret Sanger, "Statement on the American Medical Association Action," June 15, 1937, in Katz, Engelman, and Hajo, *Selected Papers* 2, 405–06 (radio quotation); Kennedy, *Birth Control in America*, 251–53; Caroline Carter Davis, "In the 'Cradle of Liberty,'" *BCR* 22 (October 1937): 6–8; "News Items: The Massachusetts Case," *Journal of Contraception* 3 (November 1938): 215; Garrow, *Liberty and Sexuality*, offers a riveting account of the Waterbury raid and ensuing legal action, in Chapter 1, 1–78.

29. NCFLBC, *New Day Dawns*, 5; Birth Control Council of America, Minutes, May 14, 1937, in *MSPME-SCC* Reel 62:13; Margaret Sanger to Robert Dickinson, July 10, 1937, and Chapter 7, Introduction, in Katz, Engelman, and Hajo, *Selected Papers* 2, 407–09, 414–15; Margaret Sanger to Edith How-Martyn, October 4, 1939, in *MSPME-CDS,* Reel 6: 1055.

30. BCFA, *Directory of Clinics and Clinical Services*, 1939, PPFA (I) Records, Sophia Smith Collection, Smith College; *Washington Post*, November 29, 1936; NCFLBC, "Summary of Polls on Birth Control," December 8, 1936, in MSP-LC Reel 69:698; Henry F. Pringle, "What Do the Women of America Think?" *Ladies' Home Journal* (March 1938): 14–15, 94–95, 97.

31. Hajo, *Birth Control on Main Street*, 135; Gordon, *Moral Property of Women*, 217; Johanna Schoen, *Choice and Coercion: Birth Control, Sterilization and Abortion in Public Health and Welfare* (Chapel Hill: University of North Carolina Press, 2005), 28; Kopp, *Birth Control in Practice*, 193–94; Ruth Robishaw, "A Study of 4,000 Patients Admitted for Contraceptive Practice and Treatment," *American Journal of Obstetrics and Gynecology* 31 (March 1936): 431; Consumers Union, *Analysis of Contraceptive Materials* (New York: Consumers Union, 1937), 3 (quotation).

32. Margaret Sanger, "The Status of Birth Control: 1938," *New Republic* 94 (April 20, 1938): 324–26; Rosen, "Federal Expansion," 53; *Belleville* (IL) *News Democrat*, July 23, 1921; Hajo, *Birth Control on Main Street*, 165–66.

33. Reed, *Birth Control Movement*, 241–52 (quotation on 250); D'Emilio and Freedman, *Intimate Matters*, 247; Robert Dickinson to Sanger, October 28, 1936, in Katz, Engelman and Hajo, *Selected Papers* 2, 375–78; Doone and Greer Williams, *Every Child a Wanted Child: Clarence James Gamble, M.D., and His Life in the Birth Control Movement* (Boston: Countway Library of Medicine, 1978), 118–27, 315–16.

34. Hannah Stone "Discussion of Occlusive Methods of Contraception: The Foam Powder Method," *Journal of Contraception* 2 (May 1937): 107; Margaret Sanger to Frederick Holden, January 11, 1937, in *MSPME-CDS* Reel 6:295; Reed, *Birth Control Movement*, 252–56; Schoen, *Choice and Coercion,* 34–37.

35. Margaret Sanger, Mary Reinhardt and Florence Rose, "Birth Control and the Negro," July 1939 (quotations on 3–4), Mary Lasker Papers, Columbia University Rare Book & Manuscript Library; Hazel Moore, "Birth Control for the Negro," 1937, Rose Papers; United States National Resources Committee, *The Problems of a Changing Population: Report of the Committee on Population Problems to the National Resources Committee*, Washington, DC, May 1938.

36. Margaret Sanger to Albert Lasker, November 12, 1939 and Lasker to Sanger, February 9, 1940, in *MSPME-SCC,* Reel 17: 453, 876; Jessie M. Rodrique, "The Black Community and the Birth Control Movement," in *Unequal Sisters,* ed. Carol Du Bois and Vicki Ruiz (New York: Routledge, 1990), 145–48; PPFA, "Better Health for 13,000,000," 7–30, Rose Papers; Robert E. Seibels, "A Rural Project in Negro Maternal Health," *Human Fertility* 6 (April 1941): 42–44; "Preliminary Annual Report of the Division of Negro Service," January 7, 1942, in *MSPME-SCC*, Reel 62: 459.

37. Dorothy Boulding Ferebee, "Planned Parenthood as a Public Health Measure for the Negro Race," *Human Fertility* 7 (February 1942): 7–10; Hannah M. Stone, "Clinical Experiences with the Foam-Powder Method," *Journal of Contraception* 3 (January 1938): 3–6; Don Wharton, "Birth Control: The Case for the State," *Atlantic Monthly* 164 (October 1939): 463–67 (quotation); Schoen, *Choice and Coercion*, 59 (quotation); McCann, *Birth Control Politics*, 168–73.

38. Gilbert W. Beebe and Murray Geisler, "A Contraceptive Service among the Migrants of the Southwest," January 14, 1941, PPFA (I) Records, Sophia Smith Collection, Smith College; BCCRB, "Confidential Report of Government Projects in Cooperation with the BCCRB," 1938, Margaret Sanger Papers, Unfilmed Portion, Sophia Smith Collection, Smith College; Schoen, *Choice and Coercion*, 37–38; *New York Times*, January 17, 1940.

39. BCFA, Annual Report 1940, January 1941, *MSPME-SCC* Reel 62:425 (quotations); BCFA, "National Referendum on the Name to Be Adopted by State Leagues, Affiliated Committees, and Federation," Apr. 17, 1941; and PPFA, Board of Director Minutes, March 5, 1942, PPFA (I) Records, Sophia Smith Collection, Smith College.

40. Margaret Sanger to D. Kenneth Rose, Jan. 22, 1942, (quotation); Margaret Sanger, Twenty-fifth Anniversary Dinner Speech, Oct. 16, 1941 (quotation), in *MSPME-SCC,* Reel 20:562 and Reel 62: 350.

CONCLUSION

1. PPFA, "Planned Parenthood in Wartime," 1942, PPFA (I) Records, Sophia Smith Collection, Smith College; PPFA, Annual Reports, 1950, 1954 (quotation), 1957 (quotations), in *MSPME-SCC*, Reel 66: 614, 688, 718; PPFA, "Policy Decisions," Oct. 16, 1957, in *MSPME-SCC*, Reel 65: 300; Margaret Sanger, "Tomorrow's Children," May 3, 1944, in Esther Katz, Cathy Moran Hajo, Peter C. Engelman, eds. *The Selected Papers of Margaret Sanger,* Vol. III, *The Politics of Planned Parenthood, 1939–1966* (Urbana: University of Illinois Press, 2010), 160–69.

2. *New York Times*, February 18, 1965, May 25, 1965 (Academy quotation), November 5, 1965 (Guttmacher quotation), September 6, 1966; Johanna Schoen, *Choice and Coercion: Birth Control, Sterilization and Abortion in Public Health and Welfare* (Chapel Hill: University of North Carolina Press, 2005), 263; "President, Senator Call for Funds to Aid Local Birth Control Programs," *Planned Parenthood News* 43 (March 1966): 1.

3. Matthew Connelly, *Fatal Misconception: The Struggle to Control World Population* (Cambridge, MA: Harvard University Press, 2008), 187–89; Elaine Tyler May, *Birth Control and the Pill: A History of Promise, Peril, and Liberation* (New York: Basic Books, 2010), 35–56.

4. Rosalind Pollack Petchesky, *Abortion and Woman's Choice: The State, Sexuality, and Reproductive Freedom* (Boston: Northeastern University Press, 1990), 171; *New York Times*, June 16, 1966; Katz, Hajo, and Engelman, *Selected Papers* III, 272, 345.

5. *New York Times*, June 8, 1965 (*Griswold* quotations), May 11, 1966, and March 23, 1972 (*Eisenstadt* quotations); C. Thomas Dienes, *Law, Politics and Birth Control* (Urbana: University of Illinois Press, 1972), 46, 162–83, 189–91; Louis Brandeis and Simon Warren, "The Right to Privacy," *Harvard Law Review* 4 (December 1890): 193–220; John W. Johnson, *Griswold v. Connecticut: Birth Control and the Constitutional Right of Privacy* (Lawrence: University Press of Kansas, 2005), 198–204; Harriet F. Pilpel, "The Crazy Quilt of Our Birth Control Laws," *Journal of Sex Research* 1 (July 1965): 135–42; David J. Garrow, *Liberty and Sexuality: The Right to Privacy and the Making of Roe v. Wade* (New York: MacMillan, 1994), 517–44.

6. *Los Angeles Times*, June 22, 1966; *Washington Post*, Aug. 14, 1966; *New York Times*, October 1, 1966; Petchesky, *Abortion and Woman's Choice*, 124–25; John D'Emilio and Estelle B. Freedman, *Intimate Matters A History of Sexuality in America* (Chicago: University of Chicago Press, 1988), 310–13; Leslie J. Reagan, *When Abortion Was a Crime Women, Medicine, and Law in the United States, 1867–1973* (Berkeley: University of California Press, 1997), 244–45.

7. Peter S. Harper, *A Short History of Medical Genetics* (New York: Oxford University Press, 2008), 355–56; *New York Times*, October 1 and December 27, 1966; "Detecting Foetal Abnormalities," *British Medical Journal* 1 (April 16, 1966): 932.

8. *New York Times*, August 13, 2010; Russell Shorto, "Contra-Contraception," *New York Times Magazine* (May 7, 2006), 48–55, 68, 83; Rajesh K. Naz, "Status of Contraceptive Vaccines," *American Journal of Reproductive Immunology* 61 (January 2009): 11–18; Robert Jütte, *Contraception: A History* (Malden, MA: Polity Press, 2008), 216–20.

SELECTED BIBLIOGRAPHY

Primary and secondary sources on the birth control movement are extensive and growing. I have relied most closely on the collections of Margaret Sanger's papers that have been combined in three separate microfilm editions. They provide the richest material on the movement's early history. I have listed below the other archive and manuscript sources and publications that I found most useful. For a complete listing of sources please consult the chapter notes.

ARCHIVAL COLLECTIONS AND SOURCES

American Birth Control League Records, Houghton Library, Harvard University.

Mary Ware Dennett Papers, Schlesinger Library, Radcliffe College, Harvard University.

Mabel Dodge Luhan Papers. Yale Collection of American Literature, Beinecke Rare Book and Manuscript Library, Yale University

National Committee on Maternal Health Records. Boston Medical Library, Francis A. Countway Library of Medicine.

Planned Parenthood Federation of America (I) Records, Sophia Smith Collection, Smith College.

Planned Parenthood League of Massachusetts Records, Sophia Smith Collection, Smith College.

Florence Rose Papers, Sophia Smith Collection, Smith College.

Juliet Rublee Papers, Dartmouth College.

Margaret Sanger Papers, Unfilmed Portion, Sophia Smith Collection, Smith College.

Margaret Sanger Papers Microfilm, Library of Congress. Washington, DC, 1977.

The Margaret Sanger Papers Microfilm Edition: Collected Documents, Esther Katz, Cathy Moran Hajo, Peter C. Engelman, eds. Bethesda, MD: University Publications of America, 1997.

The Margaret Sanger Papers Microfilm Edition: Smith College Collections, Esther Katz, Peter C. Engelman, Cathy Moran Hajo, Anke Voss Hubbard, eds. Bethesda, MD: University Publications of America, 1996.

BOOKS AND PAMPHLETS

Avrich, Paul. *Anarchist Voices: An Oral History of Anarchism in America*. Princeton, NJ: Princeton University Press, 1995.

Avrich, Paul. *The Modern School Movement: Anarchism and Education in the United States*. Princeton, NJ: University Press, 1980.

Baskin, Alex, ed. *Margaret Sanger, The Woman Rebel and the Rise of the Birth Control Movement in the United States*. Stony Brook, NY: Archives of Social History, 1976.

Beisel, Nicola Kay. *Imperiled Innocents: Anthony Comstock and Family Reproduction in Victorian America*. Princeton, NJ: Princeton University Press, 1997.

Bocker, Dorothy. *Birth Control Methods*. New York: Birth Control Clinical Research Bureau, 1924.

Boyer, Paul S. *Purity in Print: The Vice-Society Movement and Book Censorship in America*. New York: Charles Scribner's Sons, 1968.

Brandt, Allan M. *No Magic Bullet: A Social History of Venereal Disease in the United States Since 1880*. New York: Oxford University Press, 1987.

Brodie, Janet Farrell. *Contraception and Abortion in 19th Century America*. Ithaca, NY: Cornell University Press, 1994.

Brownlow, Kevin. *Behind the Mask of Innocence*. New York: Alfred A. Knopf, 1990.

Bruns, Roger A. *The Damndest Radical: The Life and World of Ben Reitman, Chicago's Celebrated Social Reformer, Hobo King, and Whorehouse Physician*. Urbana: University of Illinois Press, 1987.

Buhle, Mari Jo et al., eds., *Encyclopedia of the American Left*. Urbana: University of Illinois Press, 1992.

Carlson, Elof Axel. *The Unfit: A History of a Bad Idea*. Cold Spring Harbor, NY: Cold Spring Harbor Laboratory Press, 2001.

Caron, Simone M. *Who Chooses? American Reproductive History since 1830*. Gainesville: University of Florida Press, 2008.

Carpenter, Edward. *Love's Coming of Age*. New York: Vanguard Press, 1926; first published in 1896.

Chen, Constance M. *The Sex Side of Life: Mary Ware Dennett's Pioneering Battle for Birth Control and Sex Education*. New York: The New Press: 1996.

Chesler, Ellen. *Woman of Valor: Margaret Sanger and the Birth Control Movement in America*. New York: Simon & Schuster, 1992; revised 2007.

Committee of One Hundred. *The Birth Control Movement*. New York: privately printed, 1917.

Comstock, Anthony. *Traps for the Young*. New York: Funk & Wagnalls, 1883.

Connelly, Matthew. *Fatal Misconception: The Struggle to Control World Population*. Cambridge, MA: Harvard University Press, 2008.

Consumers Union. *Analysis of Contraceptive Materials*. New York: Consumers Union, 1937.

Cooper, James F. *Technique of Contraception*. New York: Day-Nichols, Inc., 1928.

Cott, Nancy. *The Grounding of Modern Feminism*. New Haven, CT: Yale University Press, 1987.

Cottrell, Robert C. *Roger Nash Baldwin and the American Civil Liberties Union*. New York: Columbia University Press, 2000.

Davis, Angela. *Women, Race, and Class*. New York: Vintage, 1981.

Degler, Carl N. *At Odds: Women and the Family in America from the Revolution to the Present*. New York: Oxford University Press, 1980.

Degler, Carl N. *In search of Human Nature: The Decline and Revival of Darwinism in American Social Thought*. New York: Oxford University Press, 1991

D'Emilio, John and Estelle B. Freedman. *Intimate Matters: A History of Sexuality in America*. Chicago: University of Chicago Press, 1988.

Dennett, Mary Ware. *Birth Control Laws: Shall We Keep Them, Abolish Them or Change Them?* New York: Frederick H. Hitchcock, 1926.

Dennett, Mary Ware. *The Sex Side of Life: An Explanation for Young People*. New York: privately printed, 1919.

Dickinson, Robert Latou. *Techniques of Conception Control*. Baltimore, MD: Williams & Wilkins, 1942.

Dienes, C. Thomas. *Law, Politics and Birth Control*. Urbana: University of Illinois Press, 1972.

Dubofsky, Melvyn. *We Shall Be All: A History of the Industrial Workers of the World*. Urbana: University of Illinois Press, 2000.

Eastman, Max. *Love and Revolution: My Journey through an Epoch*. New York: Random House, 1964.

Ellis, Havelock. *My Life: Autobiography of Havelock Ellis*. Boston: Houghton Mifflin, 1939.

Ellis, Havelock. *Studies in the Psychology of Sex*. Vol. 1, *The Evolution of Modesty*. Philadelphia: F. A. Davis, 1910.

Ellis, Havelock. *Studies in the Psychology of Sex*. Vol. 6, *Sex in Relation to Society*. Philadelphia: F. A. Davis, 1913.

Ellis, Havelock. *The Task of Social Hygiene*. New York: Houghton Mifflin, 1913.

Engelman, Peter C. "Katharine Dexter McCormick." In *Encyclopedia of Birth Control*, edited by Vern L. Bullough, 169–71. Santa Barbara, CA: ABC-CLIO, 2001.

Engelman, Peter C. "Margaret Sanger Opens the First Birth Control Clinic in the U.S." In *Great Events from History: Human Rights*, edited by Frank Northen Magil, 184–89. Pasadena, CA: Salem Press, 1992.

Ernst, Morris L. and Alexander Lindey. *The Censor Marches On*. New York: Doubleday, 1940.

Falk, Candace et al., eds. *Emma Goldman: A Documentary History of the American Years*. Vol. 1, *Made for America, 1890–1901*. Urbana: University of Illinois Press, 2003.

Falk, Candace et al., eds. *Emma Goldman: A Documentary History of the American Years*. Vol. 2, *Making Free Speech, 1902–1909*. Urbana: University of Illinois Press, 2005.

Fryer, Peter. *The Birth Controllers*. London: Secker & Warburg, 1965.

Garrow, David J. *Liberty & Sexuality: The Right to Privacy and the Making of Roe v. Wade*. New York: MacMillan, 1994.

Geddes, Donald Porter, ed. *An Analysis of the Kinsey Reports on Sexual Behavior in the Human Male and Female*. New York: E. P. Dutton, 1954.

Goldman, Emma. *Living My Life*. 2 vols. New York: Alfred A. Knopf, 1931.

Gordon, Linda. *The Moral Property of Women: A History of Birth Control Politics in America*. Urbana: University of Illinois Press, 2002.

Grosskurth, Phyllis. *Havelock Ellis: A Biography*. New York: Alfred A. Knopf, 1980.

Guttmacher, Lenore. *Planned Parenthood Beginnings: Affiliate Histories*. New York: PPFA, 1979.

Hajo, Cathy Moran. *Birth Control on Main Street: Organizing Clinics in the United States, 1916–1939*. Urbana: University of Illinois Press, 2010.

Harper, Peter S. *A Short History of Medical Genetics*. New York: Oxford University Press, 2008.

Himes, Norman. *Medical History of Contraception*. New York: Schocken Books, 1970 (reprint of 1936 edition).

Johnson, John W. *Griswold v. Connecticut: Birth Control and the Constitutional Right of Privacy*. Lawrence: University Press of Kansas, 2005.

Jütte, Robert. *Contraception: A History*. Malden, MA: Polity Press, 2008.

Katz, Esther, Cathy Moran Hajo, and Peter C. Engelman, eds. *The Selected Papers of Margaret Sanger*. Vol. 1, *The Woman Rebel, 1900–1928*. Urbana: University of Illinois Press, 2003.

Katz, Esther, Cathy Moran Hajo, and Peter C. Engelman, eds. *The Selected Papers of Margaret Sanger*. Vol. 2, *Birth Control Comes of Age, 1928–1939*. Urbana: University of Illinois Press, 2006.

Katz, Esther, Cathy Moran Hajo, and Peter C. Engelman, eds. *The Selected Papers of Margaret Sanger*. Vol. 3, *The Politics of Planned Parenthood, 1939–1966*. Urbana: University of Illinois Press, 2010.

Kennedy, David. M. *Birth Control in America: The Career of Margaret Sanger*. New Haven, CT: Yale University Press, 1970.

Kevles, Daniel J. *In the Name of Eugenics: Genetics and the Uses of Human Heredity*. New York: Knopf, 1985.

Kinsey, Alfred C. et al. *Sexual Behavior in the Human Female*. Philadelphia: W. B. Saunders, 1953.

Kline, Wendy. *Building a Better Race: Gender, Sexuality, and Eugenics from the Turn of the Century to the Baby Boom*. Berkeley: University of California Press.

Knowlton, Charles. *Fruits of Philosophy, or, the Private Companion of Adult People*. Mt. Vernon, NY: Peter Pauper Press, 1937; reprint of 1839 edition.

Konikow, Antoinette (Pseudo. "Woman Physician"). *Voluntary Motherhood: A Study of the Physiology and Hygiene of Prevention of Conception*. Boston: privately printed, 1928.

Kopp, Marie E. *Birth Control in Practice: An Analysis of Ten Thousand Case Histories of the Birth Control Clinical Research Bureau.* New York: Robert M. McBride & Company, 1934.

Kornbluh, Joyce L. "Industrial Workers of the World." In *Encyclopedia of the American Left,* edited by Mari Jo Buhle et al., 354–59. Urbana: University of Illinois Press, 1992.

Lader, Lawrence. *The Margaret Sanger Story and the Fight for Birth Control.* New York: Doubleday, 1955.

Ledbetter, Rosanna. *A History of the Malthusian League, 1877–1927.* Columbus: Ohio University Press, 1976.

Lord, Alexandra M. *Condom Nation: The U.S. Government's Sex Education Campaign from World War I to the Internet.* Baltimore, MD: Johns Hopkins University Press, 2010.

Luhan, Mabel Dodge. *Movers and Shakers.* Albuquerque: University of New Mexico Press, 1985; reprint of 1936 edition.

Luker, Kristen. *Abortion and the Politics of Motherhood.* Berkeley: University of California Press, 1984.

Lynd, Robert and Helen Merrell. *Middletown: A Study in Contemporary American Culture.* New York: Harcourt, Brace, 1929.

MacKinnon, Janice R. and Stephen R. MacKinnon. *Agnes Smedley: The Life and Times of an American Radical.* Berkeley: University of California Press, 1988.

May, Elaine Tyler. *America and the Pill: A History of Promise, Peril, and Liberation.* New York: Basic Books, 2010.

McCann, Carole R. *Birth Control Politics in the United States, 1916–1945.* Ithaca, NY: Cornell University Press, 1994.

McLaren, Angus. *A History of Contraception from Antiquity to the Present Day.* Oxford, UK: Blackwell, 1990.

Meckel, Richard A. *Save the Babies: American Public Health Reform and the Prevention of Infant Mortality, 1850–1929.* Baltimore, MD: Johns Hopkins University Press, 1990.

Meyer, Jimmy Elaine Wilkinson. *Any Friend of the Movement: Networking for Birth Control, 1920–1940.* Columbus: Ohio State University Press, 2004.

Mohr, James C. *Abortion in America: The Origins and Evolution of National Policy.* New York: Oxford University Press, 1978.

Murphy, James S. *The Condom Industry on the United States.* Jefferson, NC: McFarland & Company, 1990.

National Committee on Federal Legislation for Birth Control. *A New Day Dawns for Birth Control.* New York, July 1937.

Noonan, John T., Jr. *Contraception: A History of Its Treatment by the Catholic Theologians and Canonists.* Cambridge, MA: Harvard University Press, 1986.

Norden, Martin F. "Birth Control." In *Censorship: A World Encyclopedia,* Vol. 4, S-Z, edited by Derek Jones, 2137–38. Chicago: Fitzroy Dearborn Publishers, 2001.

Owen, Robert Dale. *Moral Physiology; or, A Brief and Plain Treatise on the Population Question,* 10th ed. Boston: J. P. Mendum, 1875.

Parascandola, John. *Sex, Sin, and Science: A History of Syphilis in America.* Westport, CT: Praeger, 2008.

Passet, Joanne E. *Sex Radicals and the Quest for Women's Equality.* Urbana: University of Illinois Press, 2003.

Paul, Diane B. *Controlling Human Heredity, 1865 to the Present*. Amherst, NY: Humanity Books, 1995.

Pearce, Fred. *The Coming Population Crash and Our Planet's Surprising Future*. Boston: Beacon Press, 2010.

Pernick, Martin S. *The Black Stork: Eugenics and the Death of 'Defective' Babies in American Medicine and Motion Pictures since 1915*. New York: Oxford University Press, 1996.

Petchesky, Rosalind Pollack. *Abortion and Woman's Choice: The State, Sexuality, & Reproductive Freedom*. Boston: Northeastern University Press, 1990.

Porta, Donatella Della and Mario Diani. *Social Movements: An Introduction*. Malden, MA: Blackwell, 2006.

Rabban, David M. *Free Speech in Its Forgotten Years*. New York: Cambridge University Press, 1997.

Reagan, Leslie J. *When Abortion Was a Crime: Women, Medicine, and Law in the United States, 1867–1973*. Berkeley: University of California Press, 1997.

Reed, James. *The Birth Control Movement and American Society: From Private Vice to Public Virtue*. Princeton, NJ: Princeton University Press, 1978.

Roberts, Dorothy. "Margaret Sanger and the Racial Origins." In *Racially Writing the Republic: Racists, Race Rebels, and Transformations of American Identity*, edited by Bruce Baum and Duchess Harris, 196–213. Durham, NC: Duke University Press, 2009.

Robinson, Caroline. *Seventy Birth Control Clinics*. Baltimore, MD: Williams & Wilkins, 1930.

Robinson, Victor. *Pioneers of Birth Control in England and America*. New York: Voluntary Parenthood League, 1919.

Robinson, William J. *Practical Eugenics: Four Means of Improving the Human Race*. New York: Critic & Guide Co., 1912.

Rodrique, Jessie M. "The Black Community and the Birth Control Movement." In *Unequal Sisters,* edited by Carol DuBois, and Vicki Ruiz, 139–54. New York: Routledge, 1990.

Sanger, Margaret. *An Autobiography*. New York: W. W. Norton, 1938.

Sanger, Margaret. *The Case for Birth Control: A Supplementary Brief and Statement of Facts*. New York: privately printed, 1917.

Sanger, Margaret. *Dutch Methods of Birth Control*. London: privately printed, 1915.

Sanger, Margaret. *English Methods of Birth Control*. London: privately printed, 1915.

Sanger, Margaret. *Family Limitation*. New York: privately printed, 1914.

Sanger, Margaret. *Magnetation Methods of Birth Control*. London: privately printed, 1915.

Sanger, Margaret. *Motherhood in Bondage*. New York: Brentano's, 1928.

Sanger, Margaret. *My Fight for Birth Control*. New York: Farrar & Rinehart, 1931.

Sanger, Margaret. *The Pivot of* Civilization. Amherst, NY: Humanity Books; reprint of 1922 edition.

Sanger, Margaret. *Woman and the New Race*. New York: Brentano's, 1920.

Schoen, Johanna. *Choice & Coercion: Birth Control, Sterilization and Abortion in Public Health and Welfare*. Chapel Hill: University of North Carolina Press, 2005.

Schroeder, Theodore. *List of References on Birth Control*. New York: H. W. Wilson Co., 1918.

Smith-Rosenberg, Carroll. *Disorderly Conduct: Visions of Gender in Victorian America*. New York: Alfred A. Knopf, 1985.

Soloway, Richard A. *Demography and Degeneration: Eugenics and the Declining Birthrate in Twentieth Century Britain*. Chapel Hill: University of North Carolina Press, 1995.

Stansell, Christine. *American Moderns: Bohemian New York and the Creation of a New Century*. New York: Henry Holt & Co., 2000.

Starr, Kevin. *Inventing the Dream: California through the Progressive Era*. New York: Oxford University Press, 1985.

Stix, Regine K. and Frank W. Notestein. *Controlled Fertility: An Evaluation of Clinic Service*. Baltimore, MD: Williams & Wilkins, 1940.

Stone, Abraham and Norman E. Himes. *Planned Parenthood: A Practical Guide to Birth-Control Methods*. New York: Macmillan, 1951.

Stone, Hannah M. *Contraceptive Methods—A Clinical Survey*. New York: Clinical Research Department of the American Birth Control League, 1925.

Stopes, Marie. *Married Love: A New Contribution to the Solution of Sex Difficulties*. New York: G. P. Putnam's Sons, 1931.

Taussig, Frederick J. *Abortion: Spontaneous and Induced*. St. Louis: C. V. Mosby, 1936.

Tentler, Leslie Woodcock. *Catholics and Contraception: An American History*. Ithaca, NY: Cornell University Press, 2004.

Thompson, Warren S. and P. K. Whelpton. *Population Trends in the United States*. New York: McGraw-Hill Book Co., 1933.

Tilly, Charles. *Social Movements, 1768–2004*. Boulder, CO: Paradigm Publishers, 2004.

Tone, Andrea, ed. *Controlling Reproduction: An American History*. Wilmington, DE: Scholarly Resources Inc., 1997.

Tone, Andrea, ed. *Devices and Desires: A History of Contraceptives in America*. New York: Hill & Wang, 2001.

Trimberger, Ellen Kay. *Intimate Warriors: Selected Works of Neith Boyce and Hutchins* Hapgood. New York: The Feminist Press, 1991.

United States National Resources Committee. *The Problems of a Changing Population: Report of the Committee on Population Problems to the National Resources Committee*. Washington, DC, May 1938.

Ware, Susan. "Florence Jaffray Hurst Harriman." In *Notable American Women, The Modern Period*, edited by Barbara Sicherman and Carol Hurd Green, 314–15. Cambridge, MA: Harvard University Press, 1980.

Wexler, Alice. *Emma Goldman: An Intimate Life*. New York: Pantheon Books, 1984.

Williams, Doone and Greer. *Every Child a Wanted Child: Clarence James Gamble, M.D., and His Life in the Birth Control Movement*. Boston: Countway Library of Medicine, 1978.

Wolfe, Bertram. *A Life in Two Centuries*. New York: Stein & Day, 1981.

DISSERTATIONS AND UNPUBLISHED RESEARCH

Hersey, Harold B. "Margaret Sanger: The Biography of the Birth Control Pioneer." 1938 unpublished manuscript, New York Public Library.

Holz, Rosemarie Petra. "The Birth Control Clinic in America: Life within, Life without, 1923–1972." PhD diss., University of Illinois, 2002.

McClearey, Kevin E. "The Noonday Devil: Margaret H. Sanger's 1916 American Lecture Tour." 1999 manuscript in author's possession.

Rodrique, Jessie M. "The Afro-American Community and the Birth Control Movement, 1918–1942." PhD diss., University of Massachusetts, 1991.

Sanger, Alexander Campbell. "Margaret Sanger: The Early Years, 1910–1917," Senior Thesis, Princeton University, 1969.

Vreeland. Francis M. "The Process of Reform with Especial Reference to Reform Groups in the Field of Population." PhD diss., University of Michigan, 1929.

ARTICLES

"Accident of Birth," *Fortune Magazine* 17 (February 1938): 83–86, 108, 110–114.

Andrist, Ralph K. "Paladin of Purity." *American Heritage* 24 (October, 1973): 5–7, 84–89.

Benjamin, Hazel C. "Lobbying for Birth Control." *Public Opinion Quarterly* 2 (January 1938): 53–60.

Brandeis, Louis and Simon Warren. "The Right to Privacy." *Harvard Law Review* IV (December 1890): 193–220.

Brooks, Carol Flora. "The Early History of the Anti-Contraceptive Laws in Connecticut and Massachusetts." *American Quarterly* 18 (Spring 1966): 3–23.

Clarke, Gary N. "Etiology of Sperm Immunity in Women." *Fertility and Sterility* 91 (Feb. 2009): 639–43.

Davis, Katharine Bement. "A Study of the Sex Life of the Normal Married Woman." *Journal of Social Hygiene* 8 (April, 1922): 173–89.

Dawson, Deborah, et al. "Fertility Control in the United States before the Contraceptive Revolution." *Family Planning Perspectives* 12 (March–April, 1980): 76–86.

Dayton, Cornelia Hughes. "'Taking the Trade': Abortion and Gender Relations in an Eighteenth-Century New England Village." *William and Mary Quarterly* 48 (1991): 19–28, 40–49.

Dennet, Mary Ware, and Frederic H. Robinson, eds. "A Symposium on Birth Control." *Medical Review of Reviews* 25 (March 1919): 131–57.

Dickinson, Robert L. "Contraception—A Medical Review of the Situation." *American Journal of Obstetrics and Gynecology* 8 (November 1924): 583–605.

Dickinson, Robert L. "Simple Sterilization of Women by Cautery Stricture of Intra-uterine Tubal Openings." *Surgery, Gynecology and Obstetrics* 23 (1916): 185–90.

Falmino, Dolores. "The Birth of a Nation: Media Coverage of Contraception, 1915–1917." *Journalism and Mass Communication Quarterly* 75 (Autumn 1998): 560–71.

Ferebee, Dorothy Boulding. "Planned Parenthood as a Public Health Measure for the Negro Race." *Human Fertility* 7 (February 1942): 7–10.

Henshaw, Paul S. "Physiologic Control of Fertility." *Science* 117 (May 29, 1953): 572–82.

Jensen, Joan M. "The Evolution of Margaret Sanger's *Family Limitation* Pamphlet, 1914–1921." *Signs* 6 (Spring 1981): 548–67.

Katz, Esther. "The History of Birth Control in the United States." *Trends in History* 4 (1988): 81–101.

Kennedy, Anne. "History of the Development of Contraceptive Materials in the United States." *American Medicine* 41 (March 1935): 159–61.

Manley, Jared L. "Crusader." *The New Yorker* (July 4, 1936): 22.

Naz, Rajesh K. "Status of Contraceptive Vaccines." *American Journal of Reproductive Immunology* 61 (January 2009): 11–18.

Pearl, Raymond. "Contraception and Fertility in 2,000 Women." *Human Biology* 4 (September 1932): 363–407.

Pilpel, Harriet F. "The Crazy Quilt of Our Birth Control Laws." *Journal of Sex Research* 1 (July 1965): 135–42.

Pringle, Henry F. "What Do the Women of America Think?" *Ladies' Home Journal* (March 1938): 14–15, 94–95, 97.

Ray, Joyce M. and F. G. Gosling. "American Physicians and Birth Control, 1936–1947." *Journal of Social History* 18 (Spring 1985): 399–411.

Robishaw, Ruth. "A Study of 4,000 Patients Admitted for Contraceptive Practice and Treatment." *American Journal of Obstetrics and Gynecology* 31 (March 1936): 426–35.

Rosen, Robyn L. "Federal Expansion, Fertility Control, and Physicians in the United States: The Politics of Maternal Welfare in the Interwar Years." *Journal of Women's History* 10 (Autumn, 1998): 53–73.

Rosen, Robyn L. "Mary Coffin Ware Dennett." *American National Biography Online* (February 2000).

Sanger, Margaret. "The War against Birth Control." *The American Mercury* (June 1924): 231–36.

Seibels, Robert E. "A Rural Project in Negro Maternal Health." *Human Fertility* 6 (April 1941): 42–44.

Shorto, Russell. "Contra-Contraception." *New York Times Magazine* (May 7, 2006): 48–55, 68, 83.

Smith, Helena Huntington. "Birth Control and the Law." *The Outlook* 149 (August 29, 1928): 686–87, 718.

Stone, Hannah M. "The Birth Control Raid." *Eugenics* 2 (August 1929): 1–4.

Stone, Hannah M. "Clinical Experiences with the Foam-Powder Method." *Journal of Contraception* 3 (January 1938): 3–6.

Thompson, Warren S. "Race Suicide in the United States." *The Scientific Monthly* 5 (July, 1917): 22–35.

Turano, Anthony M. "Birth Control and the Law." *American Mercury* (April 1935), 466–72.

Wharton, Don. "Birth Control: The Case for the State." *Atlantic Monthly* 164 (October 1939), 463–67.

Williams, J. Whitridge. "Indication for Therapeutic Sterilization in Obstetrics." *Journal of the American Medical Association* 91 (October 27, 1928): 1240–42.

SERIALS

Please refer to the chapter notes for citations to articles in these publications and for reference to the many daily newspapers used.

Birth Control Herald
Birth Control News

Birth Control Review
The Blast
The Call
Critic and Guide
Current Opinion
Harper's Weekly
Lucifer, the Light-Bearer
Margaret Sanger Papers Project Newsletter
The Masses
Medical Times
Medical World
Modern School Magazine
Mother Earth
New Republic
Physical Culture
Pictorial Review
Survey
The Woman Rebel
The Word

INDEX

About the Author

PETER C. ENGELMAN, a freelance writer, historical editor, and archivist, is an associate editor of the Margaret Sanger Papers Project at New York University and has written widely on Margaret Sanger and the birth control movement.